Philosophy and Medicine

Volume 120

The Philosophy and Medicine series is dedicated to publishing monographs and collections of essays that contribute importantly to scholarship in bioethics and the philosophy of medicine. The series addresses the full scope of issues in bioethics, from euthanasia to justice and solidarity in health care. The Philosophy and Medicine series places the scholarship of bioethics within studies of basic problems in the epistemology and metaphysics of medicine. The latter publications explore such issues as models of explanation in medicine, concepts of health and disease, clinical judgment, the meaning of human dignity, the definition of death, and the significance of beneficence, virtue, and consensus in health care. The series seeks to publish the best of philosophical work directed to health care and the biomedical sciences.

More information about this series at http://www.springer.com/series/6414

Darian Meacham
Editor

Medicine and Society, New Perspectives in Continental Philosophy

Springer

Editor
Darian Meacham
University of the West of England
Bristol
UK

ISSN 0376-7418 ISSN 2215-0080 (electronic)
Philosophy and Medicine
ISBN 978-94-017-9869-3 ISBN 978-94-017-9870-9 (eBook)
DOI 10.1007/978-94-017-9870-9

Library of Congress Control Number: 2015936378

Springer Dordrecht Heidelberg New York London

Printed on acid-free paper

Springer Science+Business Media B.V. Dordrecht is part of Springer Science+Business Media (www.springer.com)

Acknowledgments

Thank you to Jeffery Bishop and the editorial team at Philosophy and Medicine for their patience and support of this project, and to Christopher Wilby and the team at Springer. This book would not have been possible without the support of the Royal Institute of Philosophy, which sponsored the seminar series that gave rise to this volume. Support from the University of the West of England in the form of an Early Career Researcher grant and sabbatical was also invaluable in bringing this project to fruition. Most importantly, thank you to all the authors who have contributed their efforts to this volume.

Contents

Chapter 1
Introduction

Darian Meacham

It usually falls to an introduction such as this to explain the *what* and the *why* of the volume: what is contained in the contributions and why it is important. In this instance the two are more or less the same. What distinguishes "continental" approaches to bioethics and philosophy of medicine is precisely the reason why there is value in highlighting such approaches. Before elaborating on that rather vague contention, I would first like to say something briefly about how this volume came about. In 2012 I organized, together with Havi Carel, a series of public seminars on the rather broad theme of "Medicine and Society." These took place in Bristol (UK), with the generous financial support of the Royal Institute of Philosophy and an Early Career Researcher grant that I had received from the University of the West of England. Some of the participants in that seminar series have also been kind enough to contribute to this volume: Niall Keane, Eran Dorfman, Christien van den Anker and Havi Carel. It is safe to say that the seminar series had what one might call "continental leanings," meaning that nearly all of the participants approached the issues in bioethics and philosophy of medicine that they addressed with a perspective that was at least grounded in what could loosely be called continental philosophy. To be more specific, the participants approached the subject matter(s) at hand, to a greater or lesser degree, from within the varying conceptual frameworks of the phenomenological, hermeneutic, French epistemological, and post-structuralist traditions. The positive reception that these seminars received both from fellow academics and members of the interested general public convinced me of the value of showcasing the diversity of approaches and depth of analysis with which philosophers working with a background in continental philosophy address a wide range of problems pertaining to the relations between medicine and society. I should add a disclaimer that certainly not all of the philosophers who have contributed to this volume would accept the label of "continental philosopher," but certainly all of the

D. Meacham (✉)
University of the West of England, Bristol, England
e-mail: darian.meacham@uwe.ac.uk

D. Meacham (ed.), *Medicine and Society, New Perspectives in Continental Philosophy*, Philosophy and Medicine 120, DOI 10.1007/978-94-017-9870-9_1

contributions have a grounding in continental philosophy—more on that in a moment. Happily the series editors of *Philosophy and Medicine* agreed that such a volume would be a good idea. The initial plan was to take a specific set of problems prevalent in the current Anglo-American dominated bioethics discourse and ask philosophers who approached these problems from continental perspectives to address them. It was a good plan, but getting philosophers to move in an assigned direction is like herding cats. The initial plan also allowed the structure of the volume to be determined by a set of problems and philosophical frameworks that philosophers coming from a continental approach often wished to challenge. What I ended up with is in fact much more illustrative and representative of the breadth and depth of the emerging field(s) of continental bioethics and philosophy of medicine than the plan I had initially envisioned, for this I am grateful to the un-herdable contributors. The hope for this volume is that it can provide a kind of handbook illustrating the ways in which problems in bioethics and philosophy of medicine are currently being treated from within the continental traditions. In this sense, this volume follows in the footsteps of S.K. Toombs's *Handbook of Phenomenology and Medicine* (Springer 2002), which appeared in this series over a decade ago—although the present collection has a broader scope of philosophical approaches. In doing so, this volume hopefully adds to a growing and impressive body of work in this area.

There is something of an elephant in the room that needs to be tackled before we move on: the infamous analytic-continental distinction in philosophy. This is not the place and I am not the person to be partisan about this distinction, and anyway one hopes that it carries less weight than it once did. Suffice to say that it may not be crazy to suggest that analytic philosophers might sometimes do well to pay more attention to the historical development of the problems they are working on, pay more heed to concrete social and political embeddedness of these problems, the subjects or persons they pertain to and the people that write about them, and finally, and this is a bit more specific, recognize the importance of the body in our relations with the world around us and with others—all things associated with more continental approaches. To stick with rather hackneyed distinctions, it would probably not hurt some continental philosophers to remember that they are working on problems, not reporting on a tradition. All philosophers, but perhaps especially those who consider themselves continental ones would do well to be rigorous not only in the careful attention to the historical development of problems but also in conceptual analysis and careful drawing of distinctions. The "analytic" emphasis on clear argumentation and careful clarification is of course valuable for all types of philosophy. All of the contributions here embody, I think, the best aspects of both traditions.

One area of supposed difference between continental and analytic philosophy that is of particular importance to bioethics and philosophy of medicine, as they bear such a close relation to the medical and technological sciences, is their general methodological relation to the natural sciences. Though it is by no means fair to apply this as a blanket statement, it does seem safe to say that generally speaking, analytic philosophy often sees itself as continuous with the natural sciences, which in their methodology present the most accurate manner of understanding phenomena. The task of philosophy is often understood as, if not being contiguous with the natural sciences, then being one of helping to clarify through logical analysis the methodology, goals and findings of the natural sciences. This leads into sticky situations when dealing with traditional areas of philosophy that the natural sciences cannot account for, namely consciousness and ethics, the latter of which a colleague of mine, Iain Hamilton Grant, astutely refers to as the "acceptable face of anti-scientific realism." This is not the venue for diving into the deep end of either the hard problem of consciousness or the difficulties of the various forms of ethical naturalism. What is relevant in this context is the perception that continental philosophy has a very different but not necessarily less friendly relation with the natural sciences. For example, Georges Canguilhem, whose influence is felt throughout this volume, was also a medical doctor and certainly considered himself not just a man of science but a naturalist. It does seem fair to say however that continental philosophy, generally speaking, argues that the natural sciences are grounded in pre-theoretical conditions of givenness, as in various versions of Kantian transcendentalism or phenomenological notions of the "lifeworld." The Kantian project and the phenomenological one that grew out of it both sought to locate a firm transcendental ground for the natural sciences. This idea of the need for a proper ground of the natural sciences that would account for and be aware of the various presuppositions that natural scientific inquiry often took for granted persisted through historicist, post-structuralist and also feminist encounters between science and continental philosophy. However, as Gilbert Hottois and Charles Wolfe point out in this volume, there has long been a close relation between the French "biophilosophy" of Georges Canguilhem, Gilbert Simondon and Raymond Ruyer, and the biological and medical sciences. Maurice Merleau-Ponty, perhaps the most important representative of the phenomenological tradition in relation to philosophy of medicine, owing to his phenomenological accounts of the body and the ill body in particular, was greatly influenced in his early work by the German neurologist Kurt Goldstein, and later by biologists like Jakob von Uexküll, Konrad Lorenz, and E.S. Russell as well as Ruyer. Where the continental approach perhaps differs from the analytic *vis-à-vis* the natural sciences is that rather than seeing philosophy as playing a complementary or clarifying role in relation to the findings of the natural sciences, continental approaches have seen their role as participating in the foundationalist project of the sciences, in other words establishing what is, as well as critiquing the methods of the sciences. As Canguilhem writes in his essay "Machine and Organism": "Far from coming belatedly to occupy an abandoned viewpoint, philosophy points science toward a position to take." This is the case with the phenomenological projects pursued by Edmund Husserl and Merleau-Ponty in critiquing what they took to be a naïve foundationalism that can pervade scientific discourse. It is also the case with the post-structuralist critique of knowledge one finds in Michel Foucault or feminist critiques from philosophers like Evelyn Fox Keller and Donna Haraway. As the chapters that begin (Hottois) and end (Allouche) this volume attest and implore, philosophy should not shy away from what might even be called a speculative stance *vis-à-vis* technoscience—though I am relatively certain that not all the contributors in between would agree.

What is it then that distinguishes, more specifically, continental approaches to bioethics and philosophy of medicine from the dominant Anglo-American or analytic approaches? It is of course best to let the contributions speak for themselves, but a few markers are worth pointing out. First and foremost is the emphasis on the body, and particularly the lived-body as it is developed and explored in the phenomenological tradition. Though as Slatman and Widdershoven point out in their contribution, the idea of the lived-body as developed in the phenomenological tradition can be traced back to the early nineteenth-century French philosopher Maine de Biran—something that the phenomenologists were certainly aware of. From our current perspective, the analyses in the Second Book of Edmund Husserl's two volume *Ideas Pertaining to a Pure Phenomenology and to a Phenomenological Philosophy, Studies in the Phenomenology of Constitution* ([1952] 1989) and in Merleau-Ponty's magnum opus *Phenomenology of Perception* ([1945] 1962) are particularly important here. But foundational phenomenological study of the body cannot be limited to these two thinkers. Jean-Paul Sartre's *Being and Nothingness* ([1943] 1957) contains a lengthy analysis of the body in what he calls its three ontological dimensions (my body-for-itself, my body-for-others, and myself as a body know by the other). Martin Heidegger, often criticized for ignoring the body, also offers important considerations about the role of the lived-body (see Niall Keane's and Eran Dorfman's contributions). What these studies of embodied subjectivity emphasized was that the body was anything but a passive receptor of sensory impressions controlled by a disembodied (Cartesian) subjectivity. Rather, the lived-body, the body as experienced, plays a central role in constituting how it is that the world appears to the subject. In short, the body's movement in the world is itself generative or constitutive of meaning at the most fundamental level for the subject. This has an obvious importance for the way that we think about the impact that illness and bodily impairment have on the person or subject as a whole. A change in the structure of or capacity for bodily movement brought about by illness or injury does not just affect a regional change in the subject's experience of the world. Rather the centrality of the body to the constitution of a meaningful world means that a change to the physical and hence lived-body changes the subject's world from the bottom up. Often this results in a limitation of the body's own tacit "understanding" of its range of possibilities. This is explored at length in the second part of this volume.

The importance of the body is not limited to phenomenological approaches. Georges Canguilhem, whose thinking is often separated from phenomenology as the philosophy of the concept opposed to the philosophy of experience (a perhaps overly sharp distinction made by Canguilhem's student Michel Foucault), also places emphasis on embodiment, namely on the lived experience of the patient. Canguilhem writes in his seminal work *The Normal and the Pathological* ([1943] 1966): "the life of a living being [...] only recognizes the categories of health and illness on the level of experience, which is first of all an *épreuve* in the affective sense of the term—not on the level of science." Perhaps the distance between Canguilhem's philosophy of the concept and the phenomenological philosophy of experience is not as great as it is sometimes made to seem.

The emphasis on embodiment has important consequences for the understanding of the person, the subject, and ultimately consciousness. As consciousness cannot be separated from embodiment, the subject or person cannot be abstracted out from its environment and social historical context. The autonomous rational subject—the Cartesian subject—is by this account a myth. Thinking about ethical issues in the context of medicine or any other intervention or action upon the body cannot be grounded in the idea of an autonomous rational ego or subject precisely because such an entity does not exist. The being of the subject in question is bound up not only with its embodiment but also the relations that it has with other subjects, with whom it co-constitutes a shared world, and the social and historical context that the subject is "thrown" into or inherits. It could be argued that the myth of an autonomous rational subject is in fact part of the social-historical context of our modern embodiment, but one that does not fit well with the foundational account of an embodied and indeed intersubjective subjectivity that phenomenological analysis claims to provide. This is precisely what Lisa Guenther (Chap. 13) claims that the study of persons subjected to long stints of solitary confinement illustrates to a horrifying degree. The lived-body of phenomenological analysis is of course not the last word in the embodiment story. As Corry Shores (Chap. 16) argues, it is precisely the conceptual and phenomenological investigation of embodied cognition that suggests moving from an "organic" idea of a lived-body, epistemically available only to the subject herself, to a mechanic model of the body. The questions and debates opened up and explored in this volume are far from closed and the goal here is to tap into and open up to a wider readership the rich resources that the "continental" tradition provides in exploring what are surely some of the most fascinating questions in bioethics and philosophy of medicine today.

The volume is organized into five sections that break along thematic and methodological lines. Section one, "Figures and Grounds: Continental Approaches to Bioethics and Medicine," begins with a rather personal essay by Gilbert Hottois entitled, "Defining Bioethics." Hottois is one of the pioneers of what can be called (a bit coarsely) continental approaches to bioethics. As he explains in his contribution (Chap. 2), his approach is deeply influenced by his reading of Heidegger's work on "The Question Concerning Technology" (*Die Fragenach der Technik*) as well as a general grounding in the continental tradition of philosophy. For Hottois, there can be no separation between bioethical inquiry and that surrounding the neologism "techno-science." Hottois's approach also sets him apart from much of the mainstream work in Anglo-American bioethics insofar as it is not limited to reflection on problems concerning medical practice, but has as its object a radically broader context, which includes the eventuality of the human species departing planet Earth and engaging in what he calls "cosmic-prospecting." Hottois remains nonetheless attentive to the Anglo-American traditions of bioethics. He reflects on his own development alongside critical reflection on the work of H. Tristram Englehardt and Van Rensselaer Potter, two central figures in the development of Anglophone bioethics. Hottois finds a significant degree of affinity between his own approach and Potter's, while remaining attentive to the operative differences. Widely known for his work on philosophy of technology and bioethics in the

French speaking (and Spanish speaking) world, this is the first time that Hottois's work has been translated into English. The other essays in the section critically develop the approaches taken toward bioethics and philosophy of medicine by four other extremely important philosophers in the continental tradition: Hans Jonas, Hans-Georg Gadamer, Jürgen Habermas and Jacques Derrida. Both Jonas and Gadamer were students of Heidegger prior to the outbreak of the Second World War, and were deeply influenced by his work, perhaps most significantly by the importance that Heidegger placed on *Dasein's*—what we can, not at all unproblematically, the human being's—being toward death in his fundamental ontology. Jonas's work on philosophy of technology also reflects many of Heidegger's concerns about technology not simply being a tool at human disposal, but rather becoming an all encompassing frame (*Gestell*) or structuring dimension of human existence. Michael Hauskeller's (Chap. 3) contribution carefully unpacks the ontological foundations of Jonas's ethics and then takes a closer look at Jonas's position *vis-à-vis* human technological enhancement and the imperative to protect human nature.

The Heideggerian legacy in Gadamer's writings on *The Enigma of Health* is perhaps felt most strongly in the hermeneutic method that he uses, examining the relation between the concepts of nature and health in the western tradition from Aristotle's understanding of nature as *physis*, through to modern mechanical notions of nature and statistical understandings of health. Niall Keane (Chap. 4) picks up Gadamer's reflections on the difficulty of pinning down the concept of health in its relation to nature. Keane critically examines the Platonic, Aristotelian, and also phenomenological/Heideggerian influences at work in Gadamer's thought. Keane argues for a dialectical conception of health, "accounting for it by means of what is present, that is, what remains, when it is absent," but is also critical of Gadamer's *physis*-centred approach, arguing that it "ignores something that Heidegger never did and this is that *physis* cannot be defined in terms of harmony and proportion, insofar as nature is more often than not violent, destructive, terrible, pitiless and overwhelming."

In the final chapter of the first section (Chap. 5), Mihail Evans examines the conflicting attitudes that two of the most influential post-war philosophers in Europe, Jürgen Habermas and Jacques Derrida, had toward the science of genetics. Written during the period of the Human Genome Project and the competing privately funded parallel project carried out by Craig Venter's Celera Corporation, Habermas's and Derrida's interventions in the debate both reflect on what impact the knowledge and potential technoscientific capacity created by such a detailed understanding of the human genome could have on human ethical relations and self-understanding. Evans argues that Habermas's strong critique of genetic engineering in humans amounts to an attempt to defend an untenable liberal idea of an autonomous subject. Derrida, conversely, displays a much more open attitude toward genetic technology, arguing that not only does it not threaten ethical relations in the manner that Habermas fears, but actually teaches us important lessons about the constitution of the self.

The chapters in the second section of the book, "The Experience of Illness: Phenomenological Approaches," all examine how the descriptive science of phenomenology can contribute to a better understanding of the experience of illness and ultimately to better clinical practice. Phenomenology is perhaps most simply understood as a descriptive science of how the world appears to consciousness as a world of meaning. Saying that it is about how the world appears to consciousness does not of course always mean that consciousness is explicitly aware of all of the ways that the world appears to it. Paradoxically, much of what phenomenologically speaking we would call our conscious lives happens behind the back of consciousness, so to speak: we are not always aware of the myriad manners in which we are experiencing the world and how they affect our comportment. This is especially true of the way that the body silently or passively adjusts to but also shapes its environment. The "lived-body" (a term that is taken up and developed in all of the chapters in this section) does not just passively receive the world and adjust to it, but is involved in actively shaping the meaning content of the world, often before reflective consciousness takes hold. Nowhere is this more true than in the experience of illness, where changes to the physical body have enormous impact on the lived-body's own tacit understanding of what it can and cannot do in the world. Illness goes from being a regional area of phenomenological description (what it's like to be ill) to having a global impact on the entire world as it appears to a conscious subject. In the first chapter of the section (Chap. 6), Jenny Slatman and Guy Widdershoven use a phenomenological approach to develop an "ethics of embodiment" that they argue is needed to guide medical interventions. After providing a history of phenomenological approaches to the body and the ill body in particular—tracing the development of this tradition back to the French philosopher Maine de Biran—they look at the role of phenomenological lived bodily integrity in cases of amputation and specifically mastectomy. They argue that the phenomenological analysis of lived bodily integrity has important insights to offer clinical practice. Havi Carel (Chap. 7) closely interrogates the varied experiences of illness, asking: do illness experiences share certain general features? Are these features universal or eidetic, or are they culturally-dependent? Do different illness experiences, such as the experience of acute versus chronic illness, share salient features? Do mental disorder and somatic disease have common experiential features? Drawing on a close reading of Heidegger's tool analysis, Sartre's three orders of embodiment and S.K. Toombs's analyses of the eidetic (essential) features of illness, Carel builds a conceptual phenomenological framework through which to understand the experience of illness writ large: the ill body is conspicuous, obtrusive and obstinate. Eran Dorfman (Chap. 8) returns to the phenomenological analyses of embodied subjectivity in the mutuality and intertwining of body and world implied in the notion of "flesh." Through an in-depth reading of Merleau-Ponty's work, particularly in its relation to Heidegger—thereby building on themes introduced in the previous two chapters—he engages in a critical interrogation of phenomenological methodology, asking what body is it exactly that phenomenological analysis uncovers? Is it a generalized, "primordial body" that serves as an eidetic structure of meaning constitution, or an "everyday body," the body as experienced in a quotidian manner in its oscillation between health and illness, well-being and impairment. Dorfman contends that phenomenology often moves between the two. Descriptions of the pathological body can serve to "expose tendencies that already exist in everyday life in a much less accentuated way." He argues for a hermeneutic of the body that brings pathology and everyday experience closer together and develops an ethics of the body on the basis of this proximity. This conclusion, that the difference between the pathological and the everyday lived-body is a question of degree, brings him into disagreement with Carel.

It is the subject of "The Normal and The Pathological" that drives the third section of the book, not the seminal work by Georges Canguilhem but the relation between the two concepts. Of course it is not coincidental that Canguilhem's enormously influential text (*Le Normal et le Pathologique* first published in 1943, an extended version was published in 1966) looms large in all the chapters of the section, even where his approach is rejected. In their contribution (Chap. 9), Andreas De Block and Jonathan Sholl examine several instances of what they call the "normalization view," the idea that "normality" assumes an epistemological priority and that pathology can only be understood in relation to what has been established as statistically normal. They argue that despite coming under heavy criticism this view is still widespread in both philosophy of medicine and bioethics. Through a discussion of Canguilhem and Christopher Boorse, De Block and Sholl critique the biostatistical concept of normality, arguing instead for a properly philosophical concept of normality. In doing so they explore Canguilhem's idea that normality never rests on the side of the organism alone (there are no normal organisms) but is always a question of dynamic relations between an organism and its environment.

Pieter Adriaens (Chap. 10) furthers the investigation into these concepts by examining the legitimacy and usefulness of pathologizing certain forms of sexual comportment, i.e. what he terms "paraphilias." Using the example of the American Psychiatric Association's approach to what it has termed "sexual deviance," as illustrated in the consecutive editions of its famous manual, the *Diagnostic and Statistical Manual of Mental Disorders* (DSM), and the particular episode concerning the removal of homosexuality from the seventh printing of DSM-II in 1974, Adriaens takes us back to the fundamental question of "what is a mental disorder?" He puts forth an argument that the APA not only "fails to provide an exhaustive and coherent analysis of the concept of mental disorder," but also "fails to design a classification of mental disorders that is consistent with whatever analysis it does provide."

Catherine Mills (Chap. 11) extends the discussion surrounding the concepts of normality and normativity into the debates over liberal eugenics. Mills investigates what role varying concepts of normality play in recent debates over the moral acceptability of liberal eugenics. She examines Jürgen Habermas's defense of human nature as a ground for liberal autonomy, the "normal species functioning" model offered by Allen Buchanan and the co-authors of *From Chance to Choice: Genetics and Justice* (Cambridge University Press 2000), and finally John Harris's rejection of the use of the concept in arguments about enhancement. Mills uses resources from Canguilhem to develop a conception of the normal that is salient in the debates around eugenics and enhancement, while also avoiding some of the concerns that have dogged Habermas's supposed strong attachment to the concept of human nature—see Buchanan's *Beyond Humanity* (Oxford University Press 2011) for a particularly scathing attack on Habermas's position.

The fourth section of the book addresses the question of "Life" in its biological, ethical and political forms. What is life? And does it matter to debates in philosophy of medicine, bioethics and biopolitics? The question in a sense seems stunningly naïve and obvious. Doesn't the prefix "bio" precisely indicate the important of "life" to all these areas of discourse? But perhaps the obviousness has in fact hidden the difficulties surrounding the concept of life from view in the orthodox iterations of these debates. Charles Wolfe (Chap. 12) begins by noting the pathos with which Canguilhem himself lamented the falling away of the question of life from scientific investigation. As Wolfe points out, Canguilhem "insisted on a kind of uniqueness of organisms and/or living bodies—their inherent normativity, their value-production and overall their inherent difference from mere machines." Looking at both Canguilhem and the neurologist Kurt Goldstein (who was a major influence on both Canguilhem and Merleau-Ponty), Wolfe investigates the concept of "biochauvinism," the idea that there is something inherently unique about biological entities that separates living systems from all others. Contrasting Canguilhem's position with that of Merleau-Ponty, who according to Wolfe cannot resist reverting to a "Catholic mysticism of the flesh," Hans Jonas, who Wolfe accuses of looking for a "secret way of defending human uniqueness over and against the rest of the physical universe," and more recent contributors to the debate over the nature of life like Francesco Varela and Evan Thompson, who seek to reintroduce subjectivity into biology, Wolfe makes the case that Canguilhem may best be considered a kind of naturalist-vitalist-existentialist. This position manages to avoid many of the pitfalls of other forms of biochauvinism, while still maintaining that there is something unique in life itself which any ethics or philosophy of medicine must take heed of.

Michael Lewis's contribution (Chap. 13) examines the concept of auto-immunity as it functions in the work of the philosophers Jacques Derrida, Giorgio Agamben and Roberto Esposito. The philosophical concept of auto-immunity that these thinkers develop is a strong rejoinder to notions of autonomy and individuality that continue to structure many of the contemporary bioethical debates. Lewis's essay can in a sense be read as a plea for granting priority to biopolitics over bioethics.

In "The Psychopathology of Space: A Phenomenological Critique of Solitary Confinement" (Chap. 14), Lisa Guenther launches a devastating critique of the practice of solitary confinement. Using first hand testimony and insights on embodied subjectivity from philosophers like Merleau-Ponty and Husserl, Guenther argues that solitary confinement is literally life destroying insofar as isolation and sensory deprivation pull the very subjectivity of the confined person apart at the seams. Guenther exposes the myth that solitary confinement allows for a period of cool down and reflection as based (at best) on ill conceived (Cartesian) notions of the relation between subjectivity, embodiment, movement and intersubjectivity. She makes a strong case that the often ignored widespread use of solitary confinement in the American penal system is a bioethical and indeed biopolitical issue of the highest importance, and one that invokes the question of precisely what a human life is.

The fifth and final section of the book takes up the question of eugenics again, but also looks to the horizons of developing debates over human enhancement and the therapy-enhancement distinction. Christien van den Anker (Chap. 15) addresses the legacy of eugenics in relation to what she calls the "right to be impaired." Drawing on resources from phenomenology, post-structuralism and also criticism of the dominant liberal models of social inclusion, van den Anker makes a case that the current discourse surrounding liberal eugenics retains an ethically and politically problematic residue of coercive practices and thinking on eugenics and disability from the not-so-distant past. In this light, van den Anker offers a critical reading of the 2006 UN Convention on the Rights of Persons with Disabilities and makes the case for adopting a principle of inclusion beyond contributing economically to society as emphasized in the UN Convention.

Cory Shores (Chap. 16) brings into question the standard prosthetic model of thinking on enhancement and technology applied to the body in general. This standard model, Shores argues, is grounded to a large extent in the phenomenology of the lived-body developed by Husserl and Merleau-Ponty. But, he asks, is the phenomenological "organic" view of the body really the best theoretical framework to explain how our bodies are becoming more and more technologized? Instead, Shores makes a case for reconsidering the model of the body that guides nearly all thinking on enhancement and argues instead that "[Gilles] Deleuze's and [Felix] Guattari's 'machinic' model is a more promising theoretical basis for the notion of posthuman enhancement and also for successful therapeutic prosthesis usage."

Sylvie Allouche (Chap. 17) calls into question the entire conceptual framework of the therapy-enhancement distinction and the enhancement debate. Drawing on Canguilhem, but also on more recent work by Gilbert Hottois and the French philosopher Jérôme Goffette, Allouche argues that rather than "enhancement" belonging within the broader conceptual category of medicine, both medicine and enhancement need to be rethought as domains under the umbrella concept of "*anthropotechny*"—technological intervention in and on the human body. In order to accomplish this, Allouche first sets out a sustained critique of the relation between the concepts of medicine and norm that are operative in much of the theorizing about the therapy-enhancement distinction. She then lays out a new conceptual framework for thinking these problems, introducing and developing the term "anthropotechy" and its component aspects, "anthropotechnics" (which would include cosmetic make-up and leech therapy) and "anthropotechnology" (which would include high-tech pharmaceutical doping methods and the use of pace makers).

It seems appropriate that a line of conceptual development—continental approaches to medicine and bioethics—that initially demanded that philosophy take the body and its constituting powers more seriously now in fact doubles back and brings into question the very models of embodiment that it had once actively endorsed. This conceptual sophistication and critical reflection upon its own concepts illustrates nicely the fecundity and diversity of positions and approaches to problems in philosophy of medicine and bioethics that might be called "continental." The essays in this volume do an exemplary job of illustrating just that.

Part I
Figures and Grounds

Chapter 2
Defining Bioethics: Back to the Sources

Gilbert Hottois

1 Introduction: What Is Defining?

To define is not an activity that is foreign to philosophy. Quite the contrary: it is constitutive of much of it, and has been present from its origins. Plato, through the voice of Socrates, was basically seeking definitions: what is virtue, beauty, courage, piety, philosophy…? He did not want us to respond by a series of examples of acts, or brave or virtuous men, or beautiful works. He wanted the idea itself be presented: the very essence itself of courage or beauty. He expected a definition imposed by reality itself: the one reality, perfect, immutable, universal. Put in a different manner, Plato sought an ontological definition. These types of definitions also carry a normative scope: they express the ideal and the truth-value that sensible empirical realities cannot approach.

The desire for the real, essential and necessary definition that should prevail over all can be found throughout the history of philosophy and to a certain degree in science. From Platonic idealism, this desire is perpetuated through substantialist Aristotelian essentialism, Cartesian rationalism, critical and transcendentalist Kantianism, logicism and phenomenological eideticism, etc.

I have for quite a long time distanced myself from this powerful essentialist tradition, too often dogmatic, in favor of a more empiricist approach that is more widespread in European Anglo-Saxon thought than in what is called Continental (meaning for the most part French and German) philosophy. My way of

---

Translated by D. Meacham and D. Meacham,

An earlier version of this text was published simultaneously in French and Spanish, see, Hottois (2011).

G. Hottois (✉)
Université Libre de Bruxelles, Brussels, Belgium
e-mail: ghottois@ulb.ac.be

D. Meacham (ed.), *Medicine and Society, New Perspectives in Continental Philosophy*, Philosophy and Medicine 120, DOI 10.1007/978-94-017-9870-9_2

approaching the problem of definition is, and for a long time has been, inspired by the philosophical work of Ludwig Wittgenstein. Wittgenstein takes, specifically, the example of the word "game." What is a game? For the illusory desire to free the concept or the essential meaning, Wittgenstein substitutes a more modest goal—tolerant, pluralistic and open—a family of uses.

When considering what are called "games," we can see an enormous variety of examples, cases, and contexts of use. Here it seems pointless to want to repeat the Platonic gesture which claims to see the uniqueness of an idea behind or beyond this diversity, an essential trait common to all. Between all the myriad uses of the word "game" there are of course similarities, as there are always similarities between members of a family. But these similarities are many and no one characteristic is necessary and shared by all. If A, B, C, D, E, F, etc. are examples of games, it is perfectly plausible that A, C, D and M share the characteristics alpha, beta and gamma, but only C and D have in common with D, E, F and G, the characteristics delta and epsilon, or even that D and J have in common the lambda and mu characters, and so on. A, therefore does not have a common trait with J, but is connected to J via D. Thus, the series holds together, loosely but at the same time quite firmly. It is not, Wittgenstein observes again, because a single fiber runs throughout the rope that it is resistant. It is the collection of several fibers of limited length that makes its sturdiness.[1]

Certainly, in a family, some characteristics are more common than others and it is usually possible to reach a core that is more representative of games examples, i.e. a paradigmatic core nucleus. But this by no means indicates that when one characteristic is particularly widespread, or even present everywhere, we have a clear criterion of what a game is. Suppose, for example, we could say that all games are entertaining or governed by rules. But what is it to be "entertaining"? We certainly do not all entertain ourselves in the same manner and under the same circumstances. What is a game for one is not for another. And what is a rule? There are many kinds of rules and ways to follow them: administrative, legal, moral, aesthetic, logical, mathematical, technical, and monastic. "Rules," "entertainment," "game" all are terms that correspond to families of uses, not clearly defined and unchanging concepts, and these families of usage variously intersect.

When one navigates through the uses of the word "Bioethics"[2] and the various definitions that are given, we are confronted with a similar kind of "family" in the

---

[1]On this point see Wittgenstein (2009), Philosophical Investigation no. 66.

[2]See, for example, Callahan (1973); In the first edition of the *Encyclopedia of Bioethics* (1978) the definition written by Danner Clouser is essentially a vehicle for the message that bioethics is nothing more than the application of traditional ethics to new aspects of ancient problems raised by developments in medicine: "The position taken in this article has been that the revelations and capabilities mediated by science create an urgency for moral guidance but do not require a new morality, revised in its basic principles" (vol. 1, p. 125). It mentions, very briefly, Potter, who as we will see below is an opponent of this view. Instead of defining bioethics in its essence, better to characterize it as relative to a series of questions sharing some "family resemblances." But Clouser is not content to stop at this, nor does he mention Wittgenstein. In the second edition of the Encyclopedia (1995), the entry on "Bioethics" was written by Daniel Callahan, a Catholic

sense that Wittgenstein describes. This situation does not prevent proponents of the various definitions of bioethics from claiming to present the true or the single proper definition, without realizing or wanting to admit the interested, partial, biased, subjective, normative or even outright controversial nature of their proposals. Of course, it is entirely legitimate, in specific contexts (technical, scientific, educational, etc.), to cut loose semantic tissue from clearly defined meanings and purposes. But these are normative rational decisions, whose products are largely constructed and not given by a reality or common sense that would be all encompassing, and that claims simply to discover and to explain.

In philosophy there is also another manner of revealing reveal the "true meaning" of words that is equally as old—it is found as early as Plato's *Cratylus*. This approach had a major success in the twentieth century, especially in the hermeneutics inspired by Heidegger. It seeks the original meaning of a word by tracing its history through a language or a succession of languages, as is the case for the philosophical terms: "reason," which refers to *ratio*, which in turn refers to *logos*; or "nature" which refers to *natura* which refers to *physis*; "morality," which refers to *mos*, which refers to *ethos*, etc. The hermeneutic looks at how these terms were used and what they meant in the early presocratic philosophical texts. This undertaking is of an undeniable philological and historical interest, but it also participates in an almost mythological valorization of origin (think of a Golden Age) where truth and meaning would have shined only to have faded and been lost during the subsequent history. It is a process of recovery of the past, of tradition and of nature and it may prove to be as dogmatic as essentialist idealism, because it is still pretending to read the real and unique signification without assuming active responsibility in this normative discovery.

"Bioethics" is a constructed word; a dated artifact whose paternity is known[3] and it seems to somehow evade the temptation to trace its origin very far into the past.

(Footnote 2 continued)
philosopher benefiting from a broader historical perspective. This entry is much richer than the first and illustrates the vast diversity that we find in the use of the word at the end of the twentieth-century, encompassing medical ethics, environmental ethics, social and political questions (bio-politics). Bioethics here concerns the "sciences of living." Potter is acknowledged as the inventor of the word, but only one paragraph is devoted to him. Callahan strongly insists on the inter-disciplinary character of bioethical inquiry, however he maintains that it runs primarily on insights from various branches of moral philosophy (consequentialism, deontological principalism, virtue ethics, casuistry, feminism, narrative approaches, hermeneutics, etc.), while emphasizing that a practical agreement on narrow questions does not postulate a theoretical agreement on the ultimate philosophical foundations or theological justifications. *The Birth of Bioethics* (1998) is also an essential reference for the formation and history of bioethics, both the term and the field of study. Its author, Albert R. Jonsen is close to the Georgetown group (discussed below). But again, his mention of Potter is minimal. This is a brief and incomplete account of the formation of the term and field—bioethics, but I thought it helpful to point out several significant landmarks.

[3]I have recently discover the use of the term "Bio-Ethic" by the protestant theologian Fritz Jahr in a text from 1927, but it is a hapax and did not have any influence on the history of bioethics that started in the 1970s. I do not deny the existence of a pre-history of bioethics that can be traced back to antiquity.

But the components and amalgam that it uses—Greek roots "bios" and "ethos"—are inherited from a millenary tradition. It would be an interesting and curious exercise to apply to the word "bioethics" the methodology of etymological hermeneutics in going back towards the original meanings of bios and ethos and seeking to find to what extent these words meet and are linked. This path would willingly borrow a Heideggerian ending, probably leading to the conclusion that whoever coined the word "Bioethics" did not know himself what he was doing by bringing these ancient Greek roots together to forge the neologism.

It is Van Rensselaer Potter who first developed the term "bioethics," without the hermeneutic exercise dear to certain strains of twentieth century Continental philosophy. However, simply blaming Potter's philologico-philosophical ignorance would be too pretentious and, in addition, unfair. As we shall see, Potter advanced with a clear understanding that he was constructively defining something new, for which he assumed responsibility and which aimed at the future, not the past.

2 Bioethics According to Its Inventor

Here are the first lines of Van Rensselaer Potter's book *Bioethics. Bridge to the Future* (1971) where the term "bioethics" was coined forty years ago:

> The purpose of this book is to contribute to the future of the human species by promoting the formation of a new discipline, the discipline of Bioethics. If there are "two cultures" that seem unable to speak to each other—science and the humanities—and if this is part of the reason that the future seems in doubt, then possibly, we might build a "bridge to the future" by building the discipline of Bioethics as a bridge between the two cultures. […] What we must now face up to is the fact that human ethics cannot be separated from a realistic understanding of ecology in the broadest sense. Ethical values cannot be separated from biological facts. We are in great need of a Land Ethic, a Wild Life Ethic, a Population Ethic, a Consumption Ethic, an Urban Ethic, an International Ethic, a Geriatric Ethic, and so on. All […] call for actions that are based on values and biological facts […]. (Potter 1971, pp. VII–VIII).[4]

These few lines contain crucial indications. The aim is the future: not the near future and not just any future prospects, but the survival of the human species in the long term and taking into account, which he specifies later, requirements for the quality and improvement of life.

The problem is one of "two cultures," referring to Snow's famous lecture (2001). Himself both a scientist and writer, Snow observed a very deep divide between proponents of literary disciplines and those of the technical and scientific disciplines between which there is no communication and no shared vision of the world. Associated with this harmful dichotomy that continued to widen in the twentieth century, there is another older opposition that is itself partly constitutive of modernity (see for example, Galileo, Hume): the radical separation between fact and value.

[4]The term had already appeared in an article from 1970, "Bioethics, The Science of Survival", this article was integrated into the 1971 book.

Bioethics is introduced as a response to legitimate concerns regarding the future of humanity, and it seeks to do so by building a bridge between the two cultures, denouncing their dangerous mutual ignorance and the cleavage between facts and values. Recognizing that one cannot separate individual and collective action based on values and standards on one hand, and knowledge of the laws and scientifically proven facts that shed light on the conditions and the actual consequences of the action on the other, is at the heart of the solution to the problem of the two cultures and its devastating effects. An ethics (from personal morality to politics) that inspires action cannot ignore facts that are established through biological knowledge.

Bioethics is thus defined as the discipline that builds bridges: a bridge from the present to the future by means of a bridge between two cultures, between facts and values. It is in this sense a discipline that appears therefore as inter- or multidisciplinary, and particularly broad in the range and scope of issues it addresses and the resources it uses to do so. But we must also proceed with a clear understanding that the failures stemming from the problem of "two cultures" are not just on one side, i.e. that of those in the literary and intellectual world of the Humanities who ignore the hard sciences. Scientists must share the responsibility. This is in no small part due to the hyper-specialization of which Potter himself is a lucid representative: trained as a chemist, he became a specialist in some specific aspects of certain type of cancer: "Thus, I began as a chemist, then chose biochemistry, then the biochemistry of cancer, then the biochemistry of one kind of cancer, and I am presently interested in special aspects of that biochemistry" (Potter 1971, p. 150). At the end of his *Preface,* he observes that the range of readings of a specialist is reduced as his specialization is increasingly narrowed to this absurd conclusion where we become the only expert of a hyper-specialized domain, "we read only what we write" (VIII).

Thus Potters's bioethics corresponds to what is today sometimes called "macrobioethics": it concerns human health problems, taking into account social, cultural and natural environments. It is an ecological or global approach to bioethics. The long-term survival of the human species—prior to any consideration of health—is endangered by the modern ideology of progress and unlimited growth, a thoughtless process and one that does not seem to tolerate any negative feedback which would invite it to curb or modulate its own actions or drives. More than once, Potter uses the analogy of cancer: uncontrolled human development on Earth depletes the natural substrate where it proliferates. It is like a cancer in which the cells multiply without order or limit at the expense of the host that the cancer eventually kills resulting in the same time its own end (3).

This fatal growth is global demographics associated with the unbridled exploitation of limited and vulnerable natural resources. Here, as on the issue of "two cultures," Potter reacts to a historical context which began to question the modern ideology of progress based on economic growth and the advancement of science and technology. He cites Paul and Anne Ehrlich, Rachel Carson and welcomes the advent of an Office of Technology Assessment (IX; 3), and he places his book under the aegis of Aldo Leopold. The broader historical context is obviously that of the post-war period which has finally highlighted the ambivalence of science and technology developed under the unequivocal flag of progress (58). It is in this context that Potter speaks of "dangerous knowledge."

But if he means on the one hand that science can be consciously used adversely and diverted in favor of selfish interests, he wants more specifically to say that knowledge is potentially dangerous when in the hands of narrow specialists devoid of bad intentions or even animated by intentions they believe to be good: "Knowledge can become dangerous in the hands of specialists who lack a sufficiently broad background to envisage all of the implications of their work" (69).

The first chapter of Potter's book has a title that defines bioethics on the basis of this anxiety, coupled with a sometimes apocalyptic tendency: "Bioethics, the Science of Survival." In this chapter, bioethics is a *science*; but a science of acting correctly, it is individually and collectively based on science in a more classical sense: one that examines biology and the environment together. A little further, bioethics is defined as *wisdom* in the sense that it brings "knowledge of the use of knowledge," a sort of meta-science of the good use of science and technology: a good use that would ensure "the survival of man and the improvement of quality of life" (1), for present and "future generations" (6). Bioethics is again presented here as a "new ethics," and "*interdisciplinary ethics*." "Interdisciplinary" is defined in a special way so as to include both the sciences and the humanities (4). Moreover, Potter combines these aspects meta-, inter- and multi-: wisdom is "knowledge [of] how to use science and how to balance it in relation to other knowledge" (49).

Defined as a discipline, a science, an ethic, a wisdom, a multidiscipline, bioethics is proving difficult to identify: it is science and more than science. It is a science of science or the *regulation* of science. Here, Potter's interest is carried toward the cybernetic paradigm, another salient aspect of the scientific-cultural context of the time, and mentioned above in reference to the absence of negative feedback in the modern conception of progress. I will come back to this.

And to whom is a bioethics addressed? Scientists of course and, ideally any informed individual, but perhaps first of all to university teachers and politicians (2) because they are the ones who can, through education and regulation, disseminate and enforce the measures recommended by bioethical knowledge, "explain to the public new policies that could provide a 'bridge to the future'" (2) or "make recommendations in the field of public policy" (5). From the outset, bioethics is always bio-politics founded in bio-knowledge. The knowledge it undertakes to develop is a rational knowledge which is of practical significance. The practice of bioethical rationality wants something more and indeed other than the reductive, analytical and positivist rationality that dominates the life sciences. It seeks what Potter claims a "holistic view of biology."

But here we have to be careful and not read this as an invitation to replace scientific methodology, analytical study of the facts and the intersubjective verification of objective causal laws with irrational intuition. What it takes, is more sciences (in the plural) and scientists without blinders to listen to others outside the boundaries of their own strict specializations, scientists capable of seeing the object of their study in the complexity of the relations and interactions which bind the object to its immediate context and the larger contexts that it fits into.

Potter calls himself specifically a "*mechanist*" *and not a* "*vitalist*," *but a* "*pragmatic mechanist*" (11). His invocation of holism is a way to remind the scientists: (a) to not lose sight of the complexity and the total context, in which knowledge is of course never complete or assured in anticipation of its evolution; and (b) not to forget, therefore, the limits of scientific knowledge at a given time, and recognize that we cannot master all the complexity and all the implications of something. His invocation of holism is, in reality, as much moral as epistemological: he invites us to humility, caution, and implores us away from "technological arrogance" (9).

Potter does not encourage a wisdom—vaguely philosophical or religious—which would be a conservative and contemplative holistic vision. He knows that man has always chosen to intervene in nature. Natural evolution itself has led man in a cultural evolution that is interventionist, experimental and which is at the base of the human species' success in the struggle for survival on Earth. It is not about ceasing to intervene; we must only learn to intervene more intelligently (11).

It is in this context that he proposes a conception of man inspired by the cybernetic paradigm that confirms his adherence to causal mechanism, but also to complex "reflexive," open, and prudent systems. The section "Man as an Error-Prone Cybernetic Machine" (12ff) invites us to recognize in the mechanisms of evolution, at all levels, the role of error, randomness, disorder, and the unexpected. These irruptions and interference are necessary, because they are a source of innovations and creations, without which no adaptation or evolution would be conceivable. But they are also risky, inappropriate and often destructive events. This applies both to human intervention in nature and itself. This is why we must develop the knowledge and institutions that allow us to achieve the positive products of this random mechanism and manage its dangers. Potter adheres to Darwinian evolutionism and draws on a number of crucial findings for his remarks. Evolution teaches us that: all species eventually disappear; this is duc to the fact that the mechanisms of evolution—environmental selection, random, spontaneous or induced mutation, the struggle for survival, adaptation to the environment etc.—only take account of the short term. The species that adapts best to a given environment certainly dominates but eventually disappears because of its success: its proliferation and expansion come to destroy the environment in which it lives, or its hyper-adaptation to a specified setting takes away any resilience when this environment is suddenly changed. What looks like progress then returns as a progression towards extinction (47).

The human species will not escape this evolutionary fate unless man becomes able to break away from the tyranny of the short term.[5] Man has indeed shown himself capable of developing a biological knowledge that allows him to take

[5]"Man is the sole product of evolution who knows that he has evolved and who is capable of taking steps that might help to insure survival" (Potter 1971, p. 48). In *Global Bioethics* (1988), Potter acknowledges his debt to Dobzhansky on this point: "In 1958 Dobzhansky made three important points that influenced all my subsequent thinking: (1) no biological law can be relied on to insure that our species will continue to prosper, or indeed that it will continue to exist; (2) the human species is the sole product of evolution that knows it has evolved and will continue to evolve."

account of the long term and not only of immediate and/or special interests. Without dwelling on it, Potter notes that materialistic civilization oriented toward unlimited growth and guided by capitalist laissez-faire ideology is only a kind of vulgar transposition of short-sighted evolution. More generally, the economy, politics and R&D that these civilizations deploy do not go in the direction of caution and conscious foresight of the long-term (47ff).

At the conclusion of Chap. 3 Potter turns his attention to Teilhard de Chardin, who he salutes as a man who has a vision of the long term and a concern for the articulation of the sciences and the *humanities*. Potter however distances himself from *eschatological* evolutionism of Teilhard who believes that enlightened by Christian faith, man knows where he is going: "I think, with other contemporary evolutionists, that the ultimate destiny of mankind is unknown and unpredictable, and that no path can be declared assured of success. All we can hope to do is keep the way open and allow several pathways to be followed" (30).

Potter attaches as much importance to cultural evolution as he does to natural evolution, noting that the former should not be modeled on the latter, as is too much the case in our current dominant short-term conceptions of design and unilateral progress:

> The scientific-philosophic concept of progress which places its emphasis on large-range wisdom is the only kind of progress that can lead to survival. It is a concept that places the destiny of mankind in the hands of men and charges them with the responsibility of examining the feedback mechanisms and short-sighted processes of natural selection at biological and cultural levels, and of deciding how to circumvent the natural processes that have led to the fall of every past civilization. (52)

Potter is a rigorous evolutionist who takes seriously Darwinism and its consequences for all living species. But at the same time he considers evolution as it has taken place so far to not have been inevitable. The human species, with its knowledge of Darwinism can intervene in its own evolution. It is up to bioethics to illuminate this intervention. Clarifying the scope of biopolitics in his thought, Potter devotes a whole chapter (Chap. 7) to the idea of a "Council on the Future": "A proposal to cope with the gulf between scientific knowledge and political direction" (75). It is interesting to summarize how he defines this Council:

- Its mission is to "predict the consequences and interactions that can result from applying new knowledge" (77) and "consider the consequences of major research programs" (78);
- It is "above politics and not responsible for political action" (77–78);
- It has no legislative power but should be able to recommend legislation in a published report (78);
- Its composition should be interdisciplinary in the broadest sense; and this "professional group" could be balanced by a "democratic forum" (78).

It is easy to recognize in this outline the well designed anticipation of what will be or should be bioethics committees at the national and international levels.

Although, as a researcher in oncology, Potter is close to the medical world, medicine and medical ethical problems are not at the center of bioethics as he designs it. It is not that he underestimates their importance; rather he wants to break with the specialized and individualistic approach. Thus, for example, all the difficult and controversial issues associated with assisted human reproduction (contraception, abortion, etc.) or end of life (euthanasia, futile medical care) are to be considered in light of the more general problems of demography and economics, technology and limited biological resources (grafts of tissues and organs), without excessive focus on only the individuals at stake. The same shoud be said of the issues, at the time much more speculative than today, concerning the improvement of the human species by biological means (genetic) and cultural (education, habits, life, legal, legislation, information, etc.) that bioethics currently faces. Potter clearly favors the cultural approach—which includes the development of bioethics itself—over experimental or future enterprises of biological improvement (see Chap. 12 "Science and Biological Man"). Eugenics, cloning, and the like are at this stage considered "dangerous knowledge" and certainly not priorities (153ff; 157).

Though a defender of science, Potter does not share the technoscientific futuristic optimism displayed by many scientists proclaiming: "Give us the laboratories and we will give you the future" (151). Neither optimistic nor pessimistic, he advocates an "informed realism that includes humility [...]. [A] humility that causes us to listen in order to utilize the thoughts of others" (151). This means that encouraging "pluralistic approaches to social problems" founded on the recognition that no one person can predict the future with certainty will give us a greater chance of being on the right side of the future (150).

These problems must be identified and then we must be careful not to choose the wrong priorities. Potter lists these in order "population, peace, poverty, politics and progress" (151). The complex problem of demographic control, the solution to which culture (education), the economy (the end of poverty) and technology must all work clearly comes out on top. As he says: "Acquiescence to uncontrolled fertility will in my opinion lead to war, pollution, poverty, and pestilence beyond the point of no return. As a moral philosopher I therefore say such acquiescence is immoral" (159).

The penultimate chapter returns to the cybernetic paradigm to make "Biocybernetics, the key to the science of the environment" and therefore an essential foundation of bioethics. It should overcome the hard opposition between ecology and economy, both candidates for driving political conduct in public affairs. Economists believe that the only valid criterion for assessing technology is economic growth and the extent in which it serves the economic interests and institutions of those who decide to use it or not (165; 167). However, evaluation should also be made in terms of species survival. For that, you need control mechanisms including the negative feedback and inhibitors indispensable for control and stability. In a system that knows only positive feedback, the acceleration of the process will become such that the system will eventually explode or implode after exhausting all available resources (169). The biocybernetic approach should help achieve “an ecosystem running optimally with a level of human population surviving indefinitely” providing a satisfactory life for all and improving quality (180). To this end, we must guide R&D, including “in deciding what proportion of scientists will be free to pursue pure research and how much will be paid to seek solutions to the problems of society” (184).

In the last chapter “Survival as a Goal for Wisdom,” Potter calls for a “common system of values for the future” (184): an axiological shared platform on which the various religions and philosophies informed by scientific information and maintaining the same concern about the survival of the human species and the same attention to the quality of life of future generations would agree. He relies on Kant (184ff) and goes on to formulate a “Bioethical Creed” consisting of five core beliefs associated with the five commitments arising from a profession of secular and humanist faith that he also presents as revisable (193–196) and that he does partially revise, in fact, in his later work, *Global Bioethics*.

2.1 “Global Bioethics”

Almost twenty years later, Potter published a second book entitled *Global Bioethics* (1988). This book has an interesting foreword by H. Tristram Engelhardt, who had more than once mentioned Potter in his *Foundations of Bioethics* (1986). In his foreword Engelhardt highlights that bioethics now has a history. The word has encountered extraordinary success, partly due to its vague signification and openness, permitting it to build bridges between realities, problems and issues until then treated as separate and disparate: “Such a word has a fruitful or strategic ambiguity” (Potter 1988, p. VI); “The word ‘Bioethics’ has rendered a brilliant service by bringing together a wide range of cultural concerns. The term has been deeply heuristic” (IX).

But this success of the word was unrewarding in relation to the original intentions according to which it had been created. The medical world had seized upon it to form a sort of updated label for medical ethics that primarily served to express a distance from medicine and traditional deontological medical ethics. Potter was well aware of this and he designated Georgetown University and its Center for Bioethics, put in place from the beginning of the seventies, as being primarily responsible for applying the term bioethics to problems only considered in narrowly medical terms. Engelhardt is close to this group which includes André Hellegers, LeRoy Walters, and Warren Reich, and his influence grew steadily, especially through the first Encyclopedia of Bioethics, which appeared in 1978.

Despite these developments, Potter lays out, in this second book, a very strong continuity with his initial approach which he sets about to bring back, deepen and justify with new arguments in *Global Bioethics*. Starting with the ecological and ecoethical dimensions of bioethics, much more than in his 1971 book, Potter emphasizes what he owes to Aldo Leopold: “Unquestionably the first bioethicist,” as he writes in his Preface (Potter 1988, p. XIII).[6] We should not underestimate that between the beginning of the seventies and the end of the next decade, environmental ethics had also vigorously developed and become independent, such that to preserve a distinct identity, bioethics was tempted to move closer to medical ethics.

Potter did not ignore the importance of medical issues in his first book. He wanted to place them in a more complete light, taking into account their complexity. He returned to the subject in 1988 with more space and attention: he devotes a whole chapter to "Dilemmas in Medical Bioethics." But he also criticizes traditional medical ethics as not being distinct from what he denounces in the ordinary approach to the problems raised by R&D within the context of economic, political and common morals: the short term vision, a vision limited to interests and the individual rights or immediate needs and a denial of the wider responsibilities (1; 74; 95; passim). And, I quote: "We can no longer consider medical options without considering the ecological science and the broader problems of society on a global scale" (2).

"Global bioethics" is an expression, all in all, *redundant*, because the first definition of bioethics places at its center this "holistic" requirement for a comprehensive global approach. But redundancy has become necessary because the initial conception of bioethics has been bypassed somehow by its identification with a revisited medical ethics which has not itself expanded and been made more complex by the consideration of global society and, especially, of the global natural environment, i.e. taking into account global demographics and questions of life-style/consumption. Potter now speaks of "global bioethics" because it is clear that the two major components of bioethics—the medical and ecological—tend more to depart from one another than to converge: "Much has been written about environmental ethics without mentioning the need for controlled fertility [which raises medical questions and medical ethics] while much has been written about the rights of individuals without discussing the need to preserve a healthy ecosystem" (75). "Global bioethics" is "a unification of medical bioethics and ecological bioethics" (75; 76). One of the characteristics of the Potter's approach is his desire for balance: "It's all a matter of balancing the options!" he notes (75). This concern seems to me, as a philosopher, although very important, not easy to support, because while we want to speak in a balanced way, we might neutralize the message or at least make it unsuitable for direct action. This risk is present unless we indicate, as Potter tries to do, in what sense there in an imbalance; but then one enters a more or less polemical discourse and there is a risk of being identified and reduced to the trend that one strives to defend because it is considered under-represented.

It should not surprise us to find at the center of Potter's concerns the question of the survival of the human species related to the uncontrolled demography: a problem he considers to be seriously underestimated, especially in the medical world (see, Potter 1988, Chaps. 3 "Human Survival" and 7 "The Control of Human

[6]Potter gives his book the sub-title *Building on the Leopold Legacy*, and dedicates the first chapter to Leopold. See Leopold (1949).

Fertility"). In addition to these fundamental concerns, there are also some interesting new themes in *Global Bioethics*. For example, linking the worries about population and demography to feminism. Potter argues that women are particularly sensitive to all matters relating to human reproduction (free choice, birth control) as well as those relating to the preservation of a healthy environment: they understand the meaning of "care" (86; 88). This sensitivity compensates for the primacy of the "macho morality" of "male domination and male independence" that is "in part the source of the belief that it is possible to find a technical solution to any technical disaster" (90).

We must be attentive not to read into this any technophobia or sciencephobia; rather the primary concern remains for the sense of balance: medicine must be informed about the societal global consequences of its technoscientific progress and drive to push always further. The cult of medical performance and the "tyranny of survival" of the individual lead to serious imbalances. Here, as elsewhere, Potter dreams of harmonious complementarity: "global bioethics must be based on a combination of rights and responsibilities in which the male and female are not seen as mutually exclusive dimensions of a bipolar continuum" (90). Potter is however not a dreamer: Much more than the first book, *Global Bioethics* takes on what we today call "biopolitics," analyzing and commenting on several legal trends, legislation and policies from the 1980s in the USA.[7]

Potter retains a philosophical bent, or rather a leaning towards a kind of practical wisdom, which is not exactly the same thing. He does not know philosophy well and only mentions it briefly so as to underline its limits ("The Limits of Philosophy", p. 80ff). In fact, Potter is and remains above all a scientist who does not conceive of ethics (and philosophy in general) as other than essentially fact-based.[8] This is also why he thinks it possible to develop a quasi "scientific" bioethics, a universal bioethics at least as far as science is universal. In this, he remains thoroughly modern. This is also an aspect that separates Potter from bioethics as it developed under the leadership of Georgetown whose major proponents are often philosophers and theologians. Engelhardt is one of these, but he offers the uniqueness of being a philosopher, physician and theologian.

So, what does Potter tell us about Engelhardt? Like Engelhardt, he sees Bioethics as secular: "a secular program," not to be confused however with "secular humanism," because this current of thought accords too dominant a place to humans within the biosphere, as if man was substituted for God in Judeo-Christianity. Bioethics cannot be based on religious dogma and the separation of Church and State is fundamental (Potter 1988, p. 146ff). Along with Engelhardt, Potter advocates tolerance. But, in addition, Potter is confident of the fact that members of the various religions could agree on key bioethical goals of survival and quality of life (152ff). Engelhardt does not share this belief.

[7]For example, the 1985 "Wisconsin Legislation" (Potter 1988, p. 145).

[8]From the first lines of his introduction he constantly reminds us that ethical values cannot be separated from biological fact (Potter 1988, pp. 1, 59, 75).

According to Potter, Engelhardt also insists much too exclusively on the principle of autonomy at the basis of medical ethics and in so doing only considers individuals and their interpersonal relationships.[9] What does that mean? It is necessary to go beyond the exclusively procedural and individualistic character of Engelhardt's bioethics, which allows for the peaceful management of religious and philosophical diversity, but which does not take account of the biological and ecological realities. Moving beyond diversity is possible from the point of view of global bioethics because it takes into account the scientifically established realities (the facts), and it still assumes a fundamental convergent interest of all when it comes to the survival of the species and the improvement of the quality of that survival. This is why the "global bioethics" approach must lead to conclusions and substantial decisions to which everyone can refer. This is what Potter thinks, believes and wants, and it is a result of his modern universalist vision, which includes the values of justice, solidarity, equality.

Unlike Engelhardt whose individualistic and communitarian positions, but also ethical and epistemological ones, are of a more postmodern trend, Potter has a sense of a global justice, with global (world) meaning (154): he seeks a balance between the desire of each person (rights and individual responsibilities) and concern for all. He wants to empower individuals in an accountable way not only vis-à-vis themselves and, where appropriate, of their community, but to all in general. And it is in this perspective that the problems of survival of the species and natural resources are essential. Engelhardt's bioethics focused on medical issues between individuals and is not concerned by these issues: "Clearly limited to the roles of health care givers and receivers, [Engelhardt's] book does not mention problems of overpopulation or changes in the environment. Nor does it embrace the concept of positive health for populations local or world-wide as a goal for medical bioethics" (156).

2.2 A Last Call

I had the honor and the pleasure to attend (via video link) the lecture where Potter spoke at the opening of the Global Congress of Bioethics at Gijón in June 2000. He died the following year. It was therefore, one of the final reflections on bioethics on the part of its initiator.[10] I was struck by a number of things: First, there was a very strong continuity in his thought, which in the meantime had found new "allies."[11]

[9]"Engelhardt's commendable vision of a peaceful, secular, pluralist society needs to be extended beyond the issues of health care for individuals, beyond the conflicting value differences of traditional religions, and into the biological realities that shaped 'The Land Ethic'." (Potter 1988, p. 121).

[10]Together with "Moving the Culture Toward More Vivid Utopias with Survival as the Goal" (Potter 2001).

[11]His principle references were to Lester Brown and his Worldwatch institute with its annual publication of the "State of the World" report and its call for a "new ethics."

Second, an insistence that "globalism" continues to concern firstly the taking into account of the natural environment for the survival and sustainable development of the human species, but references to the global society and the requirements of social justice are at least as important. In a 2001 article (Potter 2001) he calls for a "realistic balance between anthropocentrism and biocentrism" after having specified: "acceptable survival must be defined as survival that on the one hand is compatible with the continued diversity and symbiotic relations of full-blown species diversity and, on the other, compatible with diverse ethnic populations living in health and dignity in 'civil societies'." This is the vision of his utopia. Third, a continued emphasis on the fact that these problems cannot be resolved by traditional ethics and that bioethics in its broad sense is essential. The problem with traditional ethics could be coarsely summed up by saying that they do not concern themselves adequately with the future, other than in the short term, they are centered on the individual, they ignore the teachings of science and in particular biology. Finally, these last reflections from the founder of the bioethics were marked by a notable sense of urgency: we are living in a state of emergency, "for one hundred years to come, we need a bioethics *policy* with a sense of urgency."

3 A Personal Journey

I also belong to the first generation of "bioethics," in fact, to the generation of those who, coming from different disciplinary backgrounds, have discovered or invented and explored and established this new (inter-) disciplinary field. I belong to that generation of pioneers who have met *independently and following paths often very personal, the same family of questions.* I'm not saying the same questions, but questions that have a family air to them because they have an ethical dimension and are associated with the development of science and technology. My journey towards and in bioethics differs from that of Potter, whose name and existence I was totally ignorant of when these problems first started to demand my attention. We must go back in the mid-1970s when I was working on my Ph.D. thesis (1973–1976) as a philologist and a philosopher. I was at the time much more interested by the philosophy of language and philosophy of the sciences than in moral and political philosophy. But this interest was very critical of the dominant philosophy of the 1960s and 1970s whether it was French, German, or Anglo-Saxon. It is in this framework that I was led to create a new word that has, much like the term "bioethics", subsequently travelled at the discretion of those who used it: "techno (-) science." I have to speak about the introduction of this neologism to illuminate my path to bioethics.

3.1 *Techno (-) Science and (Bio) Ethics*

3.1.1 The Philosophical Context: Response to an Outdated Image of Science Conveyed by a Resigned Philosophy

I introduced the term "techno-science" giving it a range that is both positive and critical. Positively, it seemed more appropriate for describing contemporary science. Negatively, it allowed me to criticize the traditional concept of science as primarily theoretical and discursive, aiming at a symbolic representation of reality. In addition, the concept of techno-science offered a base to denounce the dominant currents of mid-twentieth century philosophy, a philosophy enclosed in its problems of language, unable to face the extra linguistic reality with all of the new questions raised by techno-science.

The first appearance of "techno-science" was in my doctoral thesis from the Université Libre de Bruxelles, *Essay on the Causes, Forms and Limitations of Inflation of Language in Contemporary Philosophy* (Hottois 1976). The thesis was published in book form in 1979 as *Inflation of Language in Contemporary Philosophy* (Hottois 1979).[12] The first sentence in which the word appears immediately indicates the scope and radical criticism of philosophy: "The hypothesis: What contemporary philosophy has excluded is techno-science, the cosmic confrontation, deprived of real illumination [*lumière*], that techno-science opens up, the universe with its transhuman possibilities. Is it a result of the increasingly extensive and complex stranglehold of techno-science on the real that philosophy has lost its ontological reference?" (Hottois 1979, p. 52).[13]

This original association between "techno-science" and "trans-human" is currently of great interest as the discourse around trans/posthumanism is increasingly raising attention and controversy. It is in the third part of the thesis (and the book), entitled "The Cosmic Wall" that the concept of techno-science becomes quite central. In it, a very critical view of philosophy is developed, with however a partial exception: Martin Heidegger, who had seen the importance of technology and what it implies in terms of putting in question—or even denying—human being, language, nature, history, the world, and even Being itself. But Heidegger strives to retrieve, to assimilate the radicality and otherness of technoscience in claiming that what matters to the thinker is not actual, physical techniques, but the essence or better, the "being" of technology, which he calls the "*Gestell*" (framing), meaning that in its essence technology frames or structures all of human existence, rather than being a simple

[12]The thesis is available from the ULB library and as there are some differences between it and the published text, most significantly in the notes, I will make reference to both here.

[13]The translation has altered significantly the form of the original passage: "*L'hypothèse: le forclos (de la philosophie contemporaine) est la techno-science, l'affrontement cosmique dépourvu d'authentique lumière qui s'y pratique, le cosmos aux possibles transhumains. Est-ce par suite de la mainmise de plus en plus étendue et complexe de la techno-science sur le réel, que la philosophie a perdu la référence ontologique*?".

instrumental means to an end.[14] However, Heidegger argues that Being unfolds in language, in words, and not in objects and processes. To understand what happened with the techno-sciences, one doesn't need to be an engineer or cyberneticist or geneticist, but a philologist and hermeneutician: query the word "technique" and its origin, as well as the words to which it is akin, and seek their original and authentic meaning in the texts of tradition dating back to the Presocratics. Despite his being aware of the importance and radicality of technology, Heidegger's solution remains part of the nebula which I later called "linguisticist idealism."

3.1.2 Characterizations of Techno-science and Its Ethically Problematic Scope

The concept of techno-science primarily emphasizes four aspects:

1. The crucial role of technology and more widely procedure (operativity) in modern and contemporary science;
2. The basic operative (and non-theoretical) relation of humankind to the cosmos itself: a relation of transformation, production, manipulation;
3. The dimension of the future as open and opaque;
4. Failure of a simply anthropological concept of techno-science: cosmic operativity (creativity), in which techno-science inscribes itself and intervenes, extends itself indefinitely before and beyond *anthropos*, to the past and to the future, and through cosmic space.

Let us develop this description somewhat along the following themes:

Techno-science and the End of Man

Techno-science is closely associated with the question of the end of man. Not in the sense of finality, but meaning the disappearance by *mutation or annihilation.* Religions and historical philosophies—from Christianity to Marxism—project the future in terms of finality, a sense of accomplishment: the human essence, present since origin but imperfect (fallen or alienated), will be carried or fulfilled out at the end of time or history. Techno-science refers to the disappearance, pure and simple, of the physical human, following some technical or cosmic cataclysm: a physical annihilation without descendants. This idea haunts the imagination of the future, but it seems to especially betray a *lack* of imagination. The idea of the *mutation* evokes not a pure and simple disappearance, but a rupture (sudden or gradual), a change of specific scope, that alters the "essence" of the human. "Techno-science" thus refers to these representations and actions in ways that raise both theoretical and practical

[14]In English *Gestell* is normally translated as "framing." In French the translations of this term in the Heideggerian context are more varied: "*arraisonnement*" (framing), "*dispositif*" (device), "structure," and "machine" are among the most common.

questions concerning the end (but not the finality) of the human species. A purely anthropological concept of techno-science misses this *transanthropologic scope.*

Techno-science and the Future

To characterize techno-science by reference to the future is a no-brainer. But my goal in emphasizing the distant and even very distant future in relation with techno-science was to evoke the strangeness and potential otherness, using the analogy of turning the temporal vector upside down. When compared to the biological, cultural and technical aspects of our present form of human life, the strangeness of the distant future might be as deep and as amazing as the strangeness of forms of terrestrial life from the first or second eras. Nothing could have allowed the inference, prediction or even imagination of our present civilization from the very distant past of paleontological eras. It is therefore not prohibited to imagine for the distant future a strangeness of the same weight if not the same content or same form.

The influence of the Darwinian evolutionary thinking on techno-science and how it conceives temporality is crucial.[15] The distant future must appear as radically *open and opaque*. We must avoid reducing these qualities to one or another prophetic projection and, in particular, to a socio-political utopianism. This kind of projection may have some value for the near future provided that it remains critical and does not aim to lock up evolution in the deadlock of a final utopia. The question about the distant future of man must remain unanswered—and especially avoid recourse to a fixed single answer—not only is this a philosophical question, it is a question that the philosopher has a responsibility to keep open. Keeping this question open and without an unequivocal answer is not without consequences for the evaluation of more concrete issues that arise today, including about techno-scientific R&D. I never forget this opening of the future when practicing and thinking in the field of bioethics.

Techno-science and Cosmic Prospecting

What I called "cosmic prospecting" is not reducible to the exploration of space, even if I do maintain that cosmic space and not terrestrial nature is, *par excellence*, the challenge of the future raised by techno-science. Indeed, in space, away from the support of the terrestrial biosphere, man is totally dependent on techno-science. The spaceship represents an absolute or nearly (insofar as it remains connected to the Earth by radio) absolute micro-technocosme. In the radical break with terrestrial nature and the cultivated historicity of a meaningful world, cosmic space is rough and endlessly opening without direction or horizon, it is delivered up to anthropotechnic adventure. It may involve the technical redesign of the humans that will

[15] Gérard Klein notes in the preface to *Histoires de Mutants*: "The Darwinian revolution introduces an even more vertiginous decentering than its precedent (the Copernican revolution) because it takes a lot of determination to reveal to a whole species the table of its origins and its probable disappearance and replacement in the world, establishing this upheaval in the natural order of things and not in the context of an eschatological global catastrophe." (Klein 1974).

undertake it: hence the idea of the cyborg that I mentioned as a (non-primarily organic) mutational possibility.

When the philosopher asserts that the (Kantian) question "what is a human being?" should be asked without end, indefinitely, this is not only to be understood in the hermeneutical sense of an explorative speculative or narrative discourse, that is in the sense of a merely symbolic practice. The question is also to be understood in the sense of techno-scientific experimentation itself. It is the exploration through operative procedures that are biophysically creative, transformative and inventive. Speech and narrative can accompany and recap, but not anticipate (or just barely) this process, and even less, substitute for it. In short, the exploration of what it is to be a human being, now and in the future, must be undertaken as more than a hermeneutic activity. It is also the activity of techno-science itself.

Futurology expresses however a vital responsibility for the future, but it provides only a "very pale light that accompanies the cosmic exploration" (Hottois 1979, p. 470). Cosmic-prospecting is technoscience running on all fronts. It is productive of the future, while at the same time all eschatology fades in its wake. Cosmic-prospecting, beyond the adventure of space travel, is the attempt at everything possible with the awareness that no particular standpoint, no discourse and no theory will allow for an account of the experience it produces. It is the questioning of man pursued operatively as well as symbolically.

I noted that the first occurrence of "techno-science" is associated with "transhuman" (17; Hottois 1976, pp. 52, 350); I also used the term "post-human" more or less synonymously with "*abhuman*" in this context because it functioned to distance these terms from any kind of mythology of the Superman. I remember having long hesitated between these three words (trans-, post-, abhuman), none seemed quite satisfactory to me. Alluding to the unqualifiable, these terms range from a lack of meaning and reference to over-determination and an arbitrary and naive polysemy. They are however at the heart of my original introduction of "techno-science". Techno-science contributes to the receding, and perhaps eventual removal of "limit-situations" (see Karl Jaspers concept of "*Grenzsituation*") specific to human finitude, declared insurmountable by most philosophies and religions, such as being born, suffering, vulnerability, aging, culpability, death…. I however expressed a reservation or a warning against this optimism, such a future is not expected in a simple and unequivocal manner: "Because effectively challenging limit-situations does not lead to any redemptive and accomplished superhumanity. It opens on the ab-human, the post-human" (Hottois 1976, p. 346, 1979, p. 457). "Attentive to the cosmic exploration, the philosopher," I wrote, "shows the inhuman or abhuman forces that work the human up to the limits of our imagination" (Hottois 1976, p. 362).

Techno-science and Ethics

Up to this point, in my account of the arguments put forth in *Inflation of Language in Contemporary Philosophy* you will have noted, there has been absolutely no question of ethics. It is not until the last section of the thesis and the book that I begin to express my hesitation and perplexity as to how to develop and formulate the new ethical issues invoked by techno-science and speculative imagination. This last section is entitled "The—ethical?—fundamental question." The question mark is quite significant.

The reason for this reluctance is that the categories of ethics appear as "human, too human." Moral sensitivity and conscience belong to the form of human life. Values and standards are historical and cultural. How could one seriously undertake to assess the future of the human species, make choices and decide about its future deliberate developments while using categories that were all internal to human life?

Being itself at stake, judge and party, can ethics do more than protect and encourage the conservation of the natural-cultural human against any deep and adventurous temptation for radical change without immediately rejecting such possibilities as immoral? Is ethics not intrinsically inclined to place "the ultimate dignity of man" in "the assumption of its nature (especially of the parameters of human finitude)" against "the audacity and the risk of the negation of this nature"? (Hottois 1976, p. 368).

I concluded, that however unsatisfactory and not devoid of risk themselves, the ethical categories appear all the same as "less inadequate" (363) to seriously addressing the issues from a philosophical point of view than the alternative of eschewing them. At the time, ethical categories had in fact begun to receive specific and concrete formulations, in particular in the fields of biomedicine and biotechnology, specifically in the form of the then-nascent bioethics in institutional form (commissions, committees of medical ethics).

The position of the French writer, Michel Butor, admirably reflects my own thinking here which I phrased as such: "I would reject the term of humanist if we saw in this idea an absolute validation of a human concept defined once and for all, in opposition to what is not human. […] any idea of man which does not push its boundaries towards the animal or machine, or more generally the abhuman and the superhuman necessarily leads to the oppression of man by himself" (368).

3.2 Evolution

The evolution of my approach to bioethics during the 1980s was decisive. During the first half of this decade, I opened up my thinking even more to ethics, including the more political aspects, but it was not centered on bioethics. What was important to me was a philosophical reflection on technology and techno-sciences, and particularly on the very problematic relation that philosophy and its history still had in the twentieth century (and continues to have) with technology, an attitude often best described as marked by ignorance or contempt (technophobia or techno-indifference). In several works from the 1980s, *Le Signe et la technique* (1984) and *Pour une éthique dans un univers technicien* (1984), I attempted to develop a general philosophy of technology with special emphasis on ethical issues. The latter book—which is a sort of an anthology of commentary and critique of important texts for thinking on technology —is also significant for somewhat broader reasons. Some texts contained in the volume do address bioethical issues, but neither biotechnology or biomedicine occupies a central place. In 1990 nearly the entire text of this small volume was integrated into a larger book published under the title *Le paradigme bioéthique* in French and Spanish at the same time (later also in Portuguese and Italian). What happened between 1984 and 1990 leading to the second publication was primarily a policy event. In 1986, the Belgian Ministry of Health organized the first big national multidisciplinary and pluralistic colloquium in Belgium on "Bioethics in the 1990s" bringing together all Belgian universities. At the time, I was one of the few professors or researchers at the ULB (Université Libre de Bruxelles) who addressed ethical questions associated with techno-scientific R&D. I was therefore asked to represent my University within this framework of bioethics debate that began to become institutionalized and also express policy issues.

It was then, during 1986–1987, that I founded Centre for Interdisciplinary Research in Bioethics (CRIB) with the help of population geneticist Charles Susanne, and I began to commit myself more and more to the field of bioethics, which up to that point I had only touched upon. Previously having been only a particular chapter within a much wider study of the philosophy of technology and techno-sciences or techno-scientific R&D, bioethics became increasingly the center of my research interests. The most productive decade of my work in bioethics extends from the beginning of the 1990s to the first years of the 21st century when I was membre of the European Group of Ethics for Science and New Technologies (EU) and the Comité Consultatif de Bioéthique de Belgique. I will mention here the most significant steps in this development.

In 1993 the first French "bioethics dictionary" with an encyclopedic aim was published: *Les mots de la bioéthique*, which I co-edited. This edition mainly brought together collaborators from CRIB and a medical ethics group at Université Laval in Quebec. In 1999, I published a collection of essays, *Essais de philosophie bioéthique et biopolitique*. The title perfectly illustrates how the focus of my interest had shifted to issues that I had first not contemplated (biopolitics) without abandoning the philosophical issues surrounding "bioethics." This work represented what might best be called a "bioethico-political" trend—what I considered to be a free, secular, and non religious approach. I also always strongly maintained a lively philosophical concern for compliance with the pluralistic and multidisciplinary methodology of bioethical discussion.

This concern expresses itself through the design and direction of the *Nouvelle Encyclopédie de Bioéthique* (Hottois and Missa 2001) and the short book *Qu'est-ce que la bioéthique*? (Hottois 2004a, b). These two works best illustrate my way of dealing with bioethics. In parallel with this ideologically and philosophically "committed" bioethical activity, I continued my independent and comprehensive philosophical reflection on technology and the techno-sciences.[16] These last few years, I started to deal in depth with the issue of the imaginary of science and

[16]Examples of this being *Simondon et la philosophie de la 'culture technique'* (1993), *Philosophies des sciences, philosophies des techniques* (2004a, b), *La science : entre valeurs modernes et postmodernité* (Hottois 2005), and *Dignité et diversité des hommes* (Hottois 2009).

technology in the twentieth century. Having looked at the development of my own approach to bioethics as well as some of the institutional developments in the French-speaking world, let us now return to the question of bioethics itself.

4 Two Bioethical Approaches

Confronting Van Renssselaer Potter's point of view with my own allows us to illuminate certain salient aspects of bioethics. We are both sensitive to the issue of the *two cultures*, although I became aware of it later and in a progressive manner. But we come from *extreme opposites*. Potter's background is as a specialized scientist: he marks off the problems, determines their priority and focuses on the solution. He never doubts that science is unitary, universal and objective. He sees technology as applied science. My background is as a philosophical generalist: the key issues are the ultimate questions, those that remain without a definitive answer. I see science as techno-science, I don't fundamentally distinguish between science and technology and I wonder about the reciprocal impact of techno-science on the ultimate questions and the latter on the former.

This does not prevent us from meeting up on a pragmatic field: when problems are scientifically or objectively established, it is necessary to resolve technical or practical measures. But Potter seems to consider these solvable problems with the conviction that everyone should be able to agree on their solution. His pragmatism is of a scientific and ecumenist orientation. I have sometimes described my own pragmatism as "speculative": I do not want to forget the unanswered questions that lurk in, above, or below issues regarded as solvable. For this reason, I am less convinced than Potter of the possibility that we might all come to agreement at the end of a genuinely pluralist discussion, during which fundamentalist voices for example, are also expressed. As bioethical problems are linked to or even grounded in often-intractable philosophical ones, I, unlike Potter, often see no definitive or consensual answer.

If there is a topic on which we share common ground, it is the importance of the future, beyond the immediate future. But Potter actually sees the future in the medium term, a future extrapolated from the noticeable trends of the present in order to anticipate the problems and risks, and to resolve them. His relation to the future is practical and pragmatic. My first interest in the future is much more speculative: it is the long-term future and even the very long-term, unanticipable, opaque, and open future that grips me philosophically. However, neither Potter nor I have eschatological beliefs concerning the end of time or history and we are not counting on any natural or divine providence.

We are both evolutionary in the sense in which we take seriously the Darwinian revolution. But above all, Potter sees a risk of extinction of the human species by an imbalance and exhaustion of its natural environment. He wants to use science and technology to avert this risk. The danger and the priority that dwarf all other considerations are there: humankind can and should intervene in evolution to escape even its natural fate of extinction. To this end, for the preservation of the human species, the number one priority is the preservation of nature. Beyond this desire for mere survival, Potter also seeks an improvement of the living conditions of humans (or even living in general). He sometimes speaks of an "optimal environment," a kind of utopia in a reconciled peaceful world, evolving perhaps, but without failures, conflicts, or serious imbalances. The danger is the destructive change of natural balances. My vision of evolution is not primarily focused on problems of conservation and preservation of nature. It further takes into account the possibilities of human self-transformation. Its emphasis is more on creativity, diversity, and growth associated with spontaneous evolutionary processes or human-induced. Techno-scientific intervention into evolutionary processes should not only aim to conserve or to preserve, but also to invent, create, innovate, whether it is nature or the human species itself. I am wary of any form of utopianism which tends to focus on the unique and universal and is considered itself the only good way forward, but which may lead to an evolutionary impasse.

If Potter is haunted by the pure and simple disappearance of the human species, which for him lurks in the foreseeable future, I am fascinated by the possible self-transformation(s) of the human species. And I do not exclude the hypothesis that in the very long term, these are better guarantees for the future of man and his offspring than approaches to preservation and conservation. I will therefore leave wide open this field of research and invention, which is absolutely not on the agenda according to Potter.

Potter identifies nature, and I want to add, the original and final universe of humankind, with Earth's natural environment. It is obviously limited in energy and other resources. Potter absolutely does not take into consideration what I call "the great nature," the cosmos, whose resources are potentially endless. He cannot imagine that man, or at least a fraction of the human species, may one day completely split from this native terrestrial nature, migrate through space and live, transformed, in extraterrestrial natures or in technocosms: entirely artificial environments.

I do not share the feeling of an almost apocalyptic urgency that mobilizes Potter. I do not deny the very serious problems, including the environment, that we face, but I think there are various ways to treat them, i.e. various socio-political and technoscientific responses. I still have more confidence in technoscientific research, technological innovations and pragmatic approaches, than in a certainly seductive wisdom that remains vague and has little effect despite its scientific references. In the range of what he calls global bioethics, Potter is more sensitive to the problems of environmental ethics. Personally, I discussed and practiced bioethics more through the issues associated with biomedical ethics.

But both of us have evolved taking still more seriously issues of "society," what could also be called "biopolitics" and "biolaw": bioethical issues approached in their actual context of formulation and discussion that is social, economic, political and legal. Within this framework, Potter straightaway welcomes a more moderate principle of autonomy which underlines risk of excesses and abuse, as well as possible negative consequences for the environment and for social equality, solidarity and justice. Personally, I have always strongly defended this principle both on the individual and community level as well that of R&D. The freedom of scientific research cannot be exclusively or excessively dependent on solving problems of society and companies (defined by the policy or/and the economy).

We agree that bioethics is multidisciplinary, pluralistic and secular. But Potter is more optimistic and positive than me with regard to the possibilities and necessities of consensus. This is because he perceives bioethics primarily as a response to *one* pressing problem or at least a set of closely related urgent problems, which he sees based on a modern vision of science that should enable overcoming differences and divergences especially in emergency situations. Bioethics will be able to solve the environmental and societal problems resulting from individual and collective human activity associated with technological development. He sees bioethics as a new *discipline* or inter-discipline, a new ethic and at the same time a new *science*, a regulatory "scientific" wisdom of science. He continues to rely on this vision while becoming more and more sensitive to the political and economic aspects, the multiplicity of the forces at play that tend to make the bioethics a nebula of ethical-political pressure, pretty far from an actual science. I myself have evolved in my vision of bioethics. But it remains for me, above all, a field of new or renewed questions raised by R&D in the fields of biotechnology and biomedicine within a multicultural civilization in the difficult process of globalization. Questions to which there are, most often, several responses and interim responses; others for which there is no answer.

From a philosophical point of view, the elaboration of these issues demands a respectful pluralism that also respects the multidisciplinary methodology of the techno-sciences with their objective operativity, as well as multiculturalism. I care for the preservation of diversity and for the non-confrontational management of this diversity allowing change, creation and evolution. I see agreements and consensus sometimes as essential and sometimes as dangerous. In fact, Potter thinks of bioethics in terms of multidisciplinarity more than pluralism, without clearly seeing that these notions are quite different. Potter is not hostile to pluralism, but his embrace of modern science does not allow him to see all the difficulties of pluralism. I am much more aware of this question of pluralism linked to the issues of postmodernity and technoscience.

Potter often compared bioethics to *wisdom* and this term connotes the virtues of humility, reserve, temperance, etc. Is it not wisdom that philosophy aims for? But it is precisely the word "philosophy" itself that reminds us that we can never reach wisdom. Wisdom is reserved for the gods. The invocation of wisdom by those who claim to possess it inspires mistrust in me, because wisdom usually goes with a paternalistic authority that combines power, truth and virtue (the good), an authority that in all good conscience presents itself as unquestionable. So I have the desire to preserve the spirit of adventure, of contradiction, of transgression, and of new frontiers to explore and conquer. It is not without risk, but the absence of any risk is not life, it is death.

In conclusion, I would say that between the design of Potter's bioethics (at least as I have understood him) and my own there are many similarities, but there are also profound differences. In a very general way, I see Potter as closer than me to the modern ideology of science and progress. Progress, following Potter, only becomes ambivalent and very perilous because of man's ignorance and lack of consciousness. I am more open in my approach to what is called postmodernism—while perceiving its excesses and by-products—and its suspicion towards the "grand narratives" of science and progress. Despite this, I retain a certain optimism. In the long run, I think more in terms of evolutions and impasses in the plural than in terms of universal and unequivocal progress. The future is full of adventures that will not go without risk. I worry that an excess of caution stifles the spirit of experimentation, research and freedom. Making references among the great names of bioethics, it seems to me that Potter is often closer to Hans Jonas than to Engelhardt.[17] However, Potter does not partake of reservations about science and modern democracy. As for me, I'm probably closer to Engelhardt than to Jonas, even though I don't agree with all Engelhardt's communitarian, neo-liberal or even libertarian choices. What I can say for certain is that in bioethics all the complexities of our era, at once modern, postmodern and pre-modern, are expressed and interact. The practice of bioethics, whatever it is, must never lose the vision of this complexity in motion, which is its wealth as much as its difficulty. Bioethics should not become a narrow specialization, simplifying problems. Let us remember that Potter had invented the word in reaction against specialization, reduction, segregation, biased simplification of issues and responses. Let the current and future (bio)ethicists not forget!

References

Callahan, D. (1973). Bioethics as a Discipline. *The Hastings Center Studies, 1*(1).

Englehardt, H. T. (1986). *The foundations of bioethics*. Oxford: Oxford University Press.

Hottois, G. (1976). *Essai sur les causes, les formes et les limites de l'inflation du langage dans la philosophie contemporaine*. Unpublished manuscript available at the library of the Université Libre de Bruxelles, Belgium.

Hottois, G. (1979). *L'inflation du langage dans la philosophie contemporaine*. Brussels: Editions de ULB.

Hottois G., & Missa, J. N. (2001). *Nouvelle Encyclopédie de Bioéthique*. Bruxelles: De Boeck.

Hottois G. (2004a). *Philosophies des sciences, philosophies des techniques*. Paris: Odile Jacob.

Hottois G. (2004b). *Qu'est-ce que la bioéthique*. Paris: Vrin.

Hottois G. (2005). *La Science: entre valeurs modernes et postmodernité*. Paris: Vrin.

Hottois G. (2009). *Dignité et diversité des hommes*. Paris: Vrin.

Hottois, G. (2011). Definir la bioetica: Retorno a los origenes/Definir la bioéthique: Retour aux sources. *Revista Colombiana de Bioética, 6*(2), 62–109.

Klein, G. (Ed.). (1974). *Histoires de mutants*. Paris: Librairie Générale Française.

Leopold, A. (1949). *The land ethic: Sand County Almanac, with other essays on conservation from Round River*. Oxford: Oxford University Press.

Potter, V. R. (1971). *Bioethics. Bridge to the future*. Upper Saddle River, NJ: Prentice-Hall.

Potter, V. R. (1988). *Global bioethics: Building on the leopold legacy*. East Lansing, MI: Michigan State University Press.

Potter, V. R. (2001). Moving the culture toward more vivid utopias with survival as the goal. *Global Bioethics, 14*(4), 19–30.

Snow, C. P. (2001[1959]). *The two cultures*. London: Cambridge University Press.

Wittgenstein, L. (2009). *Philosophical investigations* (P. M. S Hacker & J. Schulte, Eds.). Oxford: Wiley Blackwell.

[17]Hans Jonas's contribution to bioethics is explored in the next chapter—the editor.

Chapter 3
The Ontological Ethics of Hans Jonas

Michael Hauskeller

1 Introduction

The Jewish-German philosopher Hans Jonas (1903–1993) was already a "bioconservative" critic of the human enhancement project in the late 1970s, before the debate on whether or not it is a good idea to use modern technologies for "making better people" (Harris 2007) had even properly started, and especially the "richer bioethics" demanded and practiced by Kass (2003, 20) owes him a lot.

Jonas studied philosophy and theology under Edmund Husserl, Martin Heidegger, and the Lutheran theologian Rudolf Bultmann, who himself was very much influenced by Heidegger. And just as Bultmann used Heidegger's method of "existential analysis" to interpret the religious terminology and narratives of the New Testament, Jonas used it to interpret the Gnostic tradition in his first major publication (Jonas 1934/1954) and would later, despite his disillusionment with Heidegger as a person[1] and a philosopher,[2] use a similar approach to interpret the phenomenon of life and its ontological implications. Jonas left Germany in 1933 when the Nazis took over, at first for England and then for Palestine. He returned as a soldier in the Jewish Brigade of the British army to defeat the Germans, only to discover when the war was over that his mother had died in a concentration camp. He vowed never to live in Germany again, and he never did. Most of his later life was spent in the United States, where he taught philosophy at the New School of Social Research in New York City. He didn't publish very much, and most of it relatively late in life, but what he published had weight, most notably his exposition of a philosophical biology in *The Phenomenon of Life* in 1966, his *Philosophical*

[1]Cf. Jonas (2008), pp. 187–193 ("Taking Leave of Heidegger").
[2]Cf. Jonas (1966), pp. 235–261 ("Heidegger and Theology").

M. Hauskeller (✉)
Department of Sociology, Philosophy and Anthropology, Exeter University, Exeter, UK
e-mail: m.hauskeller@exeter.ac.uk

D. Meacham (ed.), *Medicine and Society, New Perspectives in Continental Philosophy*, Philosophy and Medicine 120, DOI 10.1007/978-94-017-9870-9_3

Essays in 1980, and finally his ethical masterstroke *The Imperative of Responsibility* in 1984.[3]

Jonas's philosophical work can be understood as an elaborate attack on cosmic nihilism, which is the view that ultimately nothing matters, that all values are man-made and just reflect our transitory interests, so that nothing is in itself any better or worse than anything else. *We* may care what we do, but the *world* doesn't. Nature is completely indifferent to all our endeavours. Whether we live or die, or anything else lives or dies, whether we do certain things or do not do them, whether or not there exists anything at all, all this is of no concern to the universe as a whole. Values only exist in our heads: they are part of the way things *appear* to us, but not part of what they *are*. Jonas believed that this standard view, which seemed to be required by a scientific, materialist worldview and was shared, and still is, by a great number of philosophers, is in fact mistaken. To show how and why it is mistaken, a metaphysical investigation into the nature of being was needed, which, Jonas hoped, would then provide a solid ontological foundation for ethics.

But why exactly is it important to secure such a foundation in the first place? The reason is that for the first time in history humanity has acquired power over being itself, that is, a power great enough to destroy all human life or to radically change what it means to be human, which would also be a destruction of human life, only in a different way. And there is of course also the possibility of destroying *all* life on earth, and not just humanity. At times like this it is important, perhaps crucial for our survival, to once again reflect on the old question, posed by Leibniz, why there is something rather than nothing, but with an *ethical* and hence (since being can take care of itself and is not endangered by anything we might do or not do) *biological* twist: why *should* there be *life* rather than dead, inanimate matter? Could it be that it is *better* for there to be life rather than no life? If so, what exactly would make it better? And is the existence of beings such as us perhaps part of the reason why it is better for there to be life rather than no life? Does anything depend on the *kind* of being that there is? Does anything depend on there being *humans* in the world?

To answer this last question we obviously need to know what a human being is, what defines us as humans and also what, if anything, is specifically *good* about being human. Is there some characteristic of human existence of which we would say that it *ought* to exist because it constitutes an unquestionable good? If there were, this would then, by definition, be something for which it is better to exist than not to exist, and hence something that we ought to strive to keep in existence. Jonas believed that there is indeed something particularly valuable in human existence due to the fact that we are the only beings that can appreciate value and that can take responsibility for what we find to have value. We have, in other words, the ability to recognise the good, the power both to protect and to destroy it, and the capacity to make it our business to protect it, and *that* is itself a good. If this is correct, then it follows that we have a duty to preserve both humanity and a

[3]The German original was already published in 1979.

particular way of being human (that is, both our existence as a species and our human nature). This duty can be expressed in a new categorical imperative that reflects the newly gained possibility of self-destruction: "'Act so that the effects of your action are compatible with the permanence of genuine human life'; or expressed negatively: 'Act so that the effects of your action are not destructive of the future possibility of such life'" (Jonas 1984, p. 11).

This imperative addresses the two different, though interconnected, dangers that humanity faces today: physical annihilation on the one hand and existential degeneration on the other. Human life needs to be preserved, yes, but not just in any form and at any price, only on the condition that it remain *genuine* human life. If that doesn't happen, then humanity may just as well perish. We have created weapons of mass destruction that have the potential to erase all human life, but we have also created technologies that may allow us to change ourselves in such a way that we risk losing what makes our existence valuable in the first place: through manipulation, behavioural control, or genetic reconditioning or whatever else would result in an ethical incapacitation. And that may in fact be the far greater danger. We therefore need to reflect on the *bonum humanum*, on the grounds of human dignity and integrity, and avoid changes that may endanger them, even if this means that we have to forego certain opportunities for progress.

Progress if often spurred by a certain kind of faith in the future, which we may call hope: the hope that things will work out just fine, that although problems may occur along the way, we will find means to solve them, and that no real harm will come to us. Modern technology has a way of inciting such hope. It has a natural affinity to utopian thinking.[4] But hope can easily lead us to ignore the dangers that we bring upon ourselves by putting too much trust in technology. Reason alone doesn't seem to be enough to warn us off certain paths. That is why we need to learn fear again, or more precisely replace the customary heuristic of hope with a *heuristic* of fear. Instead of dwelling on all the wonderful things that the future might hold in store and that we may be able to secure for us by a bold, unhesitant use of modern technology, we should instead focus on what we might *lose* in the process. Prompted by fear we may then realise what is truly valuable (and thus worth preserving and protecting) and why, and that value is in fact at the heart of not only our own human existence, but of the existence of all living things.

Characteristic for the existence of living things is that it is an *embodied* existence. We all live in and through our organic bodies, and that means that we are essentially dependent on our environment. This dependence makes us vulnerable. Vulnerability is thus essential to life; all life is concerned with itself, that is, with the preservation of its own existence. What Heidegger saw as the essential

---

[4]Cf. for instance the landmark report *Converging Technologies for Improving Human Performance*, commissioned by the *US National Science Foundation* and *Department of Commerce* in 2002, whose authors showed themselves convinced that the envisaged convergence of nanotechnology, biotechnology, information technology and cognitive science could only result in "world peace" and "evolution to a higher level of compassion and accomplishment" (Roco and Bainbridge 2003, p. 6).

characteristic of *human* life or *Dasein*, namely *Sorge* (i.e. concern—the fact that it matters to an entity what happens to it), Jonas sees as a characteristic of *all* life, subdued in plants, more articulate in animals, most emphatic in humans, but in some way present in all living things. We all share a common heritage, after all. There is, as Darwin has taught us, no ontological gulf between humans and all the other forms of life on earth. And life itself has, somehow, sprung from inanimate nature. Nature must therefore be conceived in such a way that it allows for the emergence of something like us, of life and consciousness and self-concern, and that means of value. The emergence of life from inanimate matter and the evolution of life from its primitive beginnings to more and more complex forms, culminating in humanity, are inexplicable within the framework of the established scientific anti-teleological worldview. We can only make sense of it by supposing that nature is in fact *not* indifferent, that there is a certain *purpose* behind the appearance and evolution of life, that life was somehow *meant* to arise and to develop, that, in other words, finality is at the essence of being, and that the existence of sentient life is in some unspecified way *better* than its absence.[5]

Life is affirmation of value and in that sense intrinsically valuable. We humans, by virtue of being alive ourselves and hence being able to recognise the value of life, are responsible for life and to life. But we live at a time when the existence of life is no longer a given. We can destroy it and also ourselves. This power makes us responsible for it and informs the imperative to protect life. We ought because we can, as Jonas puts it in a reversal of the famous Kantian dictum (1984, 128).

By attaching so much importance to the role of humanity in the world, Jonas's ethic is clearly anthropocentric, but not ruthlessly so. It revolves around the image of man, which is that of a responsible being, and as such it becomes itself an object of responsibility: humans ought to continue to exist so that responsibility does not disappear.

2 The Nature of Life

Jonas's first major philosophical work, *The Phenomenon of Life*, is an attempt to understand human nature by means of those features that, to some degree, characterise all life, and vice versa: to understand the nature of life in general in terms of features that are normally thought to be peculiar to human life. "The great contradictions which man discovers in himself—freedom and necessity, autonomy and dependence, self and world, relation and isolation, creativity and mortality—have their rudimentary traces in even the most primitive forms of life, each precariously balanced between being and not-being, and each already endowed with an internal horizon of 'transcendence'" (Jonas 1966, xxiii). This precarious balance between

[5]An argument to that effect has recently been advanced, without reference to Jonas, by Nagel (2012).

being and non-being is of the essence of life (and, as will become clear later, also what triggers human responsibility). Being and non-being, life and death, are inextricably intertwined. Before there was life, existence was a given. It couldn't be lost. Things changed, but never ceased to exist. Non-existence was simply not an option. Life introduced a separation between being and being, between self and other, and only selves, i.e. beings that have an identity as that particular thing that they are, can cease to exist. Their existence is never a given; it has always to be fought for, wrested from and defended against the indifference of being. "Profound singleness and heterogeneousness within a universe of homogeneously interrelated existence mark the selfhood of organism. An identity which from moment to moment reasserts itself, achieves itself, and defies the equalizing forces of physical sameness all around, is truly pitted against the rest of things" (83). Life, by its very nature, is thus a constantly renewed act of affirmation. With every living thing a part of being has temporarily freed itself from the rest of being, and, permanently in danger of being drawn back into it, is engaged in an unceasing fight to preserve its freedom and relative independence. We call this process *metabolism*: the matter that it is made of changes constantly, but the organism itself preserves its form and identity not despite but because of this constant change. Once it stops changing, it is dead, and there is a self no longer. In living things form is not a product, an accidental result of indifferent processes. Instead, it informs the change, which is self-integrating. Their very being is a process. Metabolism as the basic level of all organic existence is the first form of freedom.[6] All organic life has freedom, and nothing that is not alive has freedom (although it must have the potential for it, but still dormant, not awakened yet). It is part of what it means to be alive. But freedom has a price. It comes with the burden of necessity and danger, the greatest of which is the danger of annihilation. Metabolism is both ability and need: being becomes emphatic through the threat of its negation. "Its 'can' is a 'must'" (83). Polarity is essential to it: being and not-being, self and world, form and matter, freedom and necessity. Life is, for good and for bad, oriented towards the world: it is open for experience, permanently in exchange. Life transcends itself towards its other, which is an inherently risky business. For this reason, life is *essentially* mortal, not despite of what it is, but because of it.

When we ask ourselves what it means to be human, what is often overlooked is that we are *living* (and that means: embodied, striving, and existentially vulnerable) beings. Yet this may well be the most important thing about us. By accepting the fact that we have evolved from other, more primitive forms of life, we have also come to accept that humans are part of nature, that, in other words, there is no ontological separation between us and the rest of living nature. It is all a question of degree. From the perspective of the modern materialist worldview this continuity

[6] "Obviously, all consciously 'mental' connotations must at first be kept away from the concept when used for so comprehensive a principle: 'Freedom' must denote an objectively discernible mode of being, i.e., a manner of executing existence, distinctive of the organic per se and thus shared by all members but by no non-members of the class: an ontologically descriptive term which can apply to mere physical evidence at first." (Jonas 1966, p. 3).

plainly shows that there is nothing special about being human, that we are nothing but biological machines, just like any other living being. Thus Darwinism strips us of our dignity. Jonas, however, draws the opposite conclusion: far from taking dignity away from us, the fact of evolution gives dignity back to nature. Materialism has got it all wrong. Subjectivity starts with life. It must be there ("however muted its voice may be") for life and death, success and failure, to make a difference. Plants are already sensitive to stimuli. Animals gain locomotion, and with it perception and feeling (fear and desire). The newly formed gap between need and satisfaction, the "mediacy" of animal existence, is a gain in freedom and openness to the world. With it comes the ability to feel pain, which is not a defect that detracts from the ability to feel pleasure, but rather its necessary complement, because animal existence is essentially *passionate*[7] existence.

Yet if being alive involves taking an existential risk, by giving up the total security of being, then it needs to be asked why nature should take such a risk in the first place. What is there to be gained? Why and in what way is it better for there to be life rather than none, and more complex forms of life rather than simpler ones? It must be allowed to ask such questions and to seek an answer. Metaphysics is a fundamental human need. And in this case the answer must have something to do with the nature of what is being created and perpetuated. The need for survival alone is insufficient to understand the phenomenon of life. "If mere assurance of permanence were the point that mattered, life should not have started out in the first place. It is essentially precarious and corruptible being, an adventure in mortality, and in no possible form as assured of enduring as an inorganic body can be" (106). So endurance as such cannot be the point of life. Endurance of *what* is the question, and once we ask it, we can easily see that the *means* of survival, namely perception and feeling, the ever increasing grades of freedom, are themselves an essential part of what is meant to survive. In other words, they are not merely means at all, but also, and perhaps more importantly, *ends*. An existence without awareness of the world and oneself, an existence without concern, is not really worth having. That is why feeling and perceiving animals strive to preserve themselves *as* feeling and perceiving entities, and why as humans, we do not merely want to go on existing, or digesting, but also to keep sensing and thinking and making choices.

That there is something that is *meant* to survive, something that is meant to *be*, is of course an idea that is alien to Darwinism. It is allegedly random mutations together with the pressures of the environment that determine the entirely unplanned direction that the development of life forms takes. But then it would seem that all such development is in fact the product of a series of mistakes. Every mutation is an aberration, a flaw in the gene transmission process, a deformity. Through the accumulation of such deformities new kinds of organism come into existence. This development may appear as a process of enrichment to us, but the theory does not really permit this interpretation. If Darwin got it right, then all apparent "enrichment" is in fact merely "an excrescence on the original simplicity, a

[7]The German word "*leidenschaftlich*" (passionate) derives from the word "*Leiden*" (suffering).

slipping of the discipline of form multiplied over and over again under the licensing of selection; and thus the high organization of any animal or of man would appear a gigantic monstrosity into which the original amoeba has grown through a long history of disease" (51).

For Jonas this implication clearly amounts to a *reductio ad absurdum*. It is an utterly implausible view. But it seems that we can only reject it if we accept that there is some *telos* at work here, or perhaps we should better say *nisus*: an effort that is being made by nature, or something in nature, to achieve certain goals, or at least to move in a certain direction, to climb to higher stages of being, but without guarantee of success, a striving that can be, and often is, thwarted and forced to make detours, and that can even fail entirely.

The highest stage that nature has climbed so far in its effort to gain more and more freedom and openness is the human being. It is also the greatest risk that nature has taken yet. Humans are special because we have reached a new level of mediacy. We are freer than any other living being has ever been. Despite being animals, there is also something "transanimal" in us. Our exceptional freedom manifests itself in three of our most characteristic creations: the tool, the image, and the grave (Jonas 1985). A tool is something that is made for a particular, freely chosen purpose. A stone or a stick is not a tool. Neither is a spider's web. Characteristic for the tool is that its use is not biologically programmed and is not rooted in any function of the organism. Tools allow us to rebuild the world according to what we think is good. The image goes even further in liberating us from the confinement of the given, precisely because it is biologically useless: images don't change the environment or the organism. They serve other ends than mere biological ones. An image makes the absent present and thus to "some extent makes actual experience superfluous by making some of its essential content available without it" (Jonas 1966, p. 171). In the image, form is separated from matter,[8] appearance from reality, and with this separation imagination comes to guide action. *Homo pictor* thus unites *homo sapiens* and *homo faber*. Finally, the grave is even more biologically useless than the image: what it does is allow us to reflect on our own being. It opens the horizon of future and past, the death that lies ahead of us, the dead that have gone before us. Religion, ethics, and metaphysics have their roots here. All three, tool, image, and grave, transcend the immediate and thus create mediacy and freedom on a scale vastly exceeding that available to animals, so that for the first time in the history of life a living being can question its own existence and role in the world. We have become objects (of reflection) to ourselves: "In reflection upon self the subject-object split which began to appear in animal evolution reaches its extreme form. It has extended into the center of feeling

[8]Although some kind of material instantiation is needed for the image to become concretely present, so that in a certain sense form is never entirely separate from matter, the image's material substrate is only accidentally linked to the projected form. The image might be physically present as paint on a canvas, but that doesn't make it the image *of* paint on a canvas. What the image is *of* is not physically present. Thus the image gives us, say, the form of a dog without requiring its material analogue. In *that* sense, form is separated from matter.

life, which is now divided against itself. Only over the immeasurable distance of being his own object can man 'have' himself. But he does have himself while no animal does" (186). But this having is not an immediate possession, but rather an "ever-mediating relation", of which we are the "quivering product". So we keep trying to find an answer to the question that we are to ourselves, and the way we answer it is reflected in the way we live our lives. This brings us finally back to ethics.

3 Human Responsibility and the Elemental Ought

For Jonas, the ontological freedom that we enjoy entails moral responsibility for what we do; at least if what we do affects the existence of things that have value. When things have value they have a claim right[9] on us, that is, on anyone who can perceive that value. Value demands reality, it implies that it is better for it to be than not to be. We are responsible to it and for it if we have the power to harm or destroy it so that it is dependent in its existence on our collaboration. Only the vulnerable or, as Jonas puts it, "the perishable *qua* perishable" (Jonas 1984, p. 87), can be an object of responsibility. Our responsibility roots in the object, which, by virtue of its vulnerability, calls out to us and holds us accountable for what we do to it. The command comes directly from the object in question and thus bridges the Humean gap between "is" and "ought." We can resist this call, but we cannot contradict it. Jonas calls this call the "elemental 'ought'" (130).

An "ought" is elemental if it is experienced independently of social expectations and sanctions in such a way that the object of the "ought" is perceived as a good. That does not mean that we always will what we ought. On the contrary, we experience the primary "ought" as a limitation of our will, but not as a limitation that has been imposed on us by some *other* person's will. The limitation is intrinsic in the sense that we cannot disregard it and rid ourselves of the obligation. It is, in other words, impossible not to care. Phenomenologically speaking, this elemental ought, which cannot be traced back to any particular will, comes to us directly from the being of those things that are affected by our actions. The reason why we ought to do something is not that other people want us to do it. Rather we ought to do it because we cannot help thinking of it as a good, be it either that we consider the action itself as good in its own right (that is, as *intrinsically* good) or that we believe the action to be conducive to the preservation of some good or the prevention of

[9]A *claim right* is a right that I hold against somebody else who has a duty to provide me with or protect whatever it is I have a right to. Claim rights are to be distinguished from *liberty rights*, which do not correspond to anyone's duty. Thus I have a liberty right to go for a stroll in the park, but nobody has the duty to make sure that I can get to the park or that there is a park to stroll in the first place. My liberty rights do not affect anyone else's freedom in any way. If, on the other hand, I have a claim right to something, then others are no longer free to do as they please with respect to what the right is about.

some evil. In most cases the source of the primary ought is an object that by virtue of what it is (or of what we recognize it as) curtails our freedom to act by demanding that we behave towards it in certain ways and not in certain other ways. This means that in the experience of the elemental "ought" the "is" and the "ought" coincide or converge.

Jonas has described the perception of a newborn baby as a paradigmatic case of such a convergence. Jonas insists that the newborn is an object that does not permit a classification in terms of a mere "is." Its very breathing directs an "ought" to its environment, namely to take care of it. Just by looking at it we know immediately what response is required, what it needs us to do. Not very surprisingly, critics have rejected Jonas's claim as an unacceptable inference of an "ought" from an "is," that is, they have accused him of a naturalistic fallacy. From the fact that an entity is a newborn baby we cannot infer anything about how we ought to treat it (Birnbacher 1997, p. 228). However, Jonas himself foresaw this objection and argued, quite rightly, that the critic's supposed fact is nothing but a construction. There simply is no such thing as *the* fact of the newborn baby. Rather, what is presented as the facts is already the product of a particular perspective, one that does not allow for the baby to be seen as more than an interacting conglomeration of cells. To be such a conglomeration of cells is at best merely a part of the reality of the child, but certainly not the whole reality. Even if it is *also* a conglomeration of cells, it is not, as Jonas says, the "given in its fullness" (Jonas 1984, p. 131). Once we see the *newborn child*, we cannot but feel duty-bound to safeguard its existence and to attend to its well-being. Although it is possible to abscond from it, the duty is still felt as such, and it is not easy to ignore it. The newborn child, whose existence unites "the self-accrediting force of being already there and the demanding impotence of being-not-yet" and thus has to be understood as a "suspension of helpless being over not-being, which must be bridged by another causality" (134), presents itself as an entity for which support by others is, as it were, ontologically intended.

Of course we can at this point, by adopting a perspective external to the situation, again ask *why* we should give the support that, allegedly, is ontologically intended. Why, after all, should we care for the ends of being (always assuming that there are such ends in the first place)? However, the crucial point to bear in mind is that this question simply does not arise for those who see the newborn child with the ontological characteristics that Jonas describes. Looking and knowing (what to do) are then one and the same. That which unites the two is feeling: the feeling of sympathy or compassion, or simply of involvement, of not-being-able-to-extract-oneself from the situation. It is in short the feeling of *responsibility*.

Being asked why we should consider such feelings morally relevant or legitimate, we will struggle to find an answer that is more persuasive than the feeling itself. It is, after all, the feeling that puts us under a certain pressure to act by legitimising a particular action and shedding doubt on the legitimacy of alternative actions. Although it is for this reason hardly possible to give a justification that does not tacitly presuppose the very feelings that it is meant to justify, the connection of these feelings with the object to which they refer is anything but arbitrary. They have their ground in the perception of an object that, in the way it presents itself or is perceived, makes the feelings in question appear to be the only proper reaction to it. When we perceive the child *as* a child we experience ourselves as being restricted in our freedom to act, in such a way that we feel that we must treat it in a certain (namely loving and caring) way. Adequately apprehending the object, that is, apprehending it in its entirety, certain actions are suggested to us, without being logically deducible from a description of the object. As soon as we extricate ourselves from the situation and try to assess it from the perspective of an "impassive observer," a "pure, will-less, painless, timeless subject of cognition" (Schopenhauer), we will inevitably perceive a gap between "is" and "ought" that can never be closed, not even by the most sophisticated justification strategy. Once we look at the world as if from the outside, reducing it to a mere spectacle and ourselves to spectators with a merely academic interest in the events that unfold before our eyes, we will no longer be able to perceive the intimate connection between "is" and "ought" that is so obvious to anyone still within the situation.[10]

4 Human Enhancement and the Imperative to Protect Human Nature

A perhaps less obvious, but in Jonas's view equally compelling case of responsibility is the one we have towards humanity as a whole, the recognition of whose newly endangered existence and value likewise demands that we protect it and make sure that humanity will continue to exist. Here, too, the "is"—the fact that there are humans—translates directly into an "ought"—the imperative that humans ought to be. Whatever we do, this must not be endangered: "Never must the existence or the essence of man as a whole be made a stake in the hazards of action" (Jonas 1984, p. 37), which also means that "no condition of future descendants of humankind should be permitted to arise which contradicts the reason why the existence of mankind is mandatory at all" (43). Thus it is our evolved nature that must be preserved, not only because we must assume that what we are is more than the product of blind forces and that it is in fact owed to a tendency in nature to produce and increase value, but also because we cannot denigrate our own nature as defective and devoid of value without contradicting ourselves: "there is the heritage of a past evolution for us to preserve—which heritage cannot be all bad in our case, if only because it has bequeathed to its present incumbents the (self-proclaimed) capacity to be judges of what is good and what is bad" (32). To deny the value of

[10]It is interesting to see that Jonas never worries about the question that is at the centre of most bioethical discussions about the moral status of human embryos, foetuses and infants, namely whether they have a *right* to life. Whether or not they do is simply not the issue: vulnerability is, which, in contrast to many contemporary bioethicists (cf. for instance Tooley 1972; Giubilini and Minerva 2012), he regards as morally relevant.

our nature is to deny the value of the judgement that our nature has no value.[11] There is nothing wrong with change, and improvement is certainly both possible and often desirable, but it must always come second to the protection of our humanness. It is *not* our duty to make the world a better place (as, for instance, Harris (2007, p. 3) claims, not accidentally invoking Karl Marx in support). We may owe future generations that we leave the world intact for them, but we do *not* owe them that we try to make things better for them.

But what is proposed as an enhancement of human nature is not only not owed to anyone, it is often, despite the initial appeal that all simple solutions to complex problems have, detrimental to human nature. The attempt to control behaviour through biotechnological means (which seems to be one of the main ends of bio-medical enhancement) is a good example:

> Shall we induce learning attitudes in schoolchildren by the mass administration of drugs, circumventing the appeal to autonomous motivation? Shall we overcome aggression by electronic pacification of brain areas? Shall we generate sensations of happiness or pleasure or at least contentment through independent stimulation (or tranquilizing) of the appropriate centers – independent, that is, of the objects of happiness, pleasure, or content and their attainment in personal living and achieving? (Jonas 1984, p. 20).

From a utilitarian point of view this may all seem like a good idea, but not when we take into account our responsibility for preserving the integrity of human nature: "Regardless of the question of compulsion or consent, and regardless also of undesirable side-effects, each time we thus bypass the human way of dealing with human problems, short-circuiting it by an impersonal mechanism, we have taken away something from the dignity of personal selfhood and advanced a further step on the road from responsible subjects to programmed behaviour systems" (20).

The danger only increases when we make the step from the manipulation of already existing (annoyingly independent) individuals to the *engineering* of humans that are (or are at least intended to be) exactly how we want them to be. First of all, we cannot experiment with the relevant technologies until we are certain that they will actually work the way we intend them to. In order to find out what will happen we need to use those methods on actual human beings and wait and see what happens (Jonas 1980, pp. 143–145). Then there is a problem with the very power that those technologies give us, because that power is never really ours, but in actual fact always the power that some people have over others, and ultimately also the power that technology has over us by making us dependent on it (146–147).[12]

[11]It is this inconsistency that Alan Buchanan overlooks when he rejects the idea of evolution as a "master engineer" to support his claim that human enhancement is not only immensely desirable, but absolutely necessary to prevent the demise of humanity. In Buchanan's view we are nothing but "tentative, changing, perishing, cobbled-together ad hoc solutions to transient design problems," and evolution, far from being a master engineer, is "more like a morally insensitive, blind, tightly shackled tinkerer" who has no clue what he is doing (Buchanan 2011, p. 2). Although Jonas would probably agree that evolution is not a master engineer, he would insist that the product is still a considerable achievement, not accidental, and definitely worth preserving.

[12]This concern had already been raised even more forcefully by Lewis (1943), pp. 67–71.

Furthermore, do we even have the *right* to try to determine future people's make-up, and if we do have that right, are we really *wise* enough to use our power properly? And where exactly do we want to go with it? Which purpose do we want to follow? Other things can be made more useful, but they are always more or less useful to *us*, and it is unclear how we can make ourselves more useful to ourselves, according to which criteria, and to *whose* criteria. "Who will be the image-makers, by what standards, and on the basis of what knowledge?" (Jonas 1984, p. 21). It seems that the conditioners, the image-makers, must be exempt from the need for improvement. They must already be what they think others should become, so that they can be trusted to determine what is useful and what not, which purposes are worth pursuing and which not. And all the while, in focusing on usefulness, on making people fit for purpose, we grow accustomed to the idea that people ought to be useful for something and hence that they are not, as we have hitherto tended to believe, *ends in themselves*. For Jonas this is yet another disruption of the image of man.

Moreover, there are various conflicting ideals of humanity, and it is not clear at all to which we should give preference: "That diabetes, epilepsy, schizophrenia, haemophilia are undesirable, to afflicted and fellow men alike, is noncontroversial. But what is 'better'—a cool head or a warm heart, high sensitivity or robustness, a placid or a rebellious temperament, and in what proportion of distribution rather than another; who is to determine that, and based on what knowledge? The pretense to such knowledge alone should be sufficient ground to disqualify the pretender" (Jonas 1980, p. 154).

It is not even clear that standardisation, which all deliberate design will ultimately result in, is desirable. That is exactly what (undirected) evolution has so far protected us against. Our great advantage has always been that we were *not* specialised, and now we are trying to remove precisely that advantage by making ourselves more and more useful with respect to certain purposes. And do we really want or need more Mozarts and Einsteins? Aren't they one of a kind, and isn't that at least part of why we treasure them? Even in the choice of ideals we tend to be guided by a narrow and short-sighted conception of usefulness: "Nobody ever mentions Nietzsche in this connection, or Kafka, few even Beethoven or Michelangelo—a revealing symptom of the tacit eudaemonism of the whole dream: one wants his genius happy or at least serene; but most of all, edifying in his 'contribution'" (160, fn).

Yet perhaps the most important objection to the non-therapeutic use of biological engineering is that it would violate a basic right, namely the *right to ignorance*. Not knowing who we are (or meant to be) is a precondition of freedom. We all have a right to seek and find ourselves, in an open encounter with the world, and to be engineered to possess certain properties prevents us from doing that. This has nothing to do with genetic determinism. Whether we actually have those properties that others meant us to have as a result of their manipulation is irrelevant. What counts is how knowing that we have been engineered to be a certain kind of person affects the way we see ourselves, and it is important (in fact imperative) that we remain able to see ourselves as new, unprecedented, rather than as copies of someone else (in the case of cloning), or someone else's imagination (in the case of genetic manipulation). "What matters is that the sexually produced genotype is a novum in itself, unknown to all to begin with and still to reveal itself to owners and fellow men alike. Ignorance is here the precondition of freedom: the new throw of the dice has to discover itself in the guideless efforts of living its life for the first and only time, i.e., to become itself in meeting a world as unprepared for the newcomer as this is for himself" (161).[13] Knowledge can be paralysing, even if it is only apparent. It must be an open question (for ourselves and others) who we are. And so, from our responsibility for the preservation of humanity (including its evolved nature) a new ethical command ensues: "never to violate the right to that ignorance which is a condition for the possibility of authentic action; or: to respect the right of each human life to find its own way and be a surprise to itself" (165).

5 The Burden and Blessing of Mortality

Among those who find it desirable that we create and use technologies that help us overcome our present human condition, few seem to have any doubts that the (ideally indefinite) extension of our life spans is what is most urgently needed today. As long as we have to die, the utility that other enhancements have for *us* personally must appear rather limited. Yet once we no longer have to die, we can take our time with other enhancements and enjoy them in peace. For this reason radical life extension is the holy grail of the human enhancement project.

From Jonas's perspective, however, the whole idea of overcoming death is misguided right from the start, not the least because it is based on a glaring misunderstanding of what life actually is. Life and death are intertwined. They are two sides of the same process. Life confirms itself (as valuable), but it can only do so because challenged. Value comes into the world through life and death. The permanent challenge, the possibility of death, "stirs and powers the yes" (Jonas 1992, p. 36). Existence of this sort "is the sole seat of meaning in the world" (38) because it works as an incentive to "number our days and make them count" (40). Moreover, without death evolution would not have been possible. And neither would progress. Death plays a *creative* role. It promotes novelty and diversity, higher forms of life and subjectivity. Through dying we make room for new life. There is birth because there is death, and the arrival of new life is in itself of great value. It allows us to "see the world for the first time, see things with new eyes, wonder where others are dulled by habit, start out from where they had arrived" (39).

---

[13]A similar argument was much later proposed by Habermas (2003), p. 41, who suggests that "the instrumentalization of human nature" might change "the ethical self-understanding of the species in such a way that we may no longer see ourselves as ethically free and morally equal beings guided by norms and reasons." So on this account it is not so much what we are that will have changed (free or not free), but rather how we will in all likelihood view ourselves and each other (as free or not free). The change "takes place in the mind" (Habermas 2003, p. 53).

> There is no substitute for this in the greater accumulation of prolonged experience: it can never [...] relive the wonder which, according to Plato, is the beginning of philosophy; never the curiosity of the child, which rarely enough lives on as thirst for knowledge in the adult, until it wanes there too. This ever renewed beginning, which is only to be had at the price of ever repeated ending, may well be mankind's hope, its safeguard against lapsing into boredom and routine, its chance of retaining the spontaneity of life. (Jonas 1984, p. 19)

Jonas is well aware, though, that for the individual their own mortality is hard to bear. Death is in many ways a blessing, but for the individual it is also, and perhaps mostly, a burden. Thus Jonas positions himself between the extreme positions of anti-deathism, where death is cast as the greatest evil,[14] and the indifferentism famously advocated by Epicurus (Laertius 1958, p. 651). Death is neither the greatest evil nor a matter of indifference. It is simply an essential part of life: the price we pay for living and for things to matter. We should therefore accept and to a certain degree welcome it. Once we do this, we may realise that there is no ethical need to save as many lives as possible, as it is often assumed today. Saving lives is good as long as those lives are still worth living and saving them does not require sacrificing what makes them valuable in the first place. And what makes them valuable is certainly not their usefulness for others, or for society as a whole. That is why, for instance, organ donation (Jonas 1980, pp. 107–133), while it may well be desirable as a voluntary sacrifice, can never be demanded. Nobody has the right to somebody else's body. Certainly, people will die if we cannot procure a sufficient number of organs, but there is no right to be saved from a natural death by all available means, or a duty that society has to procure the organs necessary for survival. Society doesn't own one's body. That society cannot "afford" wasting those organs is nonsense. Of course it can. Society is in fact based on the natural cycle of death and birth. What society *really* cannot afford is any infraction of a human right, any miscarriage of justice, and that is exactly what would occur if society claimed a right to the use of people's bodies:[15]

> At the border between the common external world that we share with others and our own interior body, at our skin, *every* public right ends. Just as nobody, neither the state nor the suffering fellow man, has a right to one of my kidneys, and just as the organs of an irreversibly comatose patient cannot be legally taken for the purpose of saving others, public interest or the common good has no right to my metabolism, my circulation, inner secretion, neuroactivity or anything that happens within my body. This is the privatissimum of the private, the non-communal, unalienable personal space per se. (Jonas 1987, p. 126)[16]

This is also the reason why Jonas vehemently opposed the proposal made in 1968 by an ad hoc committee of the Harvard Medical School to redefine death as irreversible coma or more precisely the irreversible end of all brain activity (Jonas

[14]Cf. for instance More (1990), Bostrom (2005) and de Grey (2007, p. 36).

[15]Cf. for instance Harris (1975), or Wilkinson and Savulescu (2012).

[16]This passage is from a paragraph that is missing from the English version of Jonas's article "Philosophical Reflections on Experimenting with Human Subjects," which can be found in his *Philosophical Essays* (1980, pp. 107–133). I am citing from the German version. The translation is my own.

1980, pp. 134–142). From Jonas's point of view it is simply incorrect to declare a living being, whose metabolic processes are still working, for dead. Moreover, it is morally repugnant because the redefinition is entirely motivated by pragmatic concerns: it is meant to make it easier to harvest usable organs. It is thus a device to maximise utility, to get more organs, to lower costs, to save scarce resources, etc. The formerly dying, now dead person has the advantage of still possessing a living body that we can use for all sorts of things that a dead body would not permit, but it lacks the disadvantage of having a moral status that would put moral constraints on the way we can use it. Redefining the living as dead is an ideal solution to certain perceived needs, but it can also easily be exploited, or at least there is no reason why we should not extend the license that it gives us. If we can take the organs of the living dead, why should we stop there? We could also conduct toxicological experiments on them, infect them with certain diseases to test for possible cures, etc. Whatever strikes us as useful should be allowed in the name of the common good.

Jonas, however, does not buy into this argument. We are not dead simply because we have stopped thinking. As long as our body is alive, we are too. There is no strict separation between the mind and the body, or the brain (as the alleged seat of our personality) and the rest of our body. Every living thing, ourselves included, is one integrated whole, a psychophysical unity.

> My identity is the identity of the whole organism, even if the higher functions of personhood are seated in the brain. How else could a man love a woman and not merely her brains? How else could we lose ourselves in the aspects of a face? Be touched by the delicacy of a frame? It's this person's, and no one else's. Therefore, the body of the comatose, so long as – even with the help of art – it still breathes, pulses and functions otherwise, must still be considered a residual continuance of the subject that loved and was loved, and as such is still entitled to some of the sacrosanctity accorded to such a subject by the laws of God and men. That sacrosanctity decrees that it must not be used as a mere means. (Jonas 1980, p. 141)

The rejection of the brain-death criterion has got nothing to do with the question whether or not, or when exactly, treatment of a comatose patient can and should be stopped. We don't need to define anyone as dead before it is acceptable to leave them in peace and let them die. It is merely the prevailing fainthearted attitude to death that makes us think that. "The cowardice of modern secular society which shrinks from death as an unmitigated evil needs the assurance (or fiction) that he is already dead when the decision is to be made. The responsibility of a value-laden decision is replaced by the mechanics of a value-free routine" (141). Death, Jonas believes, has its own fitness and dignity, and that is why everyone has a right to be let die if their life is not worth living anymore. Mindless vegetating is not the kind of life that humans are meant to have, the kind of life that gives value to their existence. Thus Jonas defends the "right to die," not only in the case of the irreversibly comatose, but also in cases where we are still able to make our own choices, but do no longer consider our lives worth living (Jonas 1978). Mortality is part of our lives, and just as we all should be free to live our own lives and find out for ourselves who we are (unburdened by the preconceptions of others), we should also be allowed to come to terms with our own death in our own personal way. There are of course exceptions. Sometimes we do have obligations to others, which constrains our right to die. It is also acceptable to prevent someone from committing suicide if it is in their own power to kill themselves, because such prevention can only ever be temporary. By intervening we do not really force someone to live on, we just give them the opportunity to reconsider. Yet if somebody really wants to die, then we have no right to stop them because life must be worth living; it must be a proper human life.

However, Jonas is adamant that we do *not* have a right to be *killed*. Active euthanasia is out of the question because the healer must never become the killer. Jonas thus rejects Tooley's moral symmetry principle: there is clearly a morally important difference between killing and letting die. The patient always has the right to go away, to refuse treatment. The fact that they are no longer able to do that should not be held against them. Not forcing someone to live is not the same as killing them. It is the most vulnerable that need the most protection, and it is our responsibility to protect both their right to life and their right to die because correctly and fully understood the right to life also includes the right to die.

References

Birnbacher, D. (1997). *Ökophilosophie*. Stuttgart: Reclam.

Bostrom, N. (2005). The fable of the dragon tyrant. *Journal of Medical Ethics, 31*, 273–277.

Buchanan, A. (2011). *Beyond Humanity? The ethics of biomedical enhancement*. Oxford: Oxford University Press.

de Grey, A., & Michael Rae, M. (2007). *Ending aging*. New York: St. Martins Press.

Giubilini, A., & Minerva, F. (2012). After-birth abortion: Why should the baby live? *Journal of Medical Ethics* (online first).

Habermas, J. (2003). *The future of human nature*. Cambridge: Polity.

Harris, J. (1975). The Survival Lottery. *Philosophy*, 50, 81–87.

Harris, J. (2007). *Enhancing evolution: The ethical case for making better people*. Princeton and Oxford: Princeton University Press.

Jonas, H. (1934/1954). *Gnosis und spätantiker Geist* (vol. 2). (1958, *The Gnostic Religion*. Boston: Beacon Press, Trans.). Göttingen: Vandenhoeck und Rupprecht.

Jonas, H. (1966). *The phenomenon of life*. New York: Harper & Row Publishers.

Jonas, H. (1978). The right to die. *The Hastings Center Report, 8*(4), 31–36.

Jonas, H. (1980). *Philosophical essays*. Chicago: University of Chicago Press.

Jonas, H. (1984). *The principle of responsibility*. Chicago: University of Chicago Press.

Jonas, H. (1985). Werkzeug, Bild und Grab. *Scheidewege, 15*, 47–58.

Jonas, H. (1987). *Technik, Medizin und Ethik*. Frankfurt/M: Suhrkamp.

Jonas, H. (1992). The burden and blessing of mortality. *The Hastings Center Report, 22*(1), 34–40.

Jonas, H. (2008). *Memoirs*. Lebanon, NH: Brandeis University Press.

Kass, L. (2003). Ageless bodies, happy souls: Biotechnology and the pursuit of perfection. *The New Atlantis, 1*, 9–28.

Laertius, D. (1958). *Lives of eminent philosophers* (vol. 2) (R. D. Hicks, Trans.). London: Heinemann.

Lewis, C. S. (1943). *The abolition of man*. Oxford: Oxford University Press.

More, M. (1990). Transhumanism: A futurist philosophy. *Extropy, 6*, 6–12.

Nagel, T. (2012). *Mind and cosmos*. Oxford: Oxford University Press.
Roco, M. C., & Bainbridge, W. S. (Eds.). (2003). *Converging technologies for improving human performance*. Dordrecht: Springer.
Tooley, M. (1972). Abortion and infanticide. *Philosophy and Public Affairs, 2*(1), 37–65.
Wilkinson, D., & Savulescu, J. (2012). Should we allow organ donation euthanasia? *Bioethics, 26* (1), 32–48.

Chapter 4
On the Origins of Illness and the Hiddenness of Health: A Hermeneutic Approach to the History of a Problem

Niall Keane

1 Nature and Health: The Classical View

If health is definable as a dynamic equilibrium, then there needs to be some criterion for its re-establishment or restoration. For centuries this criterion has been identified as nature, a criterion which is not altogether unproblematic. It must be said that the adjectives "natural," "artificial," "willful," and "reasonable" appear far more robust and malleable than the nouns from which they are derived, namely, "nature," "art," "will" and "reason." If one examines these terms, it is striking that the term "natural" always contains a twofold significance.

For instance, the word "natural" is a genetic notion, referring to a particular relationship to a source or origin, and yet it is also normative, indicating a criterion for judging trends, actions and situations. Consider, for example, the antithesis of natural and artificial. Artificial or false teeth, for example, are those that, unlike natural teeth, did not grow by themselves. The goal of the dental technician, however, is that he or she produces teeth which are as natural as possible, i.e. they should be as similar as possible to those which grew or would have grown of their own accord, or in some cases even better than those natural teeth. Yet the criterion for judging what is best in this particular case must take its start from nature itself, that is, from that natural function which allows us to distinguish the good from the bad, in this case good teeth from bad teeth.

For Aristotle, self-organization or self-regulation is the decisive factor to be taken into account when distinguishing what is natural from what is not. This is clarified in Book II of the *Physics* when he writes, "If the ship-building art were in the wood, it would produce the same results by nature. If, therefore, purpose is present in art, it is present also in nature. The best illustration is a doctor doctoring himself: nature is like that. It is plain then that nature is a cause, a cause that

N. Keane (✉)
University of Limerick, Limerick, Ireland
e-mail: Niall.Keane@mic.ul.ie

D. Meacham (ed.), *Medicine and Society, New Perspectives in Continental Philosophy*, Philosophy and Medicine 120, DOI 10.1007/978-94-017-9870-9_4

operates for a purpose" (Aristotle, *Physics* II, 199b27–199b31–32). Given the above quote, the opposition between the terms "natural" and "artificial" appears to have emerged from a distinction between the "from within" and the "from without." This distinction could function in pinpointing and comparing the antithesis of "natural" and "artificial" with the antithesis "natural" and "violent." Violence, for the Greeks, is that precise movement or motion which does not follow from the nature of what is moved. It should be stated that modern physics no longer knows or operates with this difference. That said, we continue to use words in a way that the ancients would have understood, for example when we distinguish natural death from violent death. For example, the lion that devours the antelope is the natural cause of its death, yet for the antelope that is eaten by the lion the death is intensely violent. The distinction between violent and natural thus presupposes an appetite or instinct of sorts, in relation to which one can say whether something is violent or not. It should be noted that while the artificial reproduces or cooperates with nature, the violent destroys it.

Yet how can the notions of "natural" and "artificial" form an antithesis, if the artificial is more and more complete the closer it gets or approximates itself to the natural? From this perspective one can see the ambiguity of these terms, the meaning of which is in some cases genetic, while in others normative. In contemporary usage "artificial" has a predominantly genetic implication. When it comes to its normative usage, the term "artificial" more often than not carries with it a pejorative sense, usually signifying that the product is not as perfect or as functional as was desired.

Things are not altogether different when it comes to the distinction between "voluntary" and "natural." It is all too easy to forget that the voluntariness of the voluntary act appears to be natural. Only when one recognizes it as natural is the natural goal reached. Only then will the will appear to agree with itself. Arguably inspired by Zeno, the Stoics called the agreement or accord of the will with itself a "harmony with nature" (*homologoumenôs têi physei zên*) (see Cicero, *De Finibus*, III, 5). For the Stoics a harmonious life was synonymous with living in harmony with nature, and by extension with the cosmos. And this meant to think in accord with reason. However, this *homologia têi physei* is not *kata physin* pure and simple, it is not simply with or for nature and does not occur by itself. This brings us to the paradox that only where the will is totally detached from the natural in the genetic sense is it natural in the fully normative sense of the word. This indirect naturalness could be defined as the emergence of rationality.

Thus there are two different ways of understanding and speaking about *physei on*, natural beings or entities. Natural can on the one hand indicate the origin or explanatory cause of something, while on the other it can indicate a criterion of what simply conforms to nature. Hence it depends on the perspective and the interests at stake when it comes to something being defined as natural or unnatural. Once again, and depending on one's perspective, the lion devouring the antelope is the antelope's natural cause of death, as well as the violent cause of death.

Consequently, the concept "natural" can be broken down into (1) the origin or explanatory genesis of something and (2) something conforming to or being in accord with nature. The reason we do not know what is good for us often comes down to the fact that the relationship our nature has with itself is essentially indirect and mediated. As we will see later, the example Plato uses continually is health. We all have a natural interest in preserving our own health, yet it is the physician who has an insight into or explanatory knowledge of those very conditions that will allow us to restore our health.

Now beyond the claim that the human being has a given nature, there is also the issue of the nature-culture-custom phenomenon, a second nature that is mediated by education and upbringing. Yet this second nature can be assessed from the perspective of a given nature. For example, in fifth century Greece the *nomos*, those enforced customs and conventions, were subjected to critique, and it was claimed that the *nomos* should be measured against a background that would express a more original or elementary normality, namely, *physis* or nature. It is important to note that the natural and the rational cannot be thought of as simple opposites here: reason belongs constitutively to our natural endowment, allowing us to recognize what is necessary and making us adhere to various social conventions.

The naïve separation of nature and reason is supported only by those who would champion an absolute concept of freedom, which is conceived as a liberation from everything that has not been posited by freedom itself, conceived as nature's other. The radical emancipation from nature is perhaps most conceivable in the act of taking one's own life, that extreme act which annuls the very condition (life) upon which our freedom nourishes itself. It should be emphasized, however, that nature must not be conceived simply from the physical or physicalistic point of view, or as merely an instinct or drive. The human being is not simply defined by its instincts and drives. This arguably simplistic way of thinking and talking about nature first emerged in modernity with the attempt to eliminate the concept of nature, the Greek notion of *physis*, and to replace it with the mechanical or mechanistic laws of phenomenal nature.

For the Greeks, *physis* did not mean the pure and brute objectivity of inert matter, but rather an identity conceived analogously with the experience that the human being has of itself in the cosmos. *Physis* in this sense is the delimitation of a being from all the other beings, of a living being from its environment. *Physis* is, according to Aristotle, the essence of everything that has in itself a first principle, the principle of movement. In this sense *physis* is, from the very outset, a concept that is used to make distinctions and a force that makes distinctions. In the *Corpus Hippocraticum* it serves to distinguish the healthy as normal from the unhealthy as abnormal.

It should be added that normality in this case does not serve as statistical concept: if 90 % of human beings had a headache, they would not be the models of health to which the other 10 % should conform. The opposite is true. A headache, in fact, is opposed to that natural tendency inherent in every natural being towards its self-preservation and well-being.

Nonetheless, it is not incorrect to say that the free movement of a being is the movement of its nature. This differs from the violent, which is a movement against its own nature, and which it is forced to accept from without. For example, we say that someone dies a natural death if the cause of death is due to old age and not to an external, violent cause. Similarly, the growth of a tree is a natural movement, while its being knocked over by a storm or felled by a lumberjack is a violent movement against its nature or natural tendency. From the perspective of the antelope, being eaten is altogether unnatural, while for the lion that is eating the antelope it is completely natural.

Thus it is my claim that any understanding of the relation between health and illness must take its start from an analysis of the history of the concept of nature, its metaphysical lineage, and hence cannot circumvent what some might feel is the outdated reflections on nature that is found in Greek literature and philosophy. If anything, these reflections are rich, complicated and important for anyone who wants to address and understand the essence of health and illness. In a word, one must go through the Greeks and not around them. In keeping with a historical-developmental account, let me now take a look at the so-called Moderns and see how they understood nature, before returning to the Greeks and the impact the Greeks had on a contemporary dialogical approach called philosophical hermeneutics, and its founder Hans-Georg Gadamer.

2 The Modern Response: Reason and Nature

Modern physics removed the distinction between natural motion and violent motion, mainly because it eliminated nature as a concept essentially related to the internal principle of movement. Human beings interact with their surroundings precisely because they are not the windowless monads of which Leibniz spoke, monads that are impervious to and unaffected by one another, monads that have no pores or doors (see Leibniz 1989, p. 1). Yet human interaction is not based on purely mechanical laws, but rather on the reciprocal exchange inherent in communal life itself. Thus the human being does not simply undergo or suffer change determined by mechanical laws and processes, but reacts to an already meaningful world and is the rational being which expresses an understanding and interpretative tendency.

For instance, when I am hungry, I do not have to eat, in fact, I may have reasons for not doing so: I want a slice of chocolate cake but I know it's bad for me. Hunger, however, is not a neutral state of affairs that requires further premises to become the grounds for an action. One's propensities or tendencies are distinguished from other states of affairs precisely because they already move or incline us towards something.

The interpretation of or reflection on the nature of such propensities or tendencies is what one might call a rational movement. Only by way of rational reflection does nature manifests itself *as* nature. The animal feels hungry, but does not linger or dwell on the natural end of its hunger, namely self-preservation. The meaning of these propensities or tendencies reveals itself only when one takes leave of them, takes a distance from them conceptually, and then translates them into language. The self-preservation of free beings is ensured not only by a powerfully natural propensity or tendency, but is linked necessarily to a free rational act, as in eating and drinking, that is, acts which, unlike breathing, are not done *naturally*. As free acts, eating and drinking are part of a cultural context; they are cultivated and shaped by cultural norms. As Claude Levi-Strauss has shown, the preparation and consumption of food is, for many people, the paradigm of culture as such. Therefore, the seemingly basic act of eating and drinking turns into a family banquet, into public festivity, or into nuptial festivity and the natural and primary purpose of eating becomes almost invisible in these cultural transformations and expressions (see Levi-Strauss 1978, p. 483).

However, the human being does not always elevate itself above its propensities or tendencies. When in the late Roman Empire the Romans prolonged their feasts only to enter the vomitorium for the sake of being able resume eating immediately, the detachment of the cultural function of eating from the natural did not demonstrate an elevated level of reflection or understanding, but rather a lower and more hedonistic level. In a word, culture is the humanisation of nature, not the abolition of nature.

Thus, it would be incorrect to say that human reason abolishes nature and takes its place; instead reason is receptive and responsive to nature. Even Kant agreed that the human being possesses something like a natural self which is not the mere instrument of its freedom, its transcendental freedom as an idea of reason, of pure practical reason, but rather the sensible representation of its personality in the phenomenal world, albeit one which does not act freely, is causally determined and is non-moral. This is precisely the much-debated antinomy (the third antinomy) between freedom and determinism. Nonetheless, if the human being in its entirety is to be respected, then its empirical nature must also be recognized and respected. One cannot simply slap someone in the face and then immediately add that one never meant to offend the person in question. Acting on or against the human body, the empirical or phenomenal self, always means acting on or against the human being as such. The human being, as rational agent, is hence not a subject that has at its disposal a natural and empirical organism: the human body is the human being itself. And yet for Kant the noumenal self is governed by laws other than those causally determining empirical laws of nature. Because of this, the noumenal self is both free and governed by and respectful of the moral law. This noumenal self is both the lawgiver and subject to the law.

Therefore, according to Kant, the givenness of a nature, nature as conditioned and determined phenomenally, does not itself lead to the binding givenness of a duty, but rather contains only sensible inclinations or natural propensities. Only when understanding operates, only when I direct or command myself to adopt a maxim that is self-originating and to act on it, only when I cause myself to adopt one and act on it spontaneously as an imperative, can empirical nature be seen to feed into and nourish moral action. Human dignity or worth (*Würde*), therefore, is inseparably linked to our naturalness in space and time and yet not simply reducible to it. Highlighting his compatibility thesis, that is, that there is no logical contradiction between freedom and nature, Kant writes, "causality through freedom is at least not incompatible with nature" (Kant 1996, A558/B586) and hence one can state legitimately that Kant's "kingdom of ends" is inextricably bound up with the "kingdom of nature" (Kant 1998, 4: 438). Or as Kant puts it a few pages later, "Philosophy [...] cannot give up the concept of nature any more than that of freedom" (Kant 1998, 4: 456).

Following Kant's great breakthrough, one can therefore claim that the nature of the human being is not simply empirical, it is not simply reducible to those sensible experiences that assail us, but also rational and free in its naturalness, the rationality and freedom of the human person as a fused unity of body and spirit, necessarily untied without contradiction. Following Kant, then, one could claim that one is genuinely natural if and only if one recognizes the good of the person and acts on the imperative that commands respect for a person's dignity, that is, that a person is always an end and never a means to an end. Yet the question of the natural also comes down to recognizing human fragility and our ability to cope with this fragility in a community of reciprocally respectful persons. Is not this Kant's "kingdom of ends" as a "kingdom of nature"? For instance, it is natural for humans to get ill and die, but it is also natural to cure, alleviate suffering and to enable solidarity in situations of serious harm and deprivation. The former is clearly a determining aspect of our human condition, yet it is also natural to seek what is good and to respond to this negative and all too natural aspect of our humanity (Kant 1996, A850/B878).

3 Back to Antiquity

As we have noted, the Classical tradition viewed health as the psychophysical state of being in harmony with nature and the cosmos as a whole. More specifically, health was understood to be a state of natural balance in the mixture of the primary qualities of the human body. According to the teachings of Aristotle, and later Galen, the human body was said to be made up of four primary elements: fire, water, air and earth, and from these elements arise the four primary qualities: hot, moist, cold and dry. While these primary elements are not said to exist in the body, they are nonetheless characterized by what has come to be known as the four humours, namely, blood, yellow bile, black bile and phlegm. From this interpretation, health comes to be conceived as a proper balance amongst the primary qualities of a particular human body. Subsequently, it was said that when one quality prevails over the other, illness is generated.

Hence, the very possibility of illness is understood as the possibility of disharmony, precisely because illness, what Susan Sontag calls the "night-side of life" (Sontag 1978, p. 3), manifests itself as a deficiency or deprivation of sorts, as a negation of that positive element which constitutes health. Someone is said to be ill, then, when they lack something and suffer not only this lack, but suffer due to this lack, because of their awareness of and reflection on it, because they perceive it as a determining limit and subsequently look for a cure.

Illness, just like nature, is therefore a hugely complex notion, which goes beyond the notion of faultiness, which could be attributed to machines, or simple defectiveness, which can be attributed to any organic substance. The various designations by which the phenomenon of illness is indicated in antiquity reflect this ambiguous complexity. For instance, one can designate different aspects of illness: weakness, infirmity or sickness (*asthéneia* in Greek or *infirmitas* in Latin), plague or disease (*nósos* or *morbus*), and pain or suffering (*pathos* or *dolentia*).

However, with Hippocrates one witnesses the birth, or better the midwifery, of a genuine *iatrické techne*, namely, medical science. In Hippocrates' time illness was considered a privative modification of a natural equilibrium. And since *physis*, nature, always does what is best, the doctor is first and foremost a servant of nature. Accordingly, the physician must aim to achieve three main goals: (1) the facilitation of health, (2) the alleviation of suffering, and (3) the preservation of the dignity of the patient. Furthermore, this is possible only by observing three basic principles: (a) "have two special objects in view with regard to illness, namely, to do good or to do no harm" (Hippocrates, *Epidemics* I, xi), encapsulated in the famous Latin expression *primum non nocere*; (b) refrain from the impossible; and (c) engage the very root cause of the illness.

4 Gadamer's *Graecophilia*: The Recovery of Plato

For Plato, who was a contemporary of Hippocrates, the physician possesses both theoretical and practical wisdom, more akin to a contingent ethical science than to a natural science, it must be said. The physician must consider the totality of nature, which is not only the singular organism in question, but also the entire lived situation in which there is both patient and doctor. In an attempt to explain this, the German philosopher Hans-Georg Gadamer draws attention to a passage from the *Phaedrus*, in which Plato compares rhetoric, which needs to understand the nature of the soul in order to lead it to virtue, to medicine, which needs to understand the nature of the body in order to facilitate health. Both rhetoric and medicine, however, cannot proceed without an awareness of the entirety of the person in question. According to Plato, illness is the loss of equilibrium, which not only has medical and biological significance, but also biographical and social, so much so that medicine must establish itself as knowledge of the living totality of the human being.

Thus Gadamer follows Plato for whom the production of health is the establishment of the component parts of the body "in a natural relation of control and being controlled" (Plato, *Republic*, IV, 444d). Agreeing with Gadamer, one could say that, "We know, roughly, what illness is. It is that 'revolt' or rebellion which takes place when something starts to dysfunction. It thus appears as something set over against us, as an 'object' (*Gegenstand*), as that which offers resistance (*Widerstand*) and must be broken" (Gadamer 1996, p. 96), Consequently, one can examine an illness closely and evaluate its particular degree of virulence. And indeed one can do so with all the different means provided by the objectifying scientific method which we have acquired through the modern natural sciences. Yet it could be said that health itself eludes these noble methods in a unique way. Health is not something that is revealed through investigation but rather something that manifests itself precisely by virtue of eluding our attention. We are not permanently aware of health and we do not anxiously bear it as we do an illness. It is not something that invites or demands permanent attention or cries out for obsessive reflection. Rather it belongs to that miraculous capacity we have to forget ourselves, i.e. to remain oblivious of ourselves as unhindered.

It must be said that the interpretation of health that Gadamer offers is largely based on insights gleaned from various Platonic dialogues, whose definitions of health derive not only from Hippocratic medicine, but also from his various metaphysical commitments. From Hippocrates comes the notion of aiming at the "right measure": neither more nor less than is necessary. Using the image of the well-balancing tightrope walker, Gadamer takes up this idea and insists that neither too much nor too little is the definition of what is appropriate or fitting (*das Angemessene*). Thus, the right measure or proportion is the very hinge upon which the concept of health turns and equilibrium is thus that constant poise between the too little and the too much.

By dint of this, Gadamer claims the physician's task is to facilitate the restoration of the hidden equilibrium, which has been disturbed by the illness. The hidden state of good health, then, is the very thing that does the restoring or, if you will, it is itself the right measure. For Plato, and thus for Gadamer too, health is the appropriate balance of bodily forces; it *is* proportion and balance. The concepts of "proportion" and "balance," as well as the "more" or "less," are closely tied up with the concept of "measure," or, more precisely, with appropriate measure. This is one of the key concepts of Platonic metaphysics, a concept upon which health and the understanding of health as well-being depends. It depends on the "right measure," the "more" or "less," the avoidance of "excess" and "deficiency." Its definition can be established according to two different relations and then placed on two different levels: proceeding on an arithmetic basis, the more or less can be mutually proportionate, while proceeding on a more complex ontological and axiological basis, they can be proportionate only according to a mean which is far from static. A mean that is not objective.

The first type of relationship is quantitative (*poson*) in nature. However, the second type of relationship is qualitative (*poion*), that is, ontological and axiological, implying a relationship of contingent existential-ontological evaluation and self-evaluation. It is according to this second type of rapport that reality is structured and by which what is good and what is bad is distinguished; and the same holds for what is true and untrue, right and wrong. We must bear in mind here that the measurement of the "more" or "less" in light of the "appropriate measure" is a theoretical revolution brought about by Plato and inspired by the nature of measurement formulated by the arithmetic insights of Pythagoras. In fact, it is a form of measurement that is non-arithmetic, or non-quantitative, but rather qualitatively onto-axiological and harmonic. And it is precisely upon this type of measuring that the arts are founded, in this case, the art of medicine.

However, it is in the *Statesman* that Plato articulates his position or doctrine, which has implications for his understanding of medicine. Plato writes:

> We should surely suppose that it is similarly the case that all the various sorts of expertise exist, and at the same time that greater and less are measured not only in relation to each other but also in relation to the coming into being of what is in due measure. For if the latter is the case, then so is the former, and also if it is the case that the sorts of expertise exist, the other is the case too. But if one or the other is not the case, then neither of them will ever be. (Plato, *Statesman*, 284e)

Thus, for Plato, health is the appropriate measure, that natural harmony, the intrinsic accord of the body with itself and with what is other than itself. As such, and this is Gadamer's claim, Plato's understanding of health is arguably a long way from the specialized modern quantifiable approach; an instrumentalized approach that quantitatively calculates more than qualitatively deliberates.

5 The Proper Measure: Nature as a Ground Rule

Hence, we must ask ourselves: What is "measure"? I must say that I genuinely value Plato's insights here, which I would highly recommend to anyone who wants to understand what seems to be missing or at least undervalued in the world of modern medicine. In Plato's dialogue the *Statesman*, for example, a very contemporary issue is addressed, namely, the qualities that distinguish a genuine politician from a mere civil servant. Plato distinguishes two forms of measure here: the first is obtained when measuring an object by approaching it from without, while the other is assessed from within the thing itself. The Greek is as follows: *metron*, meaning measure, and *metrion*, indicating what is measured or appropriate. Yet what does "appropriate" mean here? For Plato, it clearly designates the inner or interior measure of a living totality. Thus, one can define health as harmony, something like the right fit or due measure, which is attested to by means of the open and self-forgetful potential of the healthy individual. On the other hand, in the case of illness it comes to be perceived as a disturbance of vital collaboration, the disturbed balance of one's feeling "right" or "well" and one's psycho-physical openness to the outside world. The latter is what Heidegger, perhaps influenced by Husserl, terms the open "bodying-forth" (*Leiben*) of human existence (Heidegger 2001b, p. 97). By putting the problem in these terms, *metrion*, the right measure, is accessible only by means of a qualitative lived measuring, i.e. measuring as an open and self-reflexive living through.

Gadamer takes this notion of the "right measure" as his philosophical model, but adds, perhaps influenced here more by Aristotle's *Nicomachean Ethics*, that it cannot be defined with any degree of precision or rigor (see Aristotle, *Nicomachean Ethics*, 1094b13–15). Consequently, health eludes modern medicine because it cannot be rationalized, mastered or quantified, and hence the elusive phrase "quality of life" is used to describe what is missing or away due to the disturbance. Gadamer writes:

> Modern science has come to regard the results of [its] measuring procedures as the real facts which it must seek to order and collect. But the data provided in this way only reflect conventionally established criteria brought to the phenomena from without. They are always our own criteria that we impose on the thing we wish to measure. The living body and life are things that cannot simply be measured [...]. (Gadamer 1996, p. 132)

In a key passage from the *Phaedrus*, Socrates defines health as the equilibrium of human life in its relationship with everything:

> [I]sn't the method of medicine in a way the same as the method of rhetoric? In both cases we need to determine the nature of something – of the body in medicine, of the soul in rhetoric. Otherwise, all we'll have will be an empirical and artless practice. We won't be able to supply, on the basis of an art, a body with the medicines and diet that will make it healthy and strong, or a soul with the reasons and customary rules for conduct that will impart to it the convictions and virtues we want. Do you think, then, that it is possible to reach a serious understanding of the nature of the soul without understanding the nature of the world as a whole? Consider, then, what both Hippocrates and true argument say about nature. Isn't this the way to think systematically about the nature of anything? First, we must consider whether the object regarding which we intend to become experts and capable of transmitting our expertise is simple or complex. Then, if it is simple, we must investigate its power: What things does it have what natural power of acting upon? By what things does it have what natural disposition to be acted upon? If, on the other hand, it takes many forms, we must enumerate them all and, as we did in the simple case, investigate how each is naturally able to act upon what and how it has a natural disposition to be acted upon by what. (Plato, *Phaedrus*, 270b–d)

The method of Hippocrates, that is, the careful analysis of the nature of the various types and characteristics of each and every thing, is a method that corresponds perfectly to what Plato established and applied, with extraordinary depth and deftness at the ontological level, through his dialectical method. And Gadamer is to be commended for having brought this back into the debate.

6 Body and Soul: The Person as a Unified Whole

According to Gadamer, the previous passage from the *Phaedrus* is a warning against the propensity which has become prevalent in certain strands of modern medicine, which tend to eliminate the previously discussed "natural" in favour of the "artificial." As Gadamer sees it, and this is not without its problems, real medical treatment should remain faithful to the ancient idea of nature as a ground rule. He writes in reference to the previously cited passage from the *Phaedrus*:

> *The nature of the whole that is at issue here* is not merely the unified whole of the single organism. We possess abundant evidence from Greek medicine to show us how the weather and the seasons, how temperature, water *and general* sustenance, in short how all possible climatic and environmental factors were seen to make up the concrete ontological

> constitution of what it is that the physician helps to restore, namely health […] The nature of the whole includes and involves the entire life situation of the patient, and even of the physician. Medicine is compared with the true art of rhetoric which allows the right kinds of discourse to exercise an effect on the soul in the right kinds of way. (Gadamer 1996, p. 41)

Here Gadamer is pointing out that illness, or better the loss of equilibrium with which illness manifests itself, not only refers to a biological fact, but also to a biographical and social event. The individual in question is no longer the same person as before. They have been existentially transformed by their illness. To a certain extent, they are excluded from the invisible and self-forgetful normalcy of social life. If the natural equilibrium is restored, then the miraculous phenomenon of health will return with the self-effacing equilibrium of life. Unsurprisingly, the loss of equilibrium that constitutes illness simultaneously impacts upon my relationship to the other, insofar as my equilibrium is bound up with the equilibrium of others, who sustain life and contribute to the broader equilibrium of healthiness as such. However, for Plato, the parts of the body cannot be treated in isolation from the entire body, and the entire body cannot be treated in isolation from the "soul," that is, from what one might call the entirety of the person.

As I have said, Plato uses the concept of "right measure" to explain illness, defined as the disruption of a measured harmony. And in the case of the human being, the "right measure" which is most important, that upon which the ultimate meaning of health depends, is the one that exists between body and soul, and it is the lack of measure or equilibrium between these two constitutive components which is the real cause of illness (See Plato, *Gorgias*, 504c). According to Plato, care for the body is carried out with exercise and the correct use of medicine. However, Plato seems to privilege exercise over medicine by claiming that exercise prevents illness, while medicine intervenes only after the illness has taken hold, and thus one should worry more about prevention than cure. Indeed, according to Plato, illness arises when one ignores its very prevention, which amounts to exercise and the proper movement of life.

And, Plato insists, just like those who master exercise and medicine,

> [T]he good man, the man who speaks with regard to what's best, says whatever he says not randomly but with a view to something, just like the other craftsmen, each of whom keeps his own product in view and so does not select and apply randomly what he applies, but so that he may give his product some shape? Take a look at painters for instance, if you would, or house builders or shipwrights or any of the other craftsmen you like, and see how each one places what he does into a certain organization, and compels one thing to be suited for another and to fit to it until the entire object is put together in an organized and orderly way. The other craftsmen, too, […] the ones concerned with the body, physical trainers and doctors, no doubt give order and organization to the body. (Plato, *Gorgias*, 503e–504a)

In the *Republic*, the dialogue in which Plato tackles the problem of the education of the guardians of the state, we are again given a basic ground rule: proper exercise, together with proper diet, helps one avoid all forms of psychophysical impediment. Hence, just as certain kinds of music harm the soul, kinds which are not modeled on simplicity, that is, on the "right measure," so too is it with exercise and diet. Plato tells us that complex and sophisticated music produces intemperance in the soul, while a combination of complicated exercise and a fancy diet leads to illness.

The seemingly common-sense upshot of all this is that one should both exercise and eat carefully, i.e. in the right measure and at the right time, and one must also make use of medicine in a measured way. In the *Timaeus* Plato also says that medicine should be used sparingly because, in some cases, more harm than good is done. He writes:

> We should avoid aggravating with drugs diseases that aren't particularly dangerous. Every disease has a certain makeup that in a way resembles the natural makeup of living things. In fact, the constitution of such beings goes through an ordered series of stages throughout their life [...]. Now diseases have a similar makeup, so that when you try to wipe them out with drugs before they have run their due course, the mild diseases are liable to get severe, and the occasional ones frequent. That is why you need to cater to all such diseases by taking care of yourself to the extent that you are free and *have* the time to do that. What you should not do is aggravate a stubborn irritation with drugs (Plato, *Timaeus*, 89c–d).

Clearly these observations have a lot of truth to them, especially when one thinks of the contemporary use and abuse of pharmaceutical drugs, in the very questionable belief, now quite prevalent, that our health depends on drugs that are able to eliminate almost all forms of illness. In terms of the care for the body, we must again remind ourselves that Plato claims that the body can heal properly only if the soul is taken care of. For example, looking after the body with exercise, yet without music, hardens the heart, whereas caring for the soul with music only, that is without physical exercise, makes the heart weak and soft. However, more than music being dependent on exercise, it is exercise that depends on music, and always in the right measure and at the right time (*kairos*). As Plato puts it in the *Republic*: "a god has given music and physical training to human beings not, except incidentally, for the body and the soul but for the spirited and wisdom-loving parts of the soul itself, in order that these might be in harmony with one another, each being stretched and relaxed to the appropriate degree" (Plato, *Republic*, III, 411c2–412).

As is well known, Plato's *Republic* presents another argument for the immortality of the soul. However, even if an illness, pushing the body to extreme limits, brings about its death, this is not the case for the soul, for the soul, it is said, continues to exist. Against Epicurus, the soul on Plato's reading is indestructible. In the *Phaedrus* an additional argument is offered which centres on the concept of the soul as "self-moving" and thus the instigator of all movement. The concept of soul as the principle of self-movedness and of movement as such is closely connected with the concept of soul as the principle of life, insofar as life and movement are structurally related.

Above all, Plato is concerned with the rational soul, and again he writes in the *Timaeus*:

> [W]e ought to think of the most sovereign part of our soul as god's gift to us, given to be our guiding spirit. This, of course, is the type of soul that, as we maintain, resides in the top part of our bodies. It raises us up away from the earth and toward what is akin to us in heaven. In saying this, we speak absolutely correctly. For it is from heaven, the place from which our souls were originally born, that the divine part suspends our head, i.e., our root,

> and so keeps our whole body erect […]. And to the extent that human nature can partake of immortality, he can in no way fail to achieve this: constantly caring for his divine part as he does, keeping well-ordered the guiding spirit that lives within him, he must indeed be supremely happy. Now there is but one way to care for anything, and that is to provide for it the nourishment and the motions proper to it. (Plato, *Timaeus*, 90a)

From this perspective, human life attains ultimate health, beyond the body, in its care for the soul. Hence, according to Plato, the human being must engage with the virtues, and the essence of virtue coincides with knowledge of the good and its implementation. Since the good is the measure of all things, virtue is thus the mean between excess and deficiency, namely the "right measure" between too little and too much. And since the soul has a tripartite structure, "rational," "spirited" and "appetitive," and since each of these parts has its own specific function, then the virtue of each of these parts will consist in fulfilling the task which is appropriate to it.

We have thus moved from the health of the body to health as such and by this Plato means that the cultivation of virtue or excellence amounts to the healthy and harmonious functioning of the soul. The general criterion that Plato proposes when dealing with bodies and souls is that of the right measure, which is the foundation of Platonic thought. As such, Plato's perspective is both indebted to Thales and a clear forerunner to the well-known Latin maxim *mens sana in corpore sano*.

According to Plato's therapeutic proposition, a healthy body without a healthy mind is impossible; a healthy soul is the necessary condition for a healthy body. As Plato puts it in the *Timaeus*:

> [H]uman beings have two sets of natural desires—desires of the body for food and desires of the most divine part of us for wisdom—the motions of the stronger part will predominate, and amplify their own interest. They render the functions of the soul dull, stupid and forgetful, thereby bringing on the gravest disease of all: ignorance. From both of these conditions there is in fact one way to preserve oneself, and that is not to exercise the soul without exercising the body, nor the body without the soul, so that each may be balanced by the other and so be sound. The mathematician, then, or the ardent devotee of any other intellectual discipline should also provide exercise for his body by taking part in gymnastics, while one who takes care to develop his body should in his turn practice the exercises of the soul by applying himself to the arts and to every pursuit of wisdom, if he is to truly deserve the joint epithets of "fine and good." (Plato, *Timaeus*, 88b–c)

In light of these comments, one can easily see how Plato prefigures and informs the Epicurean notion of *tetrapharmakos*, that is, the philosophical-spiritual medicine for the soul.

The phenomenological perspective considers the relationship between health and illness as a first-person human experience of which the individual seeks meaning. Even if one does not deny the objective factors that constitute illness, the emphasis always falls on the interpretation that the subject offers of their own lived situation, the transformation or transfiguration of one's relationship to one's own body, to one's own self, the hyper-reflexivity of one's modified being in the world, and the frustration involved in being unable to articulate this affective, non-relational first-person transformation.

Philosophical hermeneutics also emphasizes not only the subjective aspects of health and illness, but also, as I noted earlier, the impossibility of their objective definition. Gadamer's work *The Enigma of Health* is precisely an elaboration of this perspective.

Thus one could argue that health can be only addressed dialectically, accounting for it by means of what is present, that is, what remains, when it is absent. Put otherwise, one could say that we know only too well how illness can make us insistently aware of our bodily nature by creating a disturbance in something which normally, in its very freedom from disturbance, almost completely escapes our attention. Here it is a matter of the methodological primacy of illness over health. But of course it is the state of being healthy which possesses ontological primacy, that natural condition of life that we term well-being, in so far as we register it at all. Yet what is well-being if it is not precisely this condition of not noticing, of being obliviously unhindered, of being ready for and open to everything?

Gadamer's work then points to the impossibility of defining standards of health with precision. As he puts it:

> The fundamental fact remains that it is illness and not health which "objectifies" itself, which confronts us as something opposed to us and which forces itself on us [...]. Once again we must address the fact that the real mystery lies in the hidden character of health. Health does not actually present itself to us. Of course one can also attempt to establish standard values for health. But the attempt to impose these standard values on a healthy individual would only result in making that person ill. It lies in the nature of health that it sustains its own proper balance and proportion. The appeal to standard values which are derived by averaging out different empirical data and then simply applied to particular cases is inappropriate to determining health and cannot be forced upon it. (Gadamer 1996, p. 107)

In conclusion, health, for Gadamer, like for Plato before him, is the appropriate and necessarily inconspicuous rhythm of life, the hidden or enigmatic character of health, which shows itself in the self-effacing and hence indeterminate feeling of well-being. In the main, this harmonic indeterminacy expresses itself in terms of our openness to the new, our willingness to embark on new undertakings and, in the very self-forgetfulness that becomes synonymous with health, in our intimate being at home in the world. Health is thus not simply reducible to one's general physical condition or to how one feels in oneself at a given moment in space and time. More than this, although not seeing the former as unimportant, it is first and foremost a condition of my intersubjective engagement in the world of open-ended tasks and projects and it is the world as open to me and opened by me. To borrow from the later Heidegger, it is my self-forgetful "bodying-forth" into the tasks and projects that cry out for fulfilment and engagement.

However, not content to give Gadamer, like the devil, all the best tunes, one could also offer a critique of his work on health and illness, insofar as the art of medicine, by his own admission, seems to consist in "withdrawing itself and helping to set the other person free" (Gadamer 1996, p. 43) and thus the physician becomes a mere facilitator of equilibrium re-establishment with a nature that is completely idolized. Yet this begs the question as to whether there is room in Gadamer's work for such a thing as benevolent paternalism or a coercive intervention that is both justified and necessary. On reading Gadamer's *The Enigma of Health*, and after having been convinced by so much of what is said therein, it is perhaps true that there is a wistful nostalgia motivating his various claims that physicians ought to return to the Greek ideal of natural harmony, nature as a ground rule, and that "every treatment stands in the service of nature" and nature alone (110).

What is perchance missing in his account is the recognition of the necessity of positive interventions that are technically and calculative coercive for the sake of restoring health or alleviating suffering. Clearly under the influence of Heidegger, Gadamer's allergy to the rationalization and instrumentalization of modern science, his adoration of Platonic harmony and phronetic deliberation, and his fidelity to all things "natural," cause him to overlook the important fact that medical treatment is not always about restoring an equilibrium, but often about alleviating suffering and allowing the individual to bear their suffering with dignity. In addition to this, Gadamer's *physis*-centric approach ignores something that Heidegger never did and this is that *physis* cannot be defined in terms of harmony and proportion, insofar as nature is more often than not violent, destructive, terrible, pitiless and overwhelming (see Heidegger 2001a, pp. 159–76). Accordingly, medical treatment cannot be simply at the service of nature as a ground rule, but must also express itself as a ceaseless confrontation with nature and with its most unforgiving characteristics.

Unlike Gadamer, who has nothing but praise for Plato, Karl Jaspers, Gadamer's Heidelberg predecessor who experienced the isolating effects of illness as a child, is highly critical of the attitude towards illness that he finds in Plato's thought (Jaspers 1986, p. 534). Plato's deficient assessment of illness and health, Jaspers claims, was both unmindful of and had no interest in treating someone who could not live in a normal or optimal way, someone who "nature" might deem as surplus to requirement (see Plato, *Republic* III, 406–407). And while one should not forget the ambiguous issue of authorial intention in Platonic dialogues, in the *Republic* it is argued that is undesirable to extend lives that are good for nothing, lives that are of no benefit to the ideal city, nor is it desirable to have weak parents begetting even weaker children. For Jaspers, those who have been ill, those who have lived illness from the inside out, can only read the words of Plato with unease. In the cold superiority of Plato's words Jaspers spies the seeds of that all too common recoil or "disgust" that unfeelingly healthy human beings experience in the face of unhealthy members of their own species (see Carel 2008, p. 37). I wonder whether Gadamer's nostalgic Platonism, his potentially naïve and unapologetic *Graecophilia*, does not cause him to miss this very important point. In the end, and challenging an aspect of Gadamer's largely admirable thesis, perhaps articulating a philosophy of health based on a harmony with nature is not as easy as "riding a bike" (Gadamer 1996, p. 161).

References

Aristotle. (1996). In J. Barnes (Ed.), *The complete works of Aristotle*. Princeton, NJ: Princeton University Press.
Cicero. (1971). *De Finibus Bonorum et Malorum* (H. Rackham, Trans.). *The loeb classical library*. Cambridge: Harvard University Press.
Carel, H. (2008). *Illness: The cry of the flesh*. Stocksfield: Acumen.
Gadamer, H. G. (1996). *The enigma of health: The art of healing in a scientific age* (J. Gaiger & N. Walker, Trans.). Stanford, CA: Stanford University Press.
Heidegger, M. (2001a). *Introduction to metaphysics* (G. Fried & R. Polt, Trans.). New Haven: Yale University Press.
Heidegger, M. (2001b). In M. Boss (Ed.), *Zollikon seminars: Protocols—conversations-letters* (F. Mayr & R. Askay, Trans.). Evanston: Northwestern University Press.
Hippocrates. (1923). *Loeb Classical Library* (vol. 1, p. 165, W. H. S. Jones, Trans.). London: William Heinemann.
Jaspers, K. (1986). *Basic philosophical writings*. New Jersey: Humanities Press.
Kant, I. (1996). *Critique of pure reason* (W. S. Pluhar, Trans.). Indianapolis: Hackett.
Kant, I. (1998). *Groundwork of the metaphysics of morals* (M. Gregor, Trans.). Cambridge: Cambridge University Press.
Leibniz, G. W. (1989). The Monadology. In *Philosophical essays* (R. Ariew & D. Garber (Eds.), Trans.). Indianapolis: Hackett.
Lévi-Strauss, C. (1978). *The origin of table manners* (J. Weightman & D. Weightman, Trans.). New York: Harper & Row.
Plato. (1997). In J. M. Cooper & D. S Hutchinson (Eds.), *Complete works*. Indianapolis: Hackett.
Sontag, S. (1978). *Illness as metaphor*. London: Penguin Books.

Chapter 5
The Ethical Self After Genetics

Mihail Evans

1 Introduction

The extent to which the science of genetics presents challenges to the dominant modern conceptions of the self inaugurated by Descartes and Locke which asserts the individual as sovereign is not widely recognized. Indeed there is a general misperception, widely promulgated by the media, that theories in evolutionary biology such as that of 'the selfish gene' lend support to the latter when they do not. The liberal self that has dominated philosophy since the seventeenth century conceives the human being as fundamentally autonomous and primarily characterised by agency, yet the discovery of the genome suggests, as certain philosophers in the continental tradition have long insisted, that I am not the source or foundation of myself. There is, of course, a specificity to the revelation of genetics. There has long been, for example, a strand in philosophy which sees the subject as in various ways the product of the society into which he is thrown. The main force of the challenge made by genetics is different and, in particular, undermines both any unitary identity of the biological entity and any perception of biological uniqueness. As Jacques Derrida said in a lecture given shortly before his death:

> More than ever, and every day faster than ever, the techno-scientific and genetico-industrial intervention upon the fetal cell, the genome, the fertility process, homo- or hetero- grafts, and so on, much like the deployment of so many prosthetic structures, obligate us to reelaborate the very norms of our elementary perception as to what is an ensemble or an organic identity, the "living together" of a proper body. (Derrida 2013, p. 39)

In this paper I will look at how two of the most important European philosophers of the late twentieth century, Jacques Derrida and Jürgen Habermas, have responded to the challenges thrown up by genetics and, in particular, the ethical challenges

M. Evans (✉)
New Europe College, Bucharest, Romania
e-mail: Mihail.Evans@zoho.com

D. Meacham (ed.), *Medicine and Society, New Perspectives in Continental Philosophy*, Philosophy and Medicine 120, DOI 10.1007/978-94-017-9870-9_5

of the new technologies that science has enabled. My argument will be that while Habermas unsuccessfully attempts to shore up a version of the liberal self in the face of the challenge posed by genetics, Derrida finds that genetics reveals that the self never was as self-possessed or autonomous as has generally been believed. In particular, he makes a quasi-transcendental claim that the self is structured around an absence that is irrecuperable. As he puts it: "the self, the *autos* of legitimating and legitimated self-foundation, *is still to come*, not as a *future* reality but as that which will always retain the essential structure of a promise and as that which can only arrive as such, as *to come*" (Derrida 2002, p. 22). In suggesting the self is structured by a promise Derrida is not talking about a particular commitment made in language (the promise commonly understood) but rather about the way in which any use of language whatsoever is a relation or commitment to an other.[1] That is, I do not have an existence that could be divorced from my relations with others and existing thus I am essentially open and incomplete.

I will, first of all, turn to a recent work Habermas has devoted to the new genetic technologies before problematising his approach by taking up an earlier and neglected contribution of Derrida. I will also draw on various places in his work where Derrida challenges dominant conceptions of the self, including *The Gift of Death* where he does so through a reading of Kierkegaard as well as on some comments on cloning in the late work *Rogues*. The difference between the positions of the two will be shown to be reflective of their different conceptions of what it means to be either an "autonomous" (Habermas) or "responsible" (Derrida) being.

2 Habermas, Genetics and Rational Reconstruction

Habermas's magnum opus, *The Theory of Communicative Action*, was first published in German in 1981. His well-known argument is that the modern era opened as the classical Judeo-Christian outlook broke down in the Enlightenment. Unquestioned tradition was increasingly opened to scrutiny and the necessity for processes of consensus and agreement concomitantly increased in an age subject to self-validation and the non-coercive force of the better argument. Habermas's elders, Theodor Adorno and Max Horkheimer, the first generation of the Frankfurt School, had despaired of the extent to which the modern world had come under the grasp of instrumental and calculative thinking. But Habermas argued they had overlooked those areas where argumentatively attained agreement, intersubjectivity, rather than instrumentalism was dominant. His suggestion is that each form of reason has its own proper sphere: the rationality of the lifeworld, which is

[1]He elaborates this point elsewhere: "I do not master this language because even if I wanted to do something other than promise, I would promise. I do not master it because it is older than me; language is there before me and, at the moment I commit myself in it, I say *yes to it and to you* in a certain manner" (Derrida 1995, p. 384).

discursive, is different from that of the economy where calculative rationality is more appropriate. In the thirty years since *The Theory of Communicative Action*, Habermas has gone on to elaborate through numerous publications how communicative action might relate to questions of ethics, law and politics.

In order to understand what Habermas has to say on the ethics of recent developments in genetics we need to understand, in particular, the programme of discourse ethics that has emerged from his theory of communicative action. Habermas sets out his theory of discourse ethics in *Moral Consciousness and Communicative Action* and *Justification and Application* (Habermas 1992, 1993). His core assertion is that a norm can be demonstrated to be valid if it can be shown to embody a universal interest by being tested to see if it achieves rational agreement in discourse. McCarthy contrasts Habermas with Kant: "the emphasis shifts from what each can will without contradiction to be a universal law to what all can will in agreement to be a universal norm" (McCarthy 1978, p. 326). Habermasian ethics then concern procedure rather than concrete ethical prescriptions. They are post-conventional in that they are achieved as the result of debate, being based on the principle that "only those action norms are valid to which all possibly affected persons could agree as participants in rational discourse" (Habermas 1996, p. 107). Norms must not just be rationally achieved with the involvement of all those potentially concerned but in order to claim validity they must accord with what Habermas calls "the principle of universalizability": a valid moral norm is one that can be accepted by all affected participants in a discourse. Habermas here maintains Kant's aims but sees universalizability as demonstrated socially rather than logically and individualistically: it is dialogical not monological. This means that participants in a moral discourse must put themselves in the position of other participants and engage in an exchange of perspectives. Outhwaite suggests that "his strategy is essentially to socialize Kant's individualistic moral theory in such a way as to meet Hegelian objections, or at least to point in the direction of their resolution" (Outhwaite 1996, p. 178).

There are many things that Derrida might question about Habermas's project and the claims that he makes for it. Taking just his account of communication, we could argue that where Habermas tends to see discourse as a process that is generally transparent, Derrida shows it to have an inherent and ineradicable opaqueness, one which would draw into question the possibility of establishing unquestionable universal norms. Derrida argues that in even the simplest utterance there is something that escapes communicability which he names in late work "the secret" (there are parallels here with Levinas's distinction between "the saying" and "the said" in *Otherwise than Being*, that is between our sheer exposure to another and what we make intelligible in that encounter). "The secret" is that if I share something language is such that there always remains an unshareable residue or, put in more abstract terms, the universal always has inscribed within it a certain singularity that resists it. Derrida is certainly no opponent of those who seek rational agreement but his account of communication would suggest that what can be achieved thereby is something much more fragile than "universal norms." A similar but more elaborate argument is made by Lasse Thomassen in his important deconstructive reading of the core elements of Habermas's project. This first chapter of this finds him to concede that there are not just empirical obstacles to rational discource and rational consensus but obstacles that are inherent in the very conception of rational discource and rational consensus (Thomassen 2007). Without following or engaging in such a detailed reading here we might again illustrate it by observing the divergences between Husserl's conception of the lifeworld, which Derrida substantially shares, and that of Habermas. Husserl had introduced this concept late into his work, and partly as a response to his student Heidegger's development of a concept of 'being-in-the-world', and it marks an important concession that consciousness is imbedded in a world which exceeds it and which it can never fully appropriate. This contrasts with Habermas's characterisation of the lifeworld as primarily characterised by rationality. Derrida himself never appropriates Husserl's term as his own but, for example, in what he says in late work on "living together" (a term Husserl uses twice in defining "lifeworld" in the *Crisis*), or indeed on "the secret," there is an implicit convergence around an idea of the impossibility of complete appropriation of the horizon of experience (Derrida 2013).

Habermas addressed the question of the new genetic technologies in *The Future of Human Nature* (the English edition being composed of a text originally published in German in 2001 by *Suhrkamp Verlag* with the addition of a number of other essays on the topic). The book was one of several responses to Peter Sloterdijk's comments on the possibilities of genetic technology is his "Rules for the Human Zoo." Habermas, along with others in this debate, defends the generally conservative framework within which Germany has constrained genetic experimentation (itself usually seen as a reaction against the Nazi enthusiasm for eugenics). Habermas begins by returning to his important and problematic distinction between the "moral" and the "ethical," one which has a somewhat confusing history in his work. Habermas's early claim had been that his discourse ethics only concerns itself with the procedures for reaching agreement about norms and that it abstains from specifying those norms itself. He argues that he does not concern himself with questions of "the good life." This is underscored by the introducion in *Justification and Application* of a distinction between moral and ethical discourse (his discourse ethics confusingly concerns itself with moral discourse according to this new distinction). His argument is that the moral, the right, takes precedence over specific values, the good. Yet the moral, the communal level of the state and law, must protect the individual's autonomy and choice of values. This position of Habermas is constantly troubled by objections that norms and values, the moral and ethical, are not sharply distinguishable; a point Hilary Putnam makes against him (Putnam 2002). Indeed, even one of the most dedicated Habermasians, Thomas McCarthy, has demonstrated how in certain texts of Habermas moral norms are shown to be based on values (McCarthy 1993).

In *The Future of Human Nature* Habermas argues that the abstract morality of reason proper to subjects of human rights is itself sustained by a prior ethical self-understanding of the species which needs to be shared by those who would enter the moral realm. His argument is that "an ethical self-understanding of the species [...] is crucial for our capacity to see ourselves as the authors of our own life histories and to recognize one another as autonomous persons" (Habermas 2003, p. 25). He also phrases this in terms of a reworking of Kierkegaard's notion of "being-able-to-be oneself" as an essential precondition of discourse ethics. It is this self-understanding that "preimplantation genetic diagnoses" (PGD), where embryos are created outside the womb and are subject to genetic testing prior to being implanted with only those embryos deemed fit being implanted and the remainder discarded or frozen for later use, threatens to undermine. Habermas contends that this technology blurs the distinction between the "grown" and the "made," between what is natural and what humans have created for themselves. His worry is that if one person is able to control the genetic material of another, shaping it prior to birth into a desired configuration, the relationship between the two can never be one of freedom or equality (this implicitly raises the question of education and other processes of acculturation and I will come back to address this point).[2] Rather the relation is one of maker and product, the product always being dependent on the maker for her/his existence. He goes on to speculate on the effects this might have on the self-perception of an individual who has been the subject of PGD:

> When the adolescent learns about the design drawn up by another person for intervening in her genetic features in order to modify certain traits, the perspective of being a grown body may be superseded - in her objectivating self-perception - by the perspective of being something made. (Habermas 2003, pp. 53–54).

His concern is that such a child might be seen as part of their parents' life projects, even suggesting that the damage done is in the perception of control not in any actual changes made; although he also believes it may affect the person's ability to reflect critically (Habermas 2003, p. 60). He says that unlike education, which can give the child the capacity to say no to the very goals that the parent might encourage the child towards, genetic modification is a process that offers no resources for challenging the designer's goals. Habermas thus argues that genetic modification is a betrayal of intersubjectivity: when the parents and medical staff involved assume a causal relationship to the child via medical technology, the intersubjective relationship that would normally exist between them is perverted into an instrumental one. This leads him to further contend that genetic enhancement is incompatible with a democratic constitution because those affected by the process cannot give their free consent to the law that would allow such enhancement. I will come back to address some of these points later but I will simply observe here that Habermas' presumption that the self is, or can or should, be the sovereign author of its own life is one that Derrida would dissent from.

At a level wider than that of the individual, Habermas suggests that "how we deal with human life before birth (or with human beings after death) touches on our self-understanding as members of the species and how we see ourselves as moral agents" (Habermas 2003, pp. 81–2). He sees genetic interventions as threatening not only the individual's sense of self but also the very concept of human nature and

[2]He draws a distinction between therapeutic genetic interventions and genetic enhancements and argues that a retrospective informed consent could be imagined for the former but not the later.

potential for communicative action. Genetic technology threatens to reduce human development and adaptation to one of instrumental manipulation where previously development, he asserts, has occurred due to increased learning capacity. Habermas's concern is for autonomy, that is, for the ability to engage in rational self-legislation:

> The programmed person, being no longer certain about the contingency of the natural roots of her life history, may feel the lack of a mental precondition for coping with the moral expectation to take, even if only in retrospect, the sole responsibility for her own life. (Habermas 2003, p. 14).

The danger of genetic manipulation is that it would produce what Habermas calls self-alienation and species-alienation: it would undermine the autonomy of the self, that is, its ability to engage in rational self-legislation. He argues that some genetic interventions could be allowed so long as they maintain the species-ethic by approaching the embryo as the person it one day will be. Here, he turns to a procedure which he calls "rational reconstruction" as a way of legitimating decisions that empirically the subject has no option but of consenting to. If one can assume the consensus of the future person, he believes that the embryo is not instrumentalized or turned into an object. Yet we might note that recent campaigns against PGD by disabled activists suggest that he moves too fast in speaking of the possibility of arriving at unquestionable presumptions of consent or of unambiguously distinguishing therapeutic uses from what he calls "enhancement." Habermas's conclusion is that the state should constantly review what specific interventions could be justified by such an approach in order to prevent the development of a "liberal eugenics" where individual choices are made in a market situation.

3 Derrida and the Already Technical Self

Derrida first turned to consider the new genetic technologies almost a decade before Habermas and, in addition, has commented briefly on occasion in some of his last works. Although they don't concern PGD in particular these remarks can be used together with extrapolation from more general statements to respond to Habermas before going on to consider other problems in the ethics of genetics highlighted by Derrida. On a broad level it is important to note how Habermas's sharp distinction between strategic and communicative action, between rationalities that are either purely instrumental or purely non-instrumental, is difficult to sustain against a Derridean critique.[3] The question of "economy" was a major one in Derrida's work

[3]For an overview of the main issues in contention between Habermas and Derrida see *The Derrida-Habermas Reader* (Thomassen 2006). On the particular issue of the status of reason in Derrida's work and Habermas' mistaken characterisation of him in *The Philosophical Discourse of Modernity* as an anti-modernist see Evans (2014).

and he was highly skeptical about the possibility of escaping entirely to a realm where no form of exchange or calculation is at work. Thus, where Habermas appears to present us with a gulf between the adult who has been the subject of gene therapy and the adult who is a product of a parents, schools and a particular culture, asserting one to be the subject of instrumental action and the other to be completely free of the effects of such action, we can rather argue that such an absolute distinction is not possible. In particular, we could challenge his assertion that:

> The developing adolescent will one day be able to take responsibility for her own life history; she will be able to take possession of what she is. That is, she can relate to her process of development reflectively, work out a revisionary self-understanding, and in a probing manner retrospectively restore the balance to asymmetrical responsibility that parents have for their children's upbringing. (Habermas 2003, p. 14).

Derrida does not find the self to be an autonomous and self-contained monad but rather to be inescapeably 'founded' in alterity. It is part of the condition of possibility of any self that it is already in some sense alienated and non-autonomous (to risk the use of Habermas' terminology). Here perhaps we might identify a Derrida who finds the problems Hegel poses to Kant less easy to dismiss than Habermas does (although the most immediate influence on Derrida's ethics is a Levinasian one). I can never finally appropriate myself, he would argue, because I can only be myself on the condition of an alterity that constantly demands I respond responsibly in a situation I am cast in and have never chosen.

One way to elaborate the Derridean conception of the self would be to follow his reading of Kierkegaard in *The Gift of Death*. Following *Fear and Trembling* he suggests a situation where responsibility is something that is singular, that is, an address to a particular subject who must respond but can never fully master the situation. The self is individuated in responsibility which demands an accounting for oneself given in terms of the general which at the the same time is a response to the singularity of the other that exceeds it. This Derrida associates with silence and the secret and there is a danger, of course, that the latter lead us into irresponsibility, something that can never be finally ruled out when we do not judge according to an absolute rule. This account of responsibility results in a rethinking of the decision as that which must not be governed by duty. If we only follow what we must do there is no responsibility but rather something preprogrammed. Hence both Derrida and Kierkegaard can agree that 'the instant of the decision is madness' (Derrida 1996, p. 65). One can respond to the singularity of the other only by failing to some degree to respond to the ethical or political, to plural others, more generally. We could say that the way in which the self finds itself in and through language, and the way in which fully determinable meaning always escapes us, means that our selves are never finally appropriable. That is, my self is founded in a relation with the non-self that makes me what I am, at the same time as forever preventing me incorporating this other. Habermas' turn to a supposedly Kierkegaardian notion of 'being-able-to-be oneself' would be undermined by Derrida's revelation that the Kiekegaardian self inherently guards a secret that resists and disrupts all communication.

Returning to PGD we could then suggest that it is quite possible to envisage the possibility of a recipient of 'gene therapy' who is quite untroubled by it while another disturbed person is unable to escape their psychological formation. If this is conceded Habermas' distinction between the instrumentalized and non-instrumentalized person cannot be maintained. We can even push this argument further and suggest that a threat to communicative action could be seen to be already at work in socialization and, indeed, we would find the instrumental at work in what he considers to be 'the natural' person. My deconstructive criticism here is shared by feminists and others who object to Habermas' failure to attend to the processes of power operative in socialization (Meehan 1995).

A further argument can be elaborated by drawing on Derrida's comments on cloning. There is clearly a difference between PGD and cloning which needs to be respected but the central argument is pertinent to both situations. Indeed, Derrida turns to the issue of cloning after a discussion of the decision and on how 'the technical and the logic of the prosthesis' cannot be separated from 'the problematic of reason' (Derrida 2005a, p. 146). His point about cloning is this: 'identificatory repetition, the duplication that one claims to reject with horrified indignation, is already, and fortunately, present and at work everywhere it is a question of reproduction and of heritage, in culture, knowledge, language, education' (Derrida 2005a, p. 147). Derrida argues similarly at several other places in his work that any repetition is necessarily novel. There can be no absolutely same recurrence. Every 'I' written in the English language has its own unique occurrence, indeed every reading of each occurrence has its own singularity, even though in order to read we must of course understand this pronoun at the generic, abstract level. This is also the case with cloning: even two individuals with exactly the same genetic structure will still necessarily be two different people to at least the same extent that identical twins are. Derrida never formulates the problem in the way Habermas does, as someone else making a choice over another's genetic make-up. I would suggest he doesn't find this situation to be particularly problematic because it is not so far from the 'natural' condition: a point that emerges if we ask the question, who has ever chosen their genetic formation? To be cast in the situation of having a particularly heredity is the normal situation for humans. PGD would not for Derrida give rise to 'moral questions that are not simply difficult but are of an altogether different kind' but rather we have ethical problems that are a particular complication of a more general structure, one that can be taken to include all questions of socialization (Habermas 2003, p. 13). In particular, the issue of cloning is but another case of the decision that we must take in a situation where we cannot calculate with certainty the absolutely right course of action.

In the main Derrida's concerns about and approaches to the new genetic technologies are very different from those of Habermas. Many of them have to do with not such much the science of genetics itself as how wider social forces might misunderstand or misappropriate them. One of his worries is rather than undermining what is distinctively human, the mapping of the genome will lead to an attempt to define 'the human' and, in particular, to the use of eugenics to eliminate that which would be deemed 'subhuman'.[4] If this concern has some broad similarities with Habermas' the way in which it is posed and his response is quite different. For Derrida the ethical distinctiveness of the existence of those beings called humans is that we are entities whose very being is open for transformation (who 'has its being to be', as Heidegger would put it). His concern is that there is a danger that an interpretation of genetics as a science emerges that attempts to promote a conception of the human as fixed rather than as open. Derrida notes that such positivistic conceptions most often come from those who are not scientists and, indeed, notes how the decoding of the human genome has shown our proximity to other species and undermined previous assumptions about the distinctiveness of humans. From a Derridean point of view we might say that our humanity is 'always already' technical because it is of the nature of humans to constantly work and rework what it means to be human. This is his argument when he says, 'without this technē this body is not even born to itself as a "human" body' (Derrida 2005b, p. 219). This idea of humanity as already the subject of technical processes means that Derrida, unlike Habermas, does not overstress the novelty of the possibilities opened up by the new genetic technologies. Of course, we must not fail to respect the proper distinctions between the technics involved in the use of tools and the vastly different and more complex technics enabled by the science of genetics. That said, we do need to begin with a conception of human beings not simply as inherently technical but as reflexive in that technicity, making their own nature their subject. In saying this we must be careful though to stress that Derrida would follow Heidegger in seeing the self as 'thrown'—and indeed our genetic inheritance could be an element of the situation into which we are cast—that is, we respond to a situation in which we find ourselves to be and have only limited control over. Here I think the emphasis is very different from Habermas whose work constantly tends to present the self as sovereign in its powers of self-creation (for example, the way in which the element of education as 'formation' is downplayed in favour of a conception of it as giving one the power to respond).

On the particular issue of cloning Derrida declares in one of his last works: "I can find few rational and justifiable objections to therapeutic cloning" (Derrida 2005a, p. 147). His earlier view was that while genetics allows something novel, we are not at an "unheard of moment in the history of science or techno-science" but rather need to maintain and extend an existing vigilance (again, we might note the rhetorical distance from Habermas's moral questions "of an altogether different kind") (Derrida 2002b, p. 208). Indeed, in explicitly placing this discussion within the larger question of norms, he suggests that technology is not determining in and

[4]The very title of his paper 'The Aforementioned So-called Human Genome', a published version of his contribution to a 1992 colloquium, 'Analysis of the Human Genome: Freedoms and Responsibilities' organized by Association Descartes, hints at this second concern. Indeed, he underlines that the human genome is one that is 98 % shared with apes and 90 % with mice. Derrida's anxiety is that genetics will be used to try and isolate what is purportedly uniquely human rather than showing the difficulty of drawing a line between human and animal. The later theme more generally is an important one in his late work and is surveyed in Calacro (2008).

of itself but is conditioned by a wider context. Derrida personally has a degree of faith in the ability of those working in the field of genetics (as one of his sons does), suggesting that they have "enough historical memory to set up security measures against what, henceforth, is identifiable as the temptation of negative eugenics, normative and negative, that would seek to eliminate the alleged subhumans or to produce superhumans" (Derrida 2002b, p. 209). Rather, what he sees as the most pressing problem presented by the new genetic technologies, as calling for responsibility and decision, is the problematic distinction between an invention and a discovery. Where Habermas is quick to see the arrival of absolute novelty with the advent of the new genetic technologies, Derrida rather finds existing problems occurring in new forms, in particular an attempt to 'colonise' the genome in the name of established pharmaceutical corporations. His somewhat prescient concern (writing in 1992) is that genetic advances will mostly benefit the rich, industrialized nations and that any legal framework established in this area will be moulded according to their interests (Derrida 2002b, p. 205). He suggests that this is a problem that neither scientists nor legal professionals are equipped to deal with; his view being that the law, as its stands, is inadequate, in dating from a period when science and technology had much different contours. His worry is it is "the rich and so called developed countries that will, in fact, be the first, if not the only beneficiaries of this knowledge" and, even, that benefits might particularly be restricted to the groups within those societies that can take advantage of genetics potential as predicative medicine (Derrida 2002b, p. 212).

The ethical questions thrown up by genetic technologies offer one opportunity to contrast the ethical thought of Habermas and Derrida. Although he does not mention Habermas in his work on genetics (which in any case precedes the latter's by more than ten years), I would argue that Derrida's discussion of genetic technologies challenges Habermas's closure of the possibility of ethics through his resort to "rational" handing down of norms. Against Habermas's pursuit of a communicatively agreed closure, Derrida's concern is responsibility and the possibility of a decision that is not just the application of a rule:

> a responsibility or an ethical decision, intent on modeling itself after, or ordering itself according to, a scientific or allegedly scientific knowledge that establishes the norm or normality - that is, a responsibility or an ethical decision that would be satisfied with unfolding a theoretical program or the content of a knowledge regarding a norm - obviously would not be, in the rigorous sense of the term, an act of responsibility or freedom. (Derrida 2002b, p. 200).

Habermas attempts through his "rational reconstruction" to arrive at a definitive resolution of the ethical problems of PGD. His work focuses on defending a conception of the ethical self as grounded in autonomy, as the ability to self-legislate. In contrast, Derrida believes that ethics is primarily a response to an address from an other in a situation which I can never fully comprehend or command. The ethical self is first of all *responsible* to others who make demands of it and one responds from where one finds oneself to be. The self is constituted by its lack of closure, that is by its openness to alterity, to the very possibility of the radically new. Humans, whether the subjects of genetic technologies or not, are not ethically sovereign or autonomous and, indeed, the very possibility of ethics derives from the fact that they are not. Derrida insists that: "it is because I am not one with myself that I can speak with the other and address the other" (Derrida 1997, p. 14). The way in which the other both constitutes and exceeds me is what makes me an ethical subject, at the same time as also being what frustrates any possibility of a final knowledge that would dictate how we should act. This failure of knowledge is what calls us to responsibility, to a decision we make without ever having the full command of a situation that would allow for certainty. Habermas's conception of an ethical self as primarily autonomous, and only subsequently engaged in a world of intersubjectivity, rather than opening the possibility for responsibility and decision instead closes such a chance.

References

Calacro, M. (2008). *Zoographies: The question of the animal from Heidegger to Derrida*. New York: Columbia University Press.

Derrida, J. (1995). *Points ... Interviews 1974–1994*. Palo Alto: Stanford University Press.

Derrida, J. (1996). *The Gift of Death*. Chicago: Chicago University Press.

Derrida, J. (1997). *Deconstruction in a nutshell: A conversation with Jacques Derrida*. New York: Fordham University Press.

Derrida, J. (2002a). *Who's afraid of philosophy: Right to philosophy I*. Palo Alto: Stanford University Press.

Derrida, J. (2002b). *Negotiations: Interventions and interviews 1971–2001*. Palo Alto: Stanford University Press.

Derrida, J. (2005a). *Rogues: Two essays on reason*. Palo Alto: Stanford University Press.

Derrida, J. (2005b). *On touching, Jean-Luc Nancy*. Palo Alto: Stanford University Press.

Derrida, J. (2013). Avowing—The Impossible: "Returns", Repentance, and Reconciliation. In E. Weber (Ed.), *Living together: Jacques Derrida's communities of violence and peace*. New York: Fordham University Press.

Evans, M. (2014). Reasons and Enlightenments: Of Derrida and Habermas. In K. M. Hinneburg & G. Jurewicz (Eds.), *Das Prinzip Aufklärung Zwischen Universalismus und Partikularem Anspruch*. Wilhelm Fink: Paderborn.

Habermas, J. (1992). *Moral consciousness and communicative action*. Cambridge: Polity.

Habermas, J. (1993). *Justification and application: Remarks on discourse ethics*. Cambridge: Polity.

Habermas, J. (1996). *Between facts and norms: Contributions to a discourse theory of law and democracy*. Cambridge: MIT Press.

Habermas, J. (2003). *The future of human nature*. Cambridge: Polity.

McCarthy, T. (1978). *The critical theory of Jürgen Habermas*. Cambridge: Polity.

McCarthy, T. (1993). *Ideals and illusions: On reconstruction and deconstruction in contemporary critical theory* (pp. 181–199). Cambridge: MIT Press.

Meehan, J. (1995). *Feminists read Habermas*. London: Routledge.

Outhwaite, W. (1996). *The Habermas reader*. Cambridge: Polity.

Putnam, H. (2002). *The collapse of the fact/value dichotomy and other essays* (pp. 111–134). Cambridge: Harvard University Press.

Thomassen, L. (2006). *The Derrida-Habermas reader*. Chicago: Chicago University Press.

Thomassen, L. (2007). *Deconstructing Habermas*. London: Routledge.

Part II
The Experience of Illness: Phenomenological Approaches

Chapter 6
An Ethics of Embodiment: The Body as Object and Subject

Jenny Slatman and Guy Widdershoven

1 Introduction

Most medical interventions are aimed at the *body*: the body in pain, the sick body, the infected body, the wounded body, the old body, the dysfunctioning body, the fat body, the paralyzed body, the disfigured body, the athletic body, the pregnant body etc. Medical practices intend to cure, nurse or enhance the body—whether it is sick, impaired, at risk, or healthy. They seek to prevent, release or alleviate physical suffering. To examine these practices' usefulness, and their moral and social desirability, we need an ethics of embodiment. In medical ethics a first moral principle to prevent undesirable physical harm can be traced back to the Hippocratic *primum non nocere*, "first do no harm." A more specific value (or principle) that can morally guide us in how to approach another as an embodied person is bodily integrity. This notion indicates how to appropriately approach the body of another.

Integrity, stemming from the Latin *integrum*, literally signifies "wholeness" or "intactness." Wholeness refers to the normative counterpart of vulnerability (Zwart 2007). The vulnerable body's inviolability should be respected and not infringed upon (*in-tangere*) (Rendtorff and Kemp 2000). What is meant by bodily wholeness or inviolability is, however, not unambiguous. In this paper, we will explore its meaning while focusing on the various ways in which one experiences one's body. Endorsing a phenomenological approach to embodiment,[1] we distinguish between the experi-

[1]See Cory Shores' contribution to this volume (Chap. 16) for a critique of the phenomenological approach to embodiment.

J. Slatman (✉)
Department of Health, Ethics and Society, Maastricht University, Maastricht, The Netherlands
e-mail: jenny.slatman@maastrichtuniversity.nl

G. Widdershoven
Department of Medical Humanities, VU University Medical Center, Amsterdam, The Netherlands

D. Meacham (ed.), *Medicine and Society, New Perspectives in Continental Philosophy*, Philosophy and Medicine 120, DOI 10.1007/978-94-017-9870-9_6

ence of one's body as object and the experience of one's body as subject. This difference, we argue, results in different conceptions of bodily integrity. Drawing on historical and more contemporary philosophical texts on embodiment, we identify three different meanings of embodiment, i.e. the "body as object," the "body as subject," and the "body as subject and object," and subsequently show how these ideas of embodiment inform three different conceptions of bodily integrity.

We will start with a discussion of the (nowadays) prevalent of respect for bodily integrity, i.e. the view that a medical professional is only allowed to treat a person's body after the person has given consent to this treatment. This notion of bodily integrity, legally anchored in the procedure of informed consent, is based upon the idea that the body is an object. Indeed, according to this view, bodily integrity is guaranteed by the possibility of consenting to interventions in this "object." Following philosophical criticism on the one-sidedness of "the body as object" ontology, we will argue that the ethics of embodiment implied in the procedure of informed consent is limited. To equally respect the body's subject-side we need a notion of bodily integrity according to which wholeness also refers to a certain intactness of embodied agency. Such a notion has been put forward in various phenomenological studies. In this paper we will go one step further and present yet another idea of bodily integrity. While incorporating an example from our current research project on disfigurements we will, in the last section of this paper, develop an idea of bodily integrity that accounts for both the objective and subjective aspects of the body. This is the idea of bodily integrity in terms of embodied self-identification.

2 The Body as Object

Since the rise of Modern sciences, including medicine and anatomy, and modern philosophy in the 17th century, the body has been considered as an independent substance or "thing." Whereas classical and medieval medicine was mainly inspired by Hippocrates's and Galen's view that the body should be understood as a whole that needs to be in balance, and by the philosophical view that body and soul are necessarily intertwined in living beings, modern medicine considers the body as a self-regulating thing, comparable to a machine (Le Breton 1990). Opening up dead bodies by means of (public) anatomical dissections in the 16th century, Andreas Vesalius literally cut bodies into parts, and figuratively did away with the idea of the body as a whole (to be respected). The knife of René Descartes, although not material but philosophical, was even sharper when he, in the 17th century, definitively dissected the body from the soul. According to him, body and soul are two substances or things which are radically different, and which cannot be reduced to each other since everything belonging to the body is physical (and therefore dubitable), and everything belonging to the soul is part of one's own immaterial but indubitable stream of thoughts (Descartes 1641 [2008]). Behold the birth of Cartesian dualism.

Although Descartes' work lies nearly 400 years behind us, and although his dualism has been criticized by various philosophers, it is no exaggeration to claim that western medicine and health care are still essentially inspired by Cartesianism (Leder 1992). Whereas Descartes still presumed that there is an immaterial soul next to the body machine, his empiricist successor De Lamettrie claimed that there is nothing immaterial about human existence—man is a machine (De Lamettrie 1748). This view paved the way for mechanical and materialist explanations of the human condition, and is therefore considered as the origin of so-called Cartesian materialism—an approach which is progressively prevailing in philosophy of mind, resulting in reductionist conceptions of the mind. As Foucault claimed, the birth and existence of medical clinics can only be understood on the basis of the conviction that the human body is a machine or thing which can be thoroughly "deciphered" (Foucault 1963). The art of deciphering that started with anatomical dissections has been enormously developed since the invention of imaging technologies (such as X-rays, endoscopy, MRI-scans, PET-scans etc.) that render the body "transparent" (Van Dijck 2005; Slatman 2007, 2009a). Likewise, contemporary medical technologies such as (allograft) organ, tissue or limb transplantation are only intelligible if one is allowed to think of the body as a thing that can be divided; a body "in parts and pieces" (Le Breton 1993; Hacking 2007). Cultures in which Cartesianism is not taken for granted, and in which one's body is considered as something intrinsically related to one's soul and one's ancestors' souls, as, for instance, in Maori culture, therefore do not (or only very reluctantly) accept medical practices such as organ donation (Shaw 2010).

It is not our intention here to disqualify the Cartesian view in medicine. It would indeed be unwise to ignore the progress that medicine has achieved since the 17th century. As we see it, the greater part of this success is based upon the fact that medical scientists and physicians are allowed to consider bodies as complex machines that can be analyzed and fixed. So we are not so much interested in moral claims about the so-called predominant biomedical view of physicians. We find it much more interesting to look at the consequences of the Cartesian view for the patient's *experience* and relation to his or her body.

Let us therefore explore what kind of self-experience underlies (and affirms) the assumption that one's own body is a thing. First, while considering one's own body as a thing, it becomes an *object* of reflection. Inherent in the fact that the body can become an object of reflection is that it becomes something we are explicitly conscious of. It becomes an object of one's consciousness. This immediately implies a certain distance between oneself and one's body. As we will explain in more detail in the next section, phenomenology has shown that one experiences something as an object if it appears against a certain horizon, in a possible manifold of adumbrations (Husserl 1950). If one would totally coincide with one's body, if there were no distance between oneself and one's body, one could not experience or perceive it as an *object*. Considering one's body as an object thus involves an external view on it, or a third person perspective. It is also because of this external stance towards one's body that one does not (totally) coincide with it. The body as object, therefore, is the body that one *has*, rather than the body that one *is*.

Having a body, obviously, refers to a relation of possession. But as we will explain hereafter, *being a body* also involves a kind of bodily ownership. Possession in terms of "having one's body" is often related to legal and ethical issues. It is also rather common to view the issue of bodily integrity against the background of the question of possession. Indeed, should not the (legal) owner of a body decide about his or her own body? As we know, however, the idea of possession is not a straightforward one. Differences in religion or in worldview cause different conceptions of possession and, subsequently, different ideas of bodily integrity (Zwart and Hoffer 1998). For instance, whereas a liberal may claim that she/he is the owner of her or his body and may thus treat it any way she/he likes, a Christian may believe that her or his body—the temple of the Holy Spirit—is only given to him or her on loan. Although these two views can lead to rather different moral deliberations and choices with regard to issues such as organ donation or circumcision, they both presuppose that one's body is something that can be described in terms of possession or loan, and thus as something on which one has an external and rather instrumental view.

Because of this external view, most ethical deliberations about one's body in terms of possession boil down to the question of self-determination and autonomy. This is exactly the reason why in current bioethics respect for bodily integrity is often identified with respect for personal autonomy. Based upon respect for autonomy, respect for bodily integrity, in fact, implies a person's consent is needed prior to any intervention in his or her body, or to usage of his or her body material (such as DNA, organs, tissue), i.e. to interventions in or usage of one's body as *object*. Indeed, the one (or the I-self) who is consenting is the autonomous (and perhaps rational) subject who decides about his or her body, the body that he or she owns. Zwart (2000) convincingly argues that the current identification of bodily integrity with autonomy effectively wipes out the ethical dimension of bodily integrity as a normative principle in its own right. Similarly, we suggest that to protect the integrity or wholeness in vulnerable bodies, we should not just invoke the principle of autonomy. As we see it, to grasp the idiosyncratic normative dimension of embodiment, we should not only look at bodily wholeness such as it can be pointed at in an objectified body or a body as object. According to a phenomenological view, we experience our body not only as an object, but also as something different than an object, something that can be seen as the condition of possibility for the experience of objects and could therefore be called subject.

3 The Body as Subject

The French philosopher Merleau-Ponty became famous for developing the idea of the body as incarnated subject. For this he also used the terms *corps sujet* and *corps propre*. Before we present his ideas and his influence on the current debate, we will first briefly discuss some aspects from the work of his predecessors to explain the genesis of the notion of the embodied or incarnated subject.

In fact, the notion of the embodied subject is an ambiguous one. In modern philosophy the term subject refers to the disembodied Cartesian *Cogito* or Kantian *Ich denke*. In this sense, the subject is radically opposed to and distinguished from anything embodied. One of the first post-Kantian philosophers who criticized the idea of such a pure disembodied subject was Maine de Biran (1766–1824). To our knowledge, he was also the first philosopher who used the term *corps propre*. In his eloquent essay on Biran, Huxley (1950), makes clear that Biran's philosophical ideas on embodied subjectivity had their origin in his day-to-day worries concerning his own body. Sickness was a "poltergeist" in Biran's life: he suffered greatly from his weak and unstable nervous system. His physical suffering was also very well documented since he kept a *Journal intime*, in which he entered reflections on his state of mind, which was often instigated by the condition of his body. "Having caught a cold I am in an uncomfortable situation which increases my incapability, my unwieldiness, and my self-distrust. I am dissatisfied with everybody because I am not satisfied with myself" (1814, p. 155).[2] Still following the vocabulary of Descartes and Lammetrie, he refers to his own body as a "machine": "With a vulnerable machine which is nearly always sick, I can hardly go out and see other people. I am thus turned inward onto myself, surveying the vicissitudes at the heart of my own existence" (1794, p. 133). These reflections on himself and his vulnerable "machine," however, do not result in an external instrumental view on his body. His distressing body propelled him to constantly explore his own existence, leading to a rather introspective psychological analysis of himself. Unlike Descartes' introspective meditations, Biran's self-reflections do not retrieve the realm of the mind, the *res cogitans*. They rather lead to a sort of theory of embodied self-consciousness.

Biran's later philosophical work centers around the question of self-consciousness (Maine de Biran 1812 [2001]). According to him consciousness is constituted by the sentiment or sensation of one's own existence, and we experience ourselves because we are a "*force agissante*"—an acting power; our existence consists of the fact that we always have the possibility to act, and to act does not only imply physical actions, but also intended agency. Hence, the act of willing something is already an expression of our being as "*force agissante*." Biran thus transforms Descartes' ego from an "I think" (*je pense*) into an "I will" (*je veux*). As Maine de Biran knew all too well, the force of the will always met with the resistance of the body resulting in the sensation of effort in which we feel our own existence. Human existence consists, in essence, of doing or willing something and of the will meeting resistance: it is activity and relation. Self-consciousness is therefore consciousness of one's own activity, or it is the sensation of effort (*sensation d'effort*). And this sensation is not just a mental feeling, rather it is an embodied one, a physical feeling: it is like the sensing of oneself while one is sensing something. The body is not only sensing something, rather it also senses its own sensing.

The 20th century phenomenologist and existentialist Sartre (1943) provided a critique of Biran's idea of the "sensation of effort." As he puts it: "It is true that I can see and touch my legs and hands [...] but I cannot 'see the seeing' [...] Similarly I see my hand touching objects, but do not *know* it in its aspect of touching them" (329). The rejection of the "feeling of feeling," or the "sensation of

[2]A selection of entries from the *Journal Intime* is included in Naville's study (1857). Fragments are translated by JS.

effort" is inherent to Sartre's idea of consciousness. According to him consciousness is not something, not an object of reflection; it is nothing or, as he puts it, "nothingness" (*néant*, and therefore it is not possible to be (explicitly) conscious of consciousness. The usage of the French present participle form—*ant*, underlines that *le néant* involves an activity, more precisely, the activity of negation (in a Hegelian sense).

In a nice example Sartre (355–360) provides a phenomenological description of what happens if one turns one's conscious reflection from the world outside to one's own body. While reading a book, the object of one's consciousness is this book and its story. The moment one feels pain in one's eyes, consciousness shifts from the book to one's own body. While being absorbed by the book one had no reflexive consciousness of one's body or oneself; at that point one's body was only present to oneself in an un-reflexive and non-thematic way. Pain disturbs this. However, the experience of pain does not yet objectify one's body, since pain is not intentional. In the experience of pain, there is no distinction between the act of experience and the object of experience. It is also therefore that we say that "my finger hurts" and not that "I have a pain in my finger." Sartre would say: my finger is pain. Like the experience of nausea, the experience of pain is part of our existence without distance (*sans distance*) toward our consciousness.

A distance between one's existence and one's consciousness is created at the moment that experience of pain becomes more explicit or, as Sartre says, when it becomes reflexive. Pain becomes discomfort (*le mal*). By means of this experience the body becomes objectified, it becomes an intentional *object*. The transition from pain to discomfort is caused by reflection. Consciousness of pain is still an unreflexive consciousness; this means that consciousness has not taken itself as an object of consciousness. So according to Sartre, the difference between pain and discomfort is that in the latter one not only experiences pain, but also explicitly experiences that it is oneself who is having this experience. This reflexive consciousness differs radically from Biran's "sensation of an effort": whereas Biran presupposes that we can be conscious of our own consciousness as an activity, Sartre claims that the reflection of one's own consciousness cancels out consciousness as an activity—it turns oneself into a thing or object.

In fact, Sartre's analysis follows the Husserlian logic that consciousness involves transcendence, meaning that consciousness is always directed to something else than itself, that it is always "going somewhere else"—which is indeed the literal translation of the Latin verb *transcendere* (Levinas 1965 [1988]). It is exactly this transcendence that is lacking in Biran's idea of consciousness. The "sensation of an effort" implies immanence: a total coincidence of consciousness with itself. One of the few philosophers who have taken up the idea of consciousness as immanence is Henry (2000). Following Biran's philosophy, he claims that embodied self-consciousness is constituted by consciousness that ceaselessly affects itself (*s'auto-impressionner*) (231). This means, in fact, an exclusive first person perspective on or a pure introspection of one's own bodily being. As we will explain in the next section, such an account of embodied self-experience cannot allow for the body's double-sided ontology.

Although Sartre's idea of transcendence still remains rather disembodied, for it is consciousness that does the transcending and not the body, his phenomenology of the human condition does teach us some interesting things about the body. His reflection on embodied self-experience makes visible two different modes of experience: one experiences one's own body either as something implicitly conscious (as in pain), or as something explicitly self-conscious (as in discomfort). According to the first mode, the body is not experienced as an object; according to the second mode, it is. For Sartre the objectifying mode has a negative undertone because it is a form of self-alienation. The objectified body is separated from the self or self-consciousness for, indeed, self-consciousness is the opposite or negation of an object. Although Sartre introduces two different kinds of embodied self-experiences, his strict dialectics between object (*en soi*) and consciousness (*pour soi*)—i.e. that they mutually exclude each other—makes it impossible to understand how these two experiences relate to each other. Merleau-Ponty, by contrast, claims that our existence should not be understood in terms of a strict negating dialectics between consciousness or subject (*pour soi*) and object (*en soi*), but in terms of an incarnated subject, which involves being both subject and object at once, yet without a total coincidence between to two. Merleau-Ponty thus declines both Biran's and Sartre's view. To make clear this position, we will first draw on Husserl's analysis of embodied self-experience, which forms the basis for Merleau-Ponty's idea of *corps propre* or *corps vécu*.

4 The Body as Subject and Object

Husserl (1912 [1952]) claims that if one touches one's left hand with one's right hand, the left hand can be experienced in two different ways. Firstly, it can be experienced as a thing with a certain extension and with certain properties. In this case, the left hand is the physical thing: a *Körper*. It is the intentional objective correlate of the right hand's touching. In fact, *Körper* coincides with the idea of the body as an object, a thing extended in space (*res extensa*), as described in the first section. But secondly, the left hand is also experienced as the localization of sensations. The moment one touches one's left hand, one finds a series of touch-sensations in this hand, and since these sensations do not constitute physical properties such as smoothness or roughness, they do not constitute the physical thing "left hand." Rather, they constitute the experience that one feels in one's left hand that it is touched.

Husserl coins the term *Empfindnisse* (sensings) to indicate a typical form of sensations (*Empfindungen*), i.e. localized sensations. These specific sensations include touch sensations; sensations of hot and cold, of one's posture (proprioception) and of one's movements (kinesthetic sensations) as well as pain sensations. And it is by means of these *Empfindnisse* that the body is experienced as a *Leib*. We call this the experience of "me-ness," or "own-ness." The localized non-intentional sensations affirm that this is one's own body. Yet, this experience of own-ness does not necessarily mean that one "agrees" with one's body; the experience of pain, for instance, is often considered as an experience that may lead to alienation of oneself, and is often seen as a "negative" or "bad" experience or appearance of one's body—a *dys*-appearance (Leder 1990; Zeiler 2010). What we mean by own-ness, however, is that it is by means of these kinds of localized sensations that we cannot but affirm that it is *my* body that is affected; it is my body that I experience from a first person perspective. In this respect it is interesting to refer to Cole's study on people who suffer from tetraplegia (paralysis of arms, legs and trunk due to a spinal cord injury). These people do not feel their bodies; it is as if their heads are floating, but they do have experiences of pain, due to spasms and dysreflexia. Although these pain experiences are really troublesome and in the case of dysreflexia, potentially life-threatening, some of the interviewed people say that they prefer this experience over the experience of feeling nothing, since it "anchors" them in their body (Cole 2004). One interviewee says pain is "almost my friend," because "it puts me in touch with my body" (89). In these cases, pain thus reclaims the absent body.

The *Leib* experience, the experience of "this is my body, this is me," does not automatically go together with an instrumental and objectified view on one's body (Legrand 2006; Slatman 2009b). The sense of ownership involved in this experience therefore differs from the form of possession in terms of *having one's body*, discussed above, since it cannot be equated to being the governor of one's body. Because of its typical spatiality, the *Leib* is not just a thing amongst other things and property.

The body's spatiality should be understood against the background of the idea of adumbrations (*Abschattungen*) that lies at the heart of the phenomenological theory of appearance. Phenomenal reality appears as a reality with real properties. It is not given at once; rather, it is always given through a manifold of adumbrations and sensuous schemes. This means that one and the same thing is presented in different horizons and perspectives, and that no single perspective can exhaust its possibilities of appearing. If we perceive, for example, a table, there is always one of its sides that we cannot actually perceive, and yet we still perceive one and the same table (Husserl 1950, pp. 92–93). The perceived table is never fully present to consciousness: its rear sides are what Husserl calls co-present to what is given intuitively and immediately in the flesh of an actual perceptual adumbration. The same holds for one's hand. If one's left hand appears as the thing, left hand, it appears through the constantly changing manifolds of adumbrations.

The sensings (*Empfindnisse*) of one's left hand, however, are not given through adumbrations or schematization. This means that one's body as one's own, as *Leib*, is given without any perspective, and is thus entirely present. Consequently, the *Leib* bears in itself the "zero point" of all orientations (Husserl 1912 [1952]). It is thus not an intentional object; rather it is pre-intentional, pre-objective or non-intentional, or even a "non-thing" (Waldenfels 1989). It is therefore not surprising that it is hard to find a proper translation of the German word *Leib* that emphasizes the lived-through experience of oneself instead of one's physical appearance.

In his influential study *Phenomenology of Perception* (1945), Merleau-Ponty uses the terms *corps propre*, *corps sujet* and *corps vécu* to translate *Leib*. He defines the *corps propre* first of all while exploring the ontological presuppositions of the characteristics provided by classical psychology: (1) permanence; (2) double sensations; (3) being an affective object; and (4) self-movement (90–97). In his discussion of the double sensations and the body as affective object he refers, implicitly, to the specific localized sensations which constitute the body as an embodied experience of here and now. While discussing the body's permanence, he writes that because "my body is never absent to me," the body is a condition of possibility for the permanence of other things. The permanence of the body is therefore more fundamental than the permanence of other things. Also, while discussing self-movement Merleau-Ponty in fact refers to the transcendental status of the body. One's own body is not moved by something else, but is moving itself. It is exactly in this self-movement that it opens up a field of orientation in perception and action. The body, therefore, is not just a thing amongst other things, but it is the condition of possibility of the appearance of other things. "The body is our general medium for having a world" (Merleau-Ponty 1945, p. 146).

Merleau-Ponty's analysis of embodiment in *Phenomenology of Perception* notably consists of exploring the meaning of the body as incarnated subject, as a transcendental condition of possibility for perception and action. A key issue in his analysis is the idea of motor intentionality. It is not so much by thinking or contemplating, but by moving one's body that one endows one's world with meaning. And most of these intentional actions—such as grasping a cup, kicking a ball, driving a bike or using an instrument or tool—take place at a preconscious, prereflective level. If incorporated in one's habitual body, one does not need to "think" in order to perform intentional actions. Motility should be understood as "basic intentionality," and therefore Merleau-Ponty claims that the Cartesian "I think" should be replaced by the "I can" (*je peux*) (137).

In his later work, Merleau-Ponty (1964) became more interested in the complexity of so-called double sensations. He no longer stressed embodied subjectivity and agency, but rather emphasized that the body (as subject) always remains entangled in the world because of its own "thinghood": the body may be a subject, but at the same time, it always remains a certain object or thing. He therefore replaced the term *corps propre* by the term *chair* (flesh), which denotes at once "being part of the world" and "being a certain perspective in this world." As we have explained elsewhere, this idea of being both embodied subject and object can be understood on the basis of the difference between, and the mutual independence of *Leib* and *Körper* (Slatman 2005).

At first sight, Husserl's analysis seems to head straight for a new kind of dualism: the experience of *Körper* versus the experience of *Leib*. However, if we look closer at the example of the two touching hands, we see that things are more complicated. As said, the experience of *Leib* is constituted by localized sensations, which means that the touched hand feels itself being touched. Feeling one's own touchability is only possible if the hand is also experienced as something that can be touched. And this is only possible if the hand is also experienced as a touchable thing or *Körper*. Hence, the experience of *Leib* presupposes *and* affirms the experience of *Körper*. What Merleau-Ponty calls flesh in his later work can be interpreted as the *Leibkörper*: the experience that the body one is—the body as subject—is directly related to the body one has—the body as object.

Resuming the example of the two touching hands, Merleau-Ponty claims that we are *touchant-touché* or "sensible sentient." This view, however, does not imply a sensing of one's sensing, as Biran would have it. Although there is a reversibility between touching and being touched, they will never fully coincide:

> My left hand is always on the verge of touching my right hand touching the things, but I never reach coincidence; the coincidence eclipses at the moment of realization, and one of two things always occur: either my right hand really passes over to the rank of touched, but then its hold on the world is interrupted; or it retains its hold on the world, but then I do not really touch *it* – my right hand touching, I palpate with my left hand only its outer covering. (Merleau-Ponty 1964, pp. 147–148)

There always remains an *écart* or difference between touching and being touched, between sensing and being sensed. This idea of the "sensible sentient" (or the *Leibkörper*) eventually implies that the experience of one's own body always entails some degree of distance and strangeness, since the *Leib* experience goes together with the *Körper* experience without coinciding with it (Slatman 2014).

In short, Merleau-Ponty's philosophy of embodiment has provided us with two —related—ideas of the body. In his early work he presented the body as subject (*corps sujet* and *corps propre*), mainly as the source and origin, or the condition of possibility for perception and action. In his later work he emphasized the double-sidedness of the body, the body as both subject and object. Phenomenological analyses of medical practices often endorse his idea of the body as intentional subject to deal with the question whether specific interventions are desirable or not (Leder 1999; Toombs 1999, 2001; Slatman and Widdershoven 2010b). We believe, however, that his idea of the body as double-sided, as both subject and object, as both *voyant* and *vu*, or *touchant* and *touché* can also be helpful for normative evaluations. In certain cases, it is important to take into account that the experience of one's body as subject cannot be separated from the experience of one's body as an object. In the remainder of this paper, we will therefore present two phenomenological conceptions of bodily integrity: one that is mainly based upon the idea that body is a subject, and one that is based upon the idea that the body is both subject and object, that the experience of our own body is principally double-sided.

5 Bodily Integrity and Bodily Intentionality

On the basis of a phenomenological approach to embodiment we can distinguish two conceptions of bodily integrity which both differ from the currently dominant conception according to which respect for bodily integrity is identified with respect for autonomy: (1) integrity in terms of embodied subjective capacities; and (2) integrity in terms of bodily identity or embodied self-identification. Most analyses that provide a phenomenological approach to health care and medicine, point at the first conception. Various interpreters draw on the idea that human existence implies simultaneously having (embodied) possibilities of being engaged in one's world ("I can") and being limited in one's possibilities because of one's vulnerable body. Zeiler (2009), for instance, claims that not just any physical change will threaten the integrity of one's body. One's bodily integrity is only affected if a physical change perturbs one's engaging in the world. In the same vein, Bergoffen (2009) argues that one's bodily integrity is threatened, if one's embodied possibilities are frustrated or annulled. Leder (1992), while criticizing medicine's narrow view on embodiment, stresses motor intentionality, in terms of having possibilities in relation to one's situation or life world.

It is not surprising that many interpreters emphasize the role of embodied capacities since the "I can" forms a central idea in Merleau-Ponty's early work, and his own analysis heavily draws on a case of a person (the famous case of Schneider, a brain damaged soldier documented by Kurt Goldstein and Adhémar Gelb) who had specific brain damage which caused a loss of motor intentionality. Importantly, motor intentionality should not be identified with physical motility as such. Schneider was, for instance, very well capable of touching his nose when it was itching, but he was not able to point to his nose at someone's command. From a physiological view, both movements are virtually the same, but from a phenomenological view, they are different, since they constitute a different meaning. For Schneider the decrease of his "I can" implies a lessening of his possibilities to endow meaning to his world.

Although Merleau-Ponty does not use the term, we could say that Schneider's bodily integrity is disrupted. This idea of integrity cannot be traced back to the intactness of an "objective" body, or to biological functionality. Here the rupture of bodily integrity has to do with the breakdown of bodily intentionality, i.e. the possibilities of being engaged in projects, of initiating new projects, and thus of transcending one's actual situation. Schneider, Merleau-Ponty (1945, p. 135) writes, 'is "tied" to actuality, he "lacks liberty," that "concrete liberty which comprises the general power of putting oneself into a situation". Employing an idea of bodily integrity along these lines can provide insight into the way in which a change or loss of physical functionality can affect a person's life world.

Interestingly, this idea has been taken up by disability studies to stress the other side of the coin, i.e. that biological and functional "defects" do not necessarily lead to a rupture of one's sense of bodily integrity. Scully (2008), who has a hearing impairment, for instance, describes that her spatial orientation in the world qualitatively differs from that of hearing people (97–98). She suggests that a phenomenological approach can help us to understand the differences and variances in being in the world, instead of labeling some as normal and some as inferior. Similarly, we should not simply say that using a wheelchair impairs one's being in the world. The wheelchair may indeed go together with all kinds of hindrances, but in the intertwinement of body and assistive device also new possibilities of action can emerge (Winance 2006).

6 Bodily Integrity and Self-identification

Next to this conception of bodily integrity that emphasizes embodied subjectivity and agency, a phenomenological approach of embodiment also yields an idea of integrity that additionally accounts for the body's object-side. This conception of bodily integrity is especially relevant in cases in which diseases (and their treatments) not only cause functional changes but also changes in appearance. A change in physical appearance, such as a scar or other visible blemish, first of all implies a change in how the body appears as an *object* to oneself and to others. And this (undesirable) change may disrupt one's experience of wholeness and integrity in another way than physical changes that primarily affect one's bodily intentionality or "I can." It is interesting to see that appearance related issues of embodiment are hardly considered from a phenomenological perspective. The only phenomenologists who seem to be interested in the external manifestation of bodies tend to be concerned with issues of gender or race (e.g. Diprose 1994; Grosz 1994; Alcoff 2005). Visible bodily difference in the field of health and illness is mainly explored by researchers in the field of social sciences such as medical sociology and disability studies, and habitually not by phenomenologists.

These studies discuss the social value that is inscribed into visible bodies, especially the value of bodies that deviate from prevailing socio-cultural norms, e.g. the body that is not able, the body that is not healthy, the body that is not slim and muscled, the body that is disfigured. And it is from this perspective that social mechanisms like exclusion, discrimination and stigmatization can be articulated (e.g. Goffman 1963). Although it is extremely important to reveal these kinds of mechanisms, we think that it would be interesting to go one step further and explore how the social dimension of embodiment is related to an individual's bodily intentionality, an individual's embodied "I can," an individual's life-world. Social studies often explain the meaning of embodiment in terms of social construction while stressing the social context of the body. This has as a result that they tend to ignore individual embodied subjectivity and agency. Phenomenology can take into account both the individual and the social dimension of embodiment since it—especially in Merleau-Ponty's later philosophy—allows for the double-sidedness of embodied self-experience (Slatman and Yaron 2014).

As described earlier, the body in the sense of "flesh" or "sensible sentient" involves the reversibility between the experience of *Leib* and the experience of *Körper*, without a coincidence between these two. This difference or *écart* at the heart of embodied self-experience is the reason that we cannot speak of an experience of bodily wholeness or integrity in terms of an undividable wholeness. More likely, experiences of wholeness can come into being through processes of self-identification.

In previous work we have described what these kinds of self-identification processes entail in cases of Body Integrity Identity Disorder (BIID), i.e. people who have a strong and persistent wish to have one of their healthy limbs (mostly a leg) amputated since they experience it as not belonging to their own body (Slatman and

Widdershoven 2009) and allograft hand transplants (Slatman and Widdershoven 2010a, b). These rather extreme and rare cases indeed invite us to reflect on bodily integrity in terms of identity. To illustrate that the issue of identification is always at stake in changes of appearance we will now focus on a more common and less extreme case: post-surgical breast cancer. As discussed elsewhere, body restoring medical interventions such as a breast reconstruction or an external breast prosthesis do not automatically restore a mastectomized woman's experience of bodily wholeness and completeness (Slatman 2011, 2012) To verify whether interventions and devices that primarily have a cosmetic purpose add to a restoration of a person's experience of wholeness we need to look at the various ways in which people respond to a physical change or the usage of a certain device. In fact, we need to explore how a change in the visible (and touchable) body (the body as object) affects the body as condition of possibility for perception and action (the body as subject).

From an interview that one of us had with a woman who has undergone breast surgery, it became clear, for instance, that the usage of a silicone external breast prosthesis incites a multiplicity of embodied self-experiences.[3] The respondent, with the fictional name "Janet," is 62 years old, single, and has had a mastectomy of her left breast. She always uses an external prosthesis, even when she is at home alone. The reason for using it is twofold: she does not want others to see her as a single-breasted woman, and she does not want to be reminded of her loss. She really dislikes not wearing her bra (for instance, at night after having taken a shower), and she literally feels the empty space at her chest when she is for instance reaching with her right hand for something at her left side. She only feels complete while being dressed and wearing the prosthesis. One could say that in her case the prosthetic device perfectly serves its purpose. It conceals her disfigurement.

But the device does more than that; it also facilitates her being in the world as a social being. And therefore we could say that it recovers her embodied "I can." This might sound a bit strange since the prosthesis is only cosmetic and has no motor function. But as Young (1990) has aptly described, our embodied intentionality or "I can" is not only dependent of motor intentionality (as Merleau-Ponty describes in the case of Schneider). It is also because of social and cultural body norms that one's "I can" can turn into an "I cannot." Janet says that she thinks that women who dare to go out without their prostheses are very powerful and strong (since they seem to resist the disapproving gazes of others). She also admits that that is something she also would like to do, but she adds, "I think that I am not able to do so"—"I cannot" she says. It is thus therefore that the prosthesis recovers her "I can." With her prosthesis she can go out and see other people.

[3]The first author has been conducting a qualitative empirical study in which she follows for approximately 10–12 months women who have undergone breast surgery [either mastectomy (N = 11) or breast-saving surgery (N = 9)]. All respondents were interviewed twice or three times with an interval of 4 months. This study aims at making explicit the various ways in which these women habituate to their changed bodies.

Although Janet is in general satisfied with her prosthetic device, she also experiences shortcomings. In fact, she is rather angry and offended about the way breast prosthetics is put in practice (in the Netherlands). If you need a breast prosthesis you have to purchase one in a specialized lingerie shop. She contends: "Don't you think it is ridiculous that you have to *shop* for your breast prosthesis? If you need an artificial leg you won't go shopping but you will be referred to a specialist in the hospital." Her surprise and dissatisfaction about the normal procedure of purchasing a breast prosthesis points, in fact, to some typical presuppositions concerning the female breast. The breast, so it seems, is considered more like an ornament or decoration than a functional integrated part of the body. Also, nearly all breast prostheses are ready-to-wear mass produced devices. Only in very rare cases breast prostheses are tailor-made. This indeed sharply contrasts with the manufacturing of limb prostheses that are always made-to-measure, and that are fitted by a medical professional, instead of a commercial shop assistant.

The most important thing about a limb prosthesis is that it facilitates one's motor intentionality—this is most successful if the device can be incorporated in one's body scheme, and this in fact means that one forgets about the device while wearing it. This functional aspect is often not taken into account in breast prosthetics, because the breast is not an acting body part like an arm or leg. Yet, it does move while "following" the movements of arms, shoulder and trunk. As Janet makes very clear: the most important feature of a well-fitting prosthesis should be that it does not bother you, like your own breast does not bother you. In that sense, the breast prosthesis should not only support a woman's "I can" in the sense of being able to face the normalizing gazes of others; it should also enable to forget about one's body all together. For indeed, the less one needs to pay attention to one's body or is distracted by one's body, the wider one's scope of agency, of possible actions, or as Merleau-Ponty would say; the stronger one's intentional arc.

Janet says that most of the time the prosthesis is satisfactory in the sense that it does not bother her. But sometimes it is not. She recalls that at a certain point when she was busy cleaning her house, only wearing a singlet because it was hot, and she was leaning down to reach for her cleaning cloth in the bucket, her bra with prosthesis did not remain attached to her body: "well, I could just look through this hole, this empty place at my chest, straight to my belly button, yeah, well these are moments that you are really aware of having lost something, then you are reminded of not having anything there anymore…." These are moment at which the prosthesis does not satisfy; it then loses its meaning of supporting one's embodied capacities, one's "I can." If the prosthesis slides off the body it in fact reinforces the feeling of being incomplete.

The way in which Janet has to deal with her prosthesis illustrates how experiences of her body as subject and as object intertwine and are interdependent. Her agency and subjectivity, i.e. her possibility to act within the world, to go out and see other people is dependent of the usage of a prosthesis, and thus dependent of how others perceive her, and thus of an external view on her body, her body as object. Conversely, the degree to which the prosthesis is able to fix her body as an object is dependent of the degree to which it is not explicitly noticed and thus to the degree to which it does not disturb her daily dealings and actions. Self-identification thus entails Janet's concurrence with her "prothetized" body, both in its appearance and its functioning.

7 Concluding Remarks

This example makes clear that a pluralistic view on the body may facilitate better care. For Janet, a prosthetic device should not only look good, but also fit well. Since these devices are primarily considered as cosmetic, much emphasis is put upon how they look, but as Janet's story shows this is not enough. She regrets it that she has not been referred to a specialist who could have designed a made-to-measure device for her. It is very likely that her experience of being whole and complete could have gained significantly from a tailored device. Janet's account, obviously, does not serve as a prototype for all women who have had a breast amputation. The most important thing a phenomenological approach on embodiment teaches us is that we have to listen carefully to each individual's multifaceted body story.

What medical professionals can learn from this is that adequate treatment of the body—subject and object—calls for multilateral attention and care. Medical practices might be improved if medical professionals would incorporate a wide range of questions about embodied self-experiences in their patient interviews, and if they subsequently would use patients "body-stories" while counselling them. We hope that our currently on-going research on disfigurements will result in findings that can serve as handles for medical professionals to accurately inform patients about the variety of impacts that a disfigurement can have, and about the possible benefits and shortcomings of different interventions and prosthetic devices.

In this paper, we have thus argued that a phenomenological approach to embodiment can provide an ethics that goes beyond present mainstream medical ethics, which puts a strong emphasis on patients' autonomy, sometimes to the detriment of other aspects of (embodied) well-being. On the basis of our analysis of how the body can be experienced, we have identified three different notions of integrity. The first one, based upon the "body as object" ontology, corresponds to the nowadays prevailing idea that bodily integrity can be respected through autonomy and thus through informed consent. If the body, alternatively, is considered as subject, respect for bodily integrity involves respect for and empowerment of people's embodied agency. The third notion of bodily integrity entails recognition of the body's double-sided ontology of both being object and subject, and as such it requires attention to on-going processes of embodied self-identification.

References

Alcoff, L. M. (2005). *Visible identities: Race, gender, and the self.* Oxford: Oxford University Press.

Bergoffen, D. (2009). Exploiting the dignity of the vulnerable body: Rape as a weapon of war. *Philosophical Papers, 38*(3), 307–325.

Cole, J. (2004). *Still lives: Narratives of spinal cord injury.* Cambridge, MA: MIT Press.

De Lamettrie, J. O. (1748). Machine man. In A. Thomson (Ed.), *Machine man and other wrtings* (A. Thomson, Trans. 1996) (pp. 1–40). Cambridge: Cambridge University Press.

Descartes, R. (1641 [2008]). *Meditations on first philosophy: With selections from the objections and replies.* Oxford: Oxford University Press.

Diprose, R. (1994). *The bodies of women. Ethics, embodiment and sexual difference.* London: Routledge.

Foucault, M. (1963). *Naissance de la clinique.* Paris: P.U.F.

Goffman, E. (1963). *Stigma: Notes on the management of spoiled identity.* London: Penguin.

Grosz, E. (1994). *Volatile bodies: Toward a corporeal feminism.* Bloomington: Indiana University Press.

Hacking, I. (2007). Our Neo-Cartesian bodies in parts. *Critical Inquiry, 34,* 78–105.

Henry, M. (2000). *Incarnation. Une philosophie de la chair.* Paris: Seuil.

Husserl, E. (1912 [1952]). *Ideas pertaining to a pure phenomenology and to a phenomenological philosophy, second book* (R. Rojcewicz & A. Schuwer, Trans. 1989). Dordrecht: Kluwer Academic Publishers.

Husserl, E. (1950). *Ideen zu einer reinen Phänomenologie und phänomenologischen Philosophie. Erstes Buch.* Husserliana III. The Hague: Matinus Nijhoff.

Huxley, A. (1950). Variations on a philosopher. In *Themes and variations* (pp. 1–152). London: Chatto and Windus.

Le Breton, D. (1990). *Anthropologie du corps et modernité.* Paris: Presses Universitaires de France.

Le Breton, D. (1993). *La chair à vif: usages médicaux et mondains du corps humain.* Paris: Editions Métailié.

Leder, D. (1990). *The absent body.* Chicago: University of Chicago Press.

Leder, D. (1992). A tale of two bodies. The Cartesian corpse and the lived body. In D. Leder (Ed.), *The body in medical thought and practice.* Dordrecht: Kluwer Academic Publishers.

Leder, D. (1999). Whose body? What body? The metaphysics of organ donation. In M. J. Cherry (Ed.), *Persons and their bodies: Rights, responsibilities, relationships* (pp. 233–264). Dordrecht: Kluwer Academic Publishers.

Legrand, D. (2006). The bodily self: The sensori-motor roots of pre-reflective self-consciousness. *Phenomenology and the Cognitive Sciences, 5,* 89–118.

Levinas, E. (1965 [1988]). Intentionalité et sensation. In *En découvrant l'existence avec Heidegger et Husserl* (pp. 145–162). Paris: Vrin.

Maine de Biran, F. P. G. (1812 [2001]). Essai sur les fondements de la psychologie. *Oeuvres de Maine de Biran Tome* VII-1 et 2. Paris: Vrin.

Merleau-Ponty, M. (1945). *Phenomenology of perception* (C. Smith, Trans. 1962). London: Routledge.

Merleau-Ponty, M. (1964). *The visible and the invisible* (Lingis, A. Trans. 1968). Evanston: Northwestern University Press.

Naville, E., & Maine de Biran, F. P. G. (1857). *Maine de Biran: sa vie et ses pensées.* Paris: Joel Cherbuliez.

Rendtorff, J. D. & Kemp, P. (2000). *Basic ethical principles in European bioethics and biolaw: Autonomy, dignity, integrity and vulnerability* (Vol. I.). Copenhagen: Centre for Ethics and Law.

Sartre, J.-P. (1943). *Being and nothingness. An essay on phenomenological ontology* (H. E. Barnes, Trans. 2007). London: Routledge.
Scully, J. L. (2008). *Disability bioethics: Moral bodies, moral difference*. Lanham, MD: Rowman and Littlefield Publishers.
Shaw, R. (2010). Organ donation in Aotearoa/New Zealand: Cultural phenomenology and moral humility. *Body and Society, 16*(3), 127–147.
Slatman, J. (2005). The sense of life: Husserl and Merleau-Ponty on touching and being touched. *Chiasmi International, 7*, 305–325.
Slatman, J. (2007). Recognition beyond Narcissism. Imaging the body's ownness and strangeness. In H. Fielding, G. Hiltmann, D. Olkowski, & A. Reichold (Eds.), *The Other. Feminist reflections in ethics* (pp. 186–204). London: Palgrave.
Slatman, J. (2009a). Transparant bodies: Revealing the myth of interiority. In R. Van de Vall & R. Zwijnenberg (Eds.), *The body within: Art, medicine and visualisation* (pp. 107–122). London: Equinox Publishing.
Slatman, J. (2009b). A strange hand: On self-recognition and recognition of another. *Phenomenology and the Cognitive Sciences, 8*(3), 321–342.
Slatman, J. (2011). The meaning of body experience evaluation in oncology. *Health Care Analysis, 19*(4), 295–311.
Slatman, J. (2012). Phenomenology of bodily integrity in disfiguring breast cancer. *Hypatia. Journal of Feminist Philosophy, 27*(2), 281–300.
Slatman, J. (2014). *Our strange body: Philosophical refelections on identity and medical interventions.* Amsterdam: Amsterdam University Press.
Slatman, J., & Widdershoven, G. (2009). Being whole after amputation. *American Journal of Bioethics, 9*(1), 48–49.
Slatman, J., & Widdershoven, G. (2010a). Hand transplants and bodily integrity. *Body and Society, 16*(3), 69–92.
Slatman, J., & Widdershoven, G. (2010b). Embodied self-identity in neuro-oncology: A phenomenological approach. *AJOB Neuroscience, 1*(3), 12–13.
Slatman, J., & Yaron, G. (2014). Towards a phenomenology of disfigurements. In K. Zeiler & L. Käll (Eds.), *Feminist phenomenology and medicine* (pp. 223–240). Albany: SUNY Press.
Toombs, S. K. (1999). What does it mean to be somebody? Phenomenological reflections and ethical quandries. In M. J. Cherry (Ed.), *Persons and their bodies: Rights, responsibilities, relationships* (pp. 73–94). Dordrecht: Kluwer Academic Publishers.
Toombs, S. K. (2001). Reflections on bodily change. The lived experience of disability. In S. K. Toombs (Ed.), *Handbook of phenomenology and medicine*. Dordrecht: Kluwer Academic Publishers.
Van Dijck, J. (2005). *The transparent body: A cultural analysis of medical imaging*. Washington: University of Washington Press.
Waldenfels, B. (1989). Körper - Leib. In J. Leenhardt & R. Picht (Eds.), *Esprit/Geist. 100 Schlüsselbegriffe für Deutsche und Franzosen* (pp. 342–345). München: Piper.
Winance, M. (2006). Trying out the wheelchair: The mutual shaping of people and devices through adjustment. *Science, Technology and Human Values, 31*(1), 52–72.
Young, I. M. (1990). *Throwing like a girl and other essays in feminist philosophy and social theory*. Bloomington: Indiana University Press.
Zeiler, K. (2009). Ethics and organ transfer: A Merleau-Pontean perspective. *Health Care Analysis, 17*(2), 110–122.
Zeiler, K. (2010). A phenomenological analysis of bodily self-awareness in the experience of pain and pleasure: on dys-appearance and eu-appearance. *Medicine, Health Care and Philosophy, 13*(4), 333–342.

Zwart, H. (2000). From circle to square: Integrity, vulnerability and digitalization. In P. Kemp, J. D. Rendtorff & N. M. Johansen (Eds.), *Bioethcis and biolaw. Four ethical principles* (Vol. II, pp. 141–153). Copenhagen: Centre for Ethics and Law.

Zwart, H. (2007). Integriteit. In M. Becker, B. Van Stokkom, P. Van Tongeren & J. P. Wils (Eds.), *Lexicon van de Ethiek* (pp. 166–169). Assen: Van Gorcum.

Zwart, H. & Hoffer, C. (1998). *Orgaandonatie en lichamelijke integriteit. Een analyse van christelijke, liberale en islamitische interpretaties* [*Organ donation and bodily integrity. An analysis of christian, liberal and islamic interpretations*]. Best: Damon.

Chapter 7
Conspicuous, Obtrusive and Obstinate: A Phenomenology of the Ill Body

Havi Carel

1 Introduction

Phenomenology can be used to describe the experience of illness by focusing on first-person accounts of what it is like to suffer from a particular illness.[1] On Merleau-Ponty's view, our experience is first and foremost an embodied experience, an experience of fleshly sensual existence (2012). Any change to the body would lead to far-reaching changes to one's experience. Thus phenomenology seems doubly suited for describing the experience of illness, which often includes a radical shift in one's embodiment: first, it provides a framework that enables detailed attention to experience; second, it takes as its starting point the centrality of embodiment and of perception. However, such an analysis is a challenging undertaking. The experience of illness is diverse and constantly changing; it is bound with cultural and personal meaning; it can be radically subjective and difficult to describe, or even unshareable, as S. Kay Toombs claims (Toombs 1993, p. 23; Carel 2008, 2013a).

And yet, such an analysis seems essential to our quest to understand illness. When we think about a phenomenological description of illness, immediate questions arise: do illness experiences share certain general features? Are these features

This paper was written during a period of research leave funded by the British Academy. It was revised during a period of research leave funded by the Wellcome Trust. I am grateful to the British Academy for awarding me a fellowship and to the Wellcome Trust for awarding me a Senior Investigator Award. I thank Darian Meacham and Greg Tuck for helpful comments on the paper.

[1] It can be used to understand any type of bodily experience, e.g. Young's phenomenological analysis of the embodied experience of pregnancy (Young 2005).

H. Carel (✉)
University of Bristol, Bristol, UK
e-mail: havi.carel@bristol.ac.uk

D. Meacham (ed.), *Medicine and Society, New Perspectives in Continental Philosophy*, Philosophy and Medicine 120, DOI 10.1007/978-94-017-9870-9_7

universal or eidetic, or are they culturally dependent? Do different illness experiences, such as the experience of acute versus chronic illness, share some of their features? Do mental disorder and somatic disease have common experiential features? By offering a general phenomenological framework through which to study illness, this chapter will begin to answer these questions. The framework consists of four themes that I bring together in order to offer a phenomenological understanding of the experience of illness. The first is Toombs' analysis of the eidetic (essential) features of illness. The second is Sartre's three orders of the body. The third is the claim that the healthy body is transparent and illness is the loss of this transparency. Finally, using Heidegger's tool analysis I will suggest that illness is a breakdown of "bodily tools."

2 The Eidetic Features of Illness

There are tens of thousands of diseases; those suffering from the same disease may be affected differently by symptoms, prognosis, pain, psychological impact and how it bears on daily life. It may therefore seem like an impossible task to try to distil the universal or shared features of illness that characterize illness experiences generally. However, the phenomenologist Toombs (1987), herself a sufferer of Multiple Sclerosis, has performed such an analysis. Toombs claims that although the experience of illness is complex, it nonetheless exhibits a typical way of being (1987, p. 228). Certain features that characterize the way of being of illness are manifest regardless of the particular disease state.[2] These, claims Toombs, are the eidetic (essential) characteristics of illness. They are essential to the illness experience itself and remain unchanged regardless of varying empirical features (228). These characteristics "transcend the peculiarities and particularities of different disease states and constitute the meaning of illness-as-lived" (229). Toombs lists five eidetic characteristics of illness: (1) loss of wholeness; (2) loss of certainty; (3) loss of control; (4) loss of freedom to act; and (5) loss of the familiar world. These are the losses that any patient, in whatever disease state, will experience and they cumulatively represent the impact of the disease on the patient's being-in-the-world. Toombs describes each type of loss in detail, enumerating the ways in which each is experienced.

She begins with the loss of wholeness. This loss arises from the perception of bodily impairment, which leads to a profound sense of loss of bodily integrity. The body can no longer be taken for granted or be seen as transparent or absent (cf. Leder 1990) as it assumes an opposing will of its own, which is beyond the control of the self. The disease usurps the body and disrupts its normal cohesion to the lived experience of that body. The ill body, now controlled by a [initially

---

[2] I use the term "disease" to refer to the objective physiological disease process and "illness" to denote the subjective experience of the disease.

intrusive (Carel 2012)] disease process, thwarts plans, impedes choices, and renders actions impossible. In addition, illness disrupts the fundamental body-self unity, and the body is now experienced as other-than-me (Toombs 1987, p. 229). Thus illness is experienced as a threat to the self, so the loss is not only of bodily integrity, but also of the integrity of the self (230).

The second kind of loss, the loss of certainty, ensues from the loss of wholeness. The patient "is forced to surrender his most cherished assumption, that of his personal indestructibility" (230–231). This forces the individual to face her own vulnerability. The recognition of vulnerability and loss of certainty causes great anxiety and worry and this deep apprehension is difficult to communicate. Illness is experienced as a "capricious interruption": an unexpected mishap in an "otherwise carefully crafted life" (230–231). This experience of illness as an unexpected calamity leads to a sense of loss of control, the third kind of loss Toombs describes. The illness in its seemingly random unfolding (will the cancer cells respond to the chemotherapy? why did I suffer the heart attack?) is experienced more like a stroke of bad luck than freely chosen life circumstances. This makes the familiar world suddenly seem inherently unpredictable and uncontrollable (231).

This leads to a further heightening of the sense of loss of control caused by the realization that the belief that medical science and technology protect us from the vagaries of ill health is nothing more than an illusion harbored by modern man (231). In addition, the ill person's ability to make rational choices is eroded because of her lack of medical knowledge and limited ability to judge whether the health professional professing to heal can in fact do so (232).

This leads to the fourth kind of loss, the loss of freedom to act. The ill person's ability to choose freely which course of action (medical treatment) to pursue is restricted by her lack of knowledge of what the best course of action may be. Moreover, in deciding whether to accept medical advice, the patient often assumes that the physician understands and shares her personal value system and takes these values on board when recommending a certain course of action. However, the physician may often feel that it is inappropriate, irrelevant or intrusive to inquire about the patient's values, and judges the clinical data alone to be sufficient for determining what is best for the patient. "Thus the patient not only loses the freedom to make a rational choice regarding his personal situation but additionally loses or abrogates the freedom to make the choice in light of his uniquely personal system of values" (233).

Finally, the fifth kind of loss, the loss of the everyday world, arises from the disharmony of illness and it being a distinct mode of being in the world (233). The ill person can no longer continue with normal activities, or participate as before in the world of work and play. Whereas friends and colleagues continue as they have in the past, the ill person's familiar world is lost through the adjustments to and demands of disease and this exacerbates the sense of loss. A large part of the familiarity of the world arises from its sharedness with other people. But this is now lost. The temporal dimension of one's world is also shaken because future plans have to be adjusted in light of a medical prognosis and the healthy past is broken off from the ill present (cf. Bury 1982). "The future is suddenly disabled, rendered impotent and inaccessible" (Toombs 1987, p. 234). And this loss of future further isolates the ill person from her hitherto familiar world.

Once shattered, all of these domains: wholeness, certainty, control, freedom and familiarity, can only tenuously be re-established. But even if the losses are restored, any such re-establishment is always accompanied by a sense of its fragility and uncertainty, a sense of tenuousness (Carel 2013b). So in many ways the process Toombs describes so intricately is irreversible, even if the disease itself is cured and health is restored. That is an additional reason why Toombs focuses on these features as fundamental to the experience of illness per se and claims that these features pertain regardless of the particular disease state of the individual. "These eidetic characteristics represent the "reality" of illness-as-lived. They reveal what illness means to the patient" (Toombs 1987, p. 234). For Toombs, this model of illness makes the primacy of the person explicit, and not secondary to an objective, abstract, disease entity, as the biomedical model has it. In this sense the phenomenological model of illness can better serve not only patients, as it would naturally seem, but also physicians, whose ultimate goal is to improve individual patients' lives, not merely treat a disease process.

I would like to make a few comments on Toombs' account. First, it seems that the loss of freedom is much broader than Toombs describes. Toombs focuses on the loss of freedom to make rational decisions on the best course of action in response to the medical facts. However, this loss of freedom is one aspect of a much broader loss of freedom brought about by illness. The loss of bodily freedom, freedom to make life plans, and freedom from anxiety about one's bodily integrity and continuity, is acute in both somatic and mental illness. Arthur Frank describes his diagnosis of cancer in these words: "What was it like to be told I had cancer? The future disappeared. Loved ones became faces I would never see again. I felt I was walking through a nightmare that was unreal but utterly real. […] *My body has become a kind of quicksand*, and I was sinking into myself, into my disease" (1991, p. 27, my emphasis).

A similar closure of the future and of the freedom to choose (to an extent) one's course of action and future goals is also a prominent theme in mental illness. John Stuart Mill, who suffered from depression, describes his illness in his autobiography: "the whole foundation on which my life was constructed fell down […] The end has ceased to charm, and how could there ever again be any interest in the means? I seemed to have nothing left to live for" (1989, p. 112). In this situation of acute dejection the freedom to pursue goals is effaced by the loss of meaning of any goal. Although he is free, Mill cannot seize any particular goal because of his underlying feeling that the realization of any goal would be pointless and would not bring him happiness. So it seems that the loss of freedom is a pervasive loss, spanning the freedom to choose one's future, but also a loss of freedom in the present, in that many routine activities easily performed are no longer possible and must be either given up or replaced by an alternative habit or a different way to perform an old task (Carel 2009).

Second, not all losses are experienced by the ill person. For example, someone in a persistent vegetative state may not know that they are incapacitated and may not experience any of the losses Toombs describes (even if in fact the losses are real).[3] Similarly, someone who is in profound denial and self-deceives herself into not experiencing the symptoms of her disease may experience none of the losses, despite the fact that she has in fact incurred them. Such examples demonstrate that the features of illness Toombs describes as eidetic, or essential, are in fact contingent upon the ill person's situation and capacities.

Third, an analogous argument can be made about cultural difference. It may be that in some cultures certain losses are not experienced because some values (e.g. freedom) do not exist in those cultures. So these features of illness should be understood in a more restrictive sense as not entirely eidetic in the Husserlian sense, but as offering a general characterization of the experience of illness as lived by cognitively normal conscious adults in Western societies. In what follows I use Toombs' helpful analysis in a more restrictive sense, taking into account these comments. This analysis will provide a framework for understanding the changes illness brings about to the life of the ill person. But we also need a rich account of the body as it is experienced by the ill person and by others. We now turn to Sartre for that.

3 The Objective Body and the Body as Lived

A useful tool for a phenomenology of illness is the distinction between the objective body (which Husserl called *Körper* and Merleau-Ponty called *le corps objectif*) and the body as lived (*Leib* and *corps propre*, respectively). The objective body is the physical body, the object of medicine: it is what becomes diseased. Sartre calls this body the "body of Others" (*le corps d'autrui*): it is the body as viewed by others, not as experienced by me (Sartre 2003).[4] The body as lived is the first person experience of this objective body, the body as experienced by the person whose body it is. And it is on this level that illness, as opposed to disease, appears.[5] This distinction is fundamental to any attempt to understand the phenomenon at hand:

[3]It is not clear whether there is an illness to speak of in this case, because there is no subjective experience of the disease (brain damage in this case). This raises the question whether the comatose person is ill if she does not know that she is ill. I think that there is a norm of bodily function against which illness is measured or experienced. So the case of the comatose person would consist of a violation of this norm, even if there is no subjective experience of this violation. I thank Darian Meacham for raising this point.

[4]Sartre breaks away from Husserl and Merleau-Ponty on this point. For the latter two, the body of the other is also a lived body. As we will see below, I can also see my body as objective, and moreover that it is both is essential to the givenness of my own body. I thank Darian Meacham for raising this point.

[5]Some authors (e.g. Twaddle 1968; Hoffmann 2002) suggest a third category, sickness, to denote the social dimension of human ailment.

the ill person is only and always the one who experiences the illness from within (although others may experience someone else's illness).

Only they can say if they feel pain or fatigue, or what a particular symptom *feels like*. Thus the experience of illness contains a measure of incommunicability that should be acknowledged (Carel 2013b). Or as Sartre put it more strongly: "the existed body is ineffable" (Sartre 2003, p. 377). Disease, on the other hand, is a process in the objective body that may be observed by any person (including myself) and may yield information that is not available through first-person reports. For example, one may have elevated cholesterol or blood pressure, or an early stage of heart or renal disease, whilst having no experience of these. Often such knowledge comes from medical tests that yield objective facts with no experiential correlate. For example, elevated blood pressure may not *feel like* anything. And it is only once it is revealed via a blood pressure test that it begins to feature in the diseased person's experience. In other words, it is possible to have a disease without an illness.

The relationship between illness and disease is not simple: the two aspects do not just mirror one another. Illness may precede one's knowledge of their disease: disease is commonly diagnosed following the appearance of symptoms experienced by the patient. These symptoms are part of her illness experience and are lived by the patient. Disease may appear without illness, as in the example above of high blood pressure with no symptoms. Or often we have both illness and disease, but the two do not perfectly cohere. For example, severe disease or disability (e.g. quadriplegia, COPD) may give rise to an illness experience that is tolerable or even experienced by the ill person as not causing severe incapacitation or suffering, due to adaptation (Carel 2009). So although the disease may be classed as "severe" on some clinical scale, the illness experience is not as correspondingly negative as might be expected. This is of clinical importance because interventions ought to address patients' lived experiences, but are often designed to restore objectively measured function, based on the tacit assumption that the two correlate more strongly than they do in reality, due to adaptation.

In other words, medical interventions aim at disease, but the relationship between disease and illness is poorly understood. It has been well documented in the literature that there is a surprising lack of correlation between disease severity and level of wellbeing patients report (Angner et al. 2009; Carel 2013a, 2009). A clear example of this is a study of renal patients undergoing haemodialysis and healthy controls (Riis et al. 2005). We would expect the renal patients who are tethered to a dialysis machine three times a week, unable to travel and often incapacitated, to be markedly less happy then the healthy controls. But in fact, both groups reported a similar level of wellbeing (6). Both the dialysis patients and the healthy controls overestimated the impact of haemodialysis on wellbeing and both focused too much on the dialysis as affecting patients' wellbeing more strongly than it actually did. Other examples abound (Angner et al. 2009; Chwalisz et al. 1988; Chaung et al. 1989; de Haes and van Knippenberg 1985). One way of accounting for this lack of correspondence between disease and illness arises from the phenomenological difference between the body as object and the body as subject.[6]

Another reason the difference between the objective body and the body-as-lived emerges in illness is that the body, in both its manifestations, is in large part habitual. It is used to performing certain tasks with ease. Routine actions can be performed expertly and efficiently because they have become habit, and form what Merleau-Ponty calls the "habitual body" (2012). While getting ready to go to work, one rarely notices the multitude of actions and the expertise required to have a shower and get dressed. It is only when we watch a novice, say, a child learning to button her shirt or tie her shoelaces, that we appreciate the complexity of the activity and the expertise it requires. The ease with which we perform habitual tasks frequently disappears in illness, where new novice-like behaviors appear, as a result of lost capacities. We can see this in many situations ranging from the minor and local to the global and severe. We might refrain from using a sore finger and use our left hand to clumsily hold scissors. Or we can think of the lengthy rehabilitation designed to enable stroke patients to re-learn to walk and talk. While possibly retaining the know-how, the ability to carry out an action is lost. The body loses its skills and these have to be replaced or modified.

Another example given by Merleau-Ponty to illustrate, among other things, the habitual body, is the phantom limb (2012). A phantom limb is the sensation emanating from a limb that has been amputated. The phantom limb feels painful or itchy, but the physical limb has been removed. Merleau-Ponty explains the phantom limb as a rift between the objective body and the lived experience of it. The objective body has no limb, but the body-as-lived feels that limb as present because the body schema which contained four limbs is still active and dominates the amputee's sensations. The phantom limb is the expression, based on years of having a body schema with four limbs, of the body as it used to be. The habitual body thus becomes a relationship to an environment and to a set of abilities that are no longer available to the amputee. "To have a phantom limb is to remain open to all of the actions of which the arm alone is capable and to stay within the practical field that one had prior to the mutilation" (2012, p. 84).

The rift between the objective body and the body-as-lived can also be seen in anorexia nervosa. If we look at the objective body, we may see a skeletal, emaciated body. This is the objective body whose thinness can be measured by weighing it or calculating its BMI. But if we ask the anorexic to describe her body, she may say that she experiences it as obese and cumbersome. Denying this experience by making an appeal to objective facts is unhelpful. In anorexia the rift between the body as it is objectively and the body as it is experienced is the crux of the disorder.

The distinction between the objective and the lived body is useful in several respects: it makes clear the fundamental difference between the two perspectives. The illness experience in its first-person form is not accessible to the physician, by

[6]Merleau-Ponty (2012) helpfully terms the latter the "body-subject," to indicate the inseparability of the body from the subject under this mode.

definition, other than via the patient's account. The physician's perspective means that they can only ever perceive the disease through an external observation. The patient is the only one to whom the subjective experience of illness is available. This of course does not deny the important role of empathy as enabling us to imagine, empathize, or even identify with an experience. It also does not entail that the other person will only ever view the patient's body as an objective body. One can view another's body as a lived body. Taking the objective perspective may lead the physician to seek to treat the disease, sometimes with little regard for and inadequate understanding of the illness, or to have little understanding of the impact of the disease on the patient's life as a whole.[7]

The patient, on the other hand, can observe the objective indicators of disease (e.g. look at blood test results or an X-ray) but also has unique access to the first-person experience of the disease, namely illness. In this sense the patient may have, at least in principle, an epistemic advantage over others due to having access to her own illness experience and to the objective knowledge about the disease. This epistemic advantage often goes unacknowledged and the patient experience may be subsumed under the medical view or discounted because the patient has no formal medical training (Carel and Kidd 2014). The unique ability to oscillate between the two perspectives gives the patient a deeper understanding of the illness experience, and potentially of the dual nature of the body, but this may also cause confusion and miscommunication.[8] As Toombs (1987) notes, the physician's focus on disease may clash with the patient's primary interest in her illness. Although they may seem to speak of the same thing, they in fact refer to two different entities and therefore have a communicative and interpretative gap that must be addressed before effective communication becomes possible.

4 Sartre's Three Orders of the Body

However, it is important to acknowledge that the physician's suggested objectivity is in fact a more complex position. The complexity stems from the fact that both the body of the physician and the body of the patient exist under both the objective (material, physical) and the subjective (experienced, first-person) orders, and moreover, that both are revealed to each other as belonging to both orders. This gives rise to a third order in which the body partakes: the order of intersubjectivity, or my body as I experience it as reflected in the experience of it by others. "I exist for myself as a body known by the other," writes Sartre (2003, p. 375). He gives the

[7]"Objective" in two senses: first as "naturalistic," the body as natural object. Second, as "external," I only ever have an external givenness of the other's internal states.

[8]Illness can be seen, from this epistemic point of view, as a process of edification, and potentially as having philosophical value. The split between the two perspectives holds a phenomenological lesson on the duality of the body.

example of feeling shy or self-conscious about one's body. This is only possible, he claims, because of this third order. The shy person is "vividly and constantly conscious of his body not as it is for him but as it is *for the Other*" (376). The uneasiness the shy person feels is "the horrified metaphysical apprehension of the existence of my body for the Others" (376). Only my body as it is for another person can embarrass me, not my body as I exist it. So when a patient feels self-conscious it is as a body experienced in this third order, the order of the body as experienced as socially perceived.

Sartre points to alienation, embarrassment, and social unease, claiming that what these have in common is that in these situations I experience my body *as it is experienced by another*, not in the natural pre-reflective way I usually experience it. This process continues: I may then begin to treat my body—or indeed to experience it—not as my pre-reflective opening to the world, but as an object that can be worked on, changed, and assessed in modes suited to objective bodies. Consider the attitude of plastic surgeons and people seeking plastic surgery to bodies designated for such surgery, which reflects this objectifying mode of self-regard: the person seeking plastic surgery is happy for the surgeon to draw on her body with a pen, marking out "excess" flesh or skin, that needs to be removed like excess clay on a sculpture. That flesh is not experienced as part of "my body as I exist it," but as inert matter that occludes "the real me," or "my real figure." But that "real" figure is, in fact, merely a projection of a social ideal—how I think I *should* look, according to some prevalent social norm. So the "real me" is in fact an internalised social norm masquerading as a personal preference. Plastic surgeons trade on this masquerade when they uncritically accept their patients' projection of fantasies of acceptance and omniscience onto the carving of their own flesh. This example demonstrates the multiple meanings of and registers in which the term "body" appears.

Not only the patient's, but also the physician's body falls under the duality captured by the disease/illness distinction, as well as by the third order of the social body articulated by Sartre. The physician may experience herself as a subject examining an object, the patient's physical body, but the object can touch back. When the physician's examining hand is "touched back" by a body responding to its touch with a quiver or a tensing of muscles, we no longer have a subject touching an object, but a subject, which is itself also an object, touching an object, which is itself also a subject (Carel and Macnaughton 2012). Following Sartre (2003), we can see that this seemingly simple situation contains within it a complex nexus of relations, which in turn give rise to the complex phenomenon of human sociality.

The recognition of myself as subject for myself and as object for others is elaborated in the next step in the dance of reciprocity: the recognition of the other as object for myself and as subject for her. I meet the other *both* in her object-making subjectivity *and* as an object (Sartre 2003, p. 377). These positions are not fixed and constrained by some a priori stipulation. On the contrary: the oscillation between perceiving myself as a subject that has been objectified (the patient) which is then re-subjectified in the act of touching back continues as long as the intersubjective interaction continues. Subjectivity is forever challenged and then reclaimed, only to be challenged again.

Similarly for the physician, to take an objective stance, only to have it punctured by subjective feelings, emotions, biases, that subjectify it, and yet need to be checked and held back, speaks to an on-going process. The objectified patient (or doctor, but more often it is the patient whose objective body is scrutinised as an object) does not experience her body as an object; instead, she experiences it as "the flight of the body which I exist" (378). The sense of discomfort, self-consciousness, alienation, does not arise from my being objectified *qua* the diseased body of a patient and thus becoming an object for myself, but from the escape, or draining away, of my being *qua* subject, which is dissipated by the objectifying medical gaze.

The complexity arises from the body's unique metaphysical position: it is "a non-thingly living flesh" which is neither purely an object nor pure consciousness (Moran 2010, p. 42). This intersubjective dimension of one's experience of oneself and of the other, as well as the other's experience of me and of herself, relies fundamentally on empathy. Husserl and Merleau-Ponty agree that intersubjectivity depends on empathy, which in turn depends on intercorporeality. Intercorporeality itself arises from my experience of my own body as partaking in the two different orders, as shown in Husserl's analysis of "double sensations" (Moran 2010, p. 41; Bernet 2013). Empathy depends on intercorporeality because fundamentally I perceive others as bodies that are similar to mine in that they, too, sense, perceive, etc., and I am perceived by others as a body that is similar to theirs. I am there for others, and this being-there "is precisely the body", writes Sartre (2003, p. 375).

However, the ways in which my body exceeds the first two orders (the objective and the subjective) and enters the third, social order, are the ways in which "my body escapes me on all sides" and returns to me as gazed upon by others (375). My body is my point of view, but it is also a point of view on which other points of view are brought to bear, including points of view I could never take (375). In other words, the body-as-lived encompasses not only one's experience but also the social aspect of one's experience of their and others' bodies, as well as how others' experience of one's own body might impact on their own experience of their body. The experience of empathy is fundamental to this exchange and requires careful examination to see whether a radically different lived body experience may modify or curtail empathy with others or even self-empathy.

To end this section, it is important to raise another possible mode of interaction between physician and patient: the second person perspective. It may be that I, as the mother of a child with chicken pox, do not have access to his itching and pain; but as someone witnessing the suffering of a loved one I am not occupying the objective observer's position. I am there in the room with you, my ill child, who I am trying to make comfortable. It is you, your suffering, not the objective registering of symptoms, I experience. Although I have no direct access to your pain, I am still able to empathize with it (e.g. through memory or imagination) and to transcend the objective position in order to come closer and share in your pain.

The demand to recognize the other's humanity and animality, their capacity for suffering and our shared mortality is present in the second person position: the I-thou relationship, or the face-to-face encounter and their ensuing ethical demands stem from the recognition of our shared humanity (Buber 2010; Levinas 1961).

The simplistic picture of the physician as subject who objectifies the patient is far more complex because of the oscillation of roles arising from our each partaking in the three orders of the body. Moreover, the acceptance of objectivity as the ideal stance of the medical practitioner should be tempered by the additional possibility of the second-person perspective available to the physician: "By recognizing each other's subjectivity both physician and patient stand to gain. The physician gains a more natural mode of expression, and the patient has a feeling of being listened to by a fellow human being who neither purports to stand in her shoes, nor to be completely objective" (Carel and Macnaughton 2012, p. 2335).

5 The Transparency of the Body

In the smooth everyday experience of a healthy body, the fundamental bodily experience is one of harmony, control, and predictability. This has led some authors to describe the healthy body as *transparent* or *silent*: we do not experience it explicitly or thematize it as an object of our attention, nor does it play centre stage in our actions, even if those actions are very physical (Leder 1990; Canguilhem 1991). In the same way that we do not pay attention to the pen as long as it is functioning, we do not normally pay attention to the hand gripping the pen and writing. Our attention is focused on the task we are engaged at: writing the cheque. Or a more explicitly embodied activity: if I prepare myself to catch a ball thrown towards me, I do not focus on my body but on the ball, trying to anticipate its trajectory and possible point of landing, and my body simply "follows me" to that point, arms stretching towards the ball.

In such normal everyday experiences, the physical body is not prised apart from the lived body, and the experienced functioning of the body is natural, pre-reflective and mostly either effortless or the effort involved is experienced as normal, even enjoyable. Sartre, Leder and Canguilhem describe the healthy body as transparent (Sartre 2003) or even absent (Leder 1990). Sartre says: "consciousness of the body is lateral and retrospective; the body is the *neglected*, the '*passed by in silence*'" (2003, p. 354). Leder writes: "while in one sense the body is the most abiding and inescapable presence in our lives, it is also essentially characterized by absence. That is, one's own body is rarely the thematic object of experience" (1990, p. 1). And Canguilhem characterizes health as "the silence of the organs" (1991, p. 118).

The healthy body is transparent, i.e. taken for granted. This transparency is the hallmark of health and normal function. We do not stop to consider any of its processes because as long as everything is going smoothly, the body remains in the background, the vehicle through which we experience, but not the thematic focus of experience. "The body tries to stay out of the way so that we can get on with our task; it tends to efface itself on its way to its intentional goal" (Gallagher and Zahavi 2008, p. 143). This does not mean that we have no experience of the body but, rather, that the sensations it constantly provides are neutral and tacit. A good example is that of the sensation of clothes against our skin. This sensation is only noticed when we draw our attention to it or when we undress (Ratcliffe 2008, p. 303).

We have many moments of explicit attention to the wellness of our body, for example, when a headache goes away or while exercising. But these are different to the global, terrifying disruption that takes place in illness (or accident) that moves the body from the background to the foreground of our attention. When functioning normally, our attention is deflected away from our body and towards our intentional goal or action. It is not that the body is absent but, rather, that our experience of it is in the background while the object of our focus is in the foreground. "The body is in no way apprehended for itself; it is a point of view and a point of departure" (Sartre 2003, p. 355). In contrast, when we become ill, our attention is drawn to the symptoms or disablement and all of a sudden they become the focus of our attention.

Leder contrasts the healthy, absent body with illness and other situations when the body becomes an explicit object of negative attention and appears as a "dys" (function) of sorts. "In contrast to the 'disappearances' that characterise ordinary functioning, I will term this the principle of *dys-appearance*. That is, the body *appears* as the thematic focus, but precisely as in a *dys* state [...]" (Leder 1990, p. 84). The body can appear as ill, disabled, aesthetically flawed or socially awkward, objectified or sexualised, or as attracting negative attention from others [e.g. shame discussed by Sartre (2003)]. A black man once described to me how when he walks down a street, people sitting in their cars roll up their car windows. He explained that this made him incredibly aware of his skin colour and the negative associations white people have with it. In these situations the body appears (after being transparent or absent) but in a negative way.[9]

I suggest that the transparency of the healthy body is somewhat idealized in philosophical descriptions of health, since it is often pierced by experiences in which the body comes to the fore, sometimes in negative ways. The first kind of experiences are social experiences of one's body as it is perceived or objectified by others. Sartre's famous analysis of the gaze (or look) as annihilating my subjectivity and objectifying my body, which becomes an object in the other's field of vision (2003, p. 276ff) itself recognizes the tension between the naïve unthematized body and the social body. Transparency is lost in any encounter in which the other's gaze posits a subjectivity within which my own subjectivity is subsumed.

This is "transcendence transcended": my own being (which Sartre characterizes) as transcendence is transcended by another consciousness. This realization—that my subjectivity can be transcended by another subjectivity—pierces my sense of

[9]The example is meant to illustrate a situation in which one suddenly becomes aware of one's body in a negative (in this case socially negative) way.

subjective existence (287).[10] "My being for others is a fall through absolute emptiness towards objectivity […] myself as object […] is an uneasiness, a lived wrenching away from the ekstatic unity of the for-itself, a limit which I can not reach and which yet I am" (298–9). And Leder writes, "a radical split is introduced between the body I live out and my object-body, now defined and delimited by a foreign gaze" (1990, p. 96). On this view, social existence of its very nature disrupts the transparent, effaced status of the body.

But even in everyday experiences where objectification is not a primary mode there are many ways in which the world resists us. Often the interaction between us and the world is smooth and automatic and regulated by well-developed behavioral repertoires. In these cases there is little need for conscious attention of the body. But even in health the world may resist this smooth articulation and require conscious awareness. For those, like me, who have no DIY talent, the inability to glue a broken vase, or hang a picture straight, and the effort and clumsiness involved in trying, is an experience of bodily limitation. Perhaps the small knocks and resistances that we encounter in little accidents, bodily failures, bodily needs, and the inability to easily learn new bodily skills, disrupt bodily transparency in minor ways.

However, importantly, these experiences are contained within a normal everyday, and are experienced on a spectrum of familiar, if frustrating, bodily failures. Illness, in contrast, creates areas of dramatic resistance in the exchange between body and environment, so is wholly different to these small knocks. So even if the transparency of the healthy body is somewhat overplayed and that transparency is frequently disturbed by social interactions and bodily failure, it is still the case that we intend towards the world through our body and it serves as a medium through which we encounter the world whilst remaining in the background. The body "plays a constitutive role in experience precisely by grounding, making possible, and yet remaining peripheral in the horizons of our conceptual awareness" (Carman 1999, p. 208). Or as Merleau-Ponty said, the body is "our general means of having a world" (2012, p. 147).

There are two ways of thinking about the healthy transparent body. One is thinking of it as equally vulnerable as the conspicuous ill body; on this view the two are on a continuum. The other way of thinking about the body in health and illness is as discontinuity. This view sees them as distinctive bodily states, in which modes of being and experience are radically different. I suggest that overall the discontinuity view is the stronger one. Although everyday experiences certainly include occasions when the body is explicitly thematized, and moreover is thematized negatively, these experiences are not the norm and do not fundamentally modify one's tacit sense of trust in one's body and do not disrupt the habitual body. These small injuries and bodily failures are experienced within a context of confidence and regularity, and these failures are experienced as benign, even if frustrating or painful.

In contrast, the ill body, which becomes conspicuous like Heidegger's (1962) broken tool, takes over one's way of being by constricting the range of possible

[10]But see also Merleau-Ponty's criticism of Sartre's analysis (2012, p. 378).

actions and hence restricting the number of projects available to choose from. It also constrains actions chosen from the ones that are still available. The activities of the healthy body enable projects, whilst the activities of the ill body disable or devalue projects. For example, if a healthy person goes sightseeing in London, they will experience hunger, fatigue and other bodily needs. But the project—seeing London—will not be shaped by these needs. They will be minor, expected and shared impediments, calling for a rest or a meal. For an ill person (e.g. a wheelchair user or someone required to carry an oxygen tank on their person) the entire possibility of sightseeing must be conceived within the constraints of the illness (which buildings have wheelchair access? how much oxygen can I carry with me and how long will it last?) and in that sense are not experienced perspicuously—as pure projects, but as projects weighed down (and sometimes outweighed by) concrete considerations and practical arrangements.

The sense of freedom, openness and ease with which the transparent body operates are of a different order to the limitations and anxieties that characterize the conspicuous body. It is not only the content of experience that is changed by illness, but its structure and existential inflection as well. Organizing the activities becomes more practically demanding, but more importantly the practical constraints limit the freedom which underpins projects.

On the other hand, even a minor headache can bring to light the tacit sense in which all projects ultimately rest on bodily abilities (Sartre 2003). In that sense minor ailments are also philosophically revealing. However, I suggest that minor ailments fall within, but do not modify, one's everyday being in the world, whereas serious illness does modify the ill person's entire way of being. A headache will make my head conspicuous, and will be experienced as the frustration of an action (reading a book is Sartre's example), but it will not permanently and radically modify my bodily and self experiences and understanding in the way serious illness does.

Let us look at Sartre's example more closely. I am reading a book and whilst doing so the body is given only implicitly. Then my eyes start hurting. The pain is not perceived separately to the project of reading. Rather:

> [T]his pain can itself be *indicated* by objects of the world; i.e., by the book that I read. It is with more difficulty that the words are detached from the undifferentiated ground which they constitute [...] consciousness exists its pain [...] pain *is precisely the eyes* in so far as consciousness "exists them" [...] pain in the eyes is *precisely my reading*. (2003, p.356; 58)

However, as Sartre himself points out, when the pain or illness recede, they disappear for good (360). Minor illness and pain rise and then subside again, without fundamentally altering the structures of consciousness or embodied experience. But a fundamental change to one's embodiment, bodily habits, and ability to plan and pursue goals, and the sense of freedom that normally accompanies such choice, is brought about by serious illness.

It is important to note that although the two modes of being (the transparent body and the conspicuous body) are distinct and indeed contrasted, they still mutually imply one another. First, the appearance of the ill body (what Leder calls "dys-appearance") is made possible because of the disappearance, or absence, of the healthy body. As Leder notes, "it is precisely because the normal and healthy body largely disappears that direct experience of the body is skewed toward times of dysfunction. These phenomenological modes are mutually implicatory […]" (1990, p. 86). Second, the contrast is not intended to deny that there are neutral and positive ways in which my body appears to me in health. The experience of dancing in front of an audience, for example, may be one in which pleasure is gleaned from the explicit thematization of the performing body. Other experiences may include having a good meal, resting after a hard day's hiking, or sexual pleasure.

In these experiences the pre-reflective experience may be accompanied by an explicit appreciation of the feeling of pleasure or restfulness. But dys-appearance is qualitatively different to these experiences, as it has the character of demand. The body does not appear simply to take note of its pleasurable state; it appears with a sense of urgency and a demand to do something about the pain, discomfort, or nausea through which the body comes to the fore. There is a heightening of bodily focus at times of illness and disruption. "It would be a mistake to equate all modes of bodily thematization with dys-appearance," Leder notes (91). But it would equally be a mistake to think that positive and negative ways of appearance have more in common than the explicit thematization of the body.

6 The Body as Tool

Heidegger's tool analysis is based on his distinction between present-at-hand entities (*vorhanden*) and ready-to-hand (*zuhanden*), or "handy" entities (1962, p. 96ff.). On this analysis, we do not perceive entities as mere objects, but as tools with which we go about our daily business or set about achieving our projects. Under normal circumstances, objects are never mere things, but handy tools and pieces of equipment which together form "equipmental totalities," such as offices (made up of desks, chairs, computers, reading lamps, telephones, etc.), farms, or hospitals. These are not just spaces in which objects are arranged, but a useful, meaningful, task-performing totality of tools that make sense to us *qua* functional interrelated tools. We know ready-to-hand entities not in an abstract way. Rather, "the hammering does not simply have knowledge about the hammer's character as equipment, but it has appropriated this equipment in a way which could not possibly be more suitable" (Heidegger 1962, p. 98). Practical activity is not epistemically blind but "has its own kind of sight," says Heidegger (98).

Tools are characterized by their inconspicuous presence. When I use a pen to write a birthday card, it is my friend who is at the forefront of my mind. The pen is a tool that under ideal conditions recedes to the background and is effaced by its function. It is only when such a tool breaks down that it becomes conspicuous. Heidegger distinguishes three modes of dysfunction: *conspicuousness*—the tool has ceased to work (the bicycle tyre has a puncture); *obstrusiveness*—the required tool is missing ("where are the matches?"); and *obstinacy*—the tool is there but is unsuitable ("not *those* keys, the house keys!") (1962, pp. 102–3). The conspicuousness arises from the fact that a ready-to-hand entity is now "unready-to-hand"; it has become present-at-hand, an entity that is perceived not through its utility but simply as an entity. The "unusability" of a tool is not discovered theoretically, but by trying, and failing, to use it. "The helpless way in which we stand before it is a deficient more of concern [practical engagement], and as such it uncovers the Being-just-present-at-hand-and-no-more of something ready-to-hand" (102–3).

This taxonomy of tool breakdown gives rise to an interesting analogy to illness. We can think of the inconspicuousness that characterizes the functional tool as also characterizing the healthy body. When my body does what I want it to do (keep my balance when I am walking, digest the food I've eaten), I do not pay attention to it or to the biological mechanisms performing bodily tasks. In fact we have no lived experience of our endocrine glands or of our kidneys filtering blood. I live in (as) my body and experience the world through it and much of the time my attention is directed away from the body as perceiving, walking, thinking, to the object or task I am engaged in. The case of the pen is similar. Attention is deflected from the pen to the contents of the writing. So far, the analogy seems to hold.

Now let us turn to the hand holding the pen. Imagine that the pen works perfectly but I cannot use my hand—it is paralyzed ("conspicuous") or amputated ("obtrusive") or I have had a stroke and can no longer remember how to write ("obstinate"). In these cases, too, I experience a failure of a tool, but this time the tool is part of my body. The duality of the body as object and as subject is useful here. Viewed as a physiological material machine, we can indeed think of the hand as a malfunctioning tool and in this case Heidegger's tool analysis holds. But if we think of the body as experienced and lived, we can see that its failure will be felt differently to the failure of the pen. Whereas we can throw out the useless pen and buy another, our hands (and bodies more generally) stand in a very different relation to us.[11]

Our bodies cannot be replaced or repaired as readily as some tools and bodily dysfunction is experienced very differently to tool breakdown. My head with a headache remains attached to me and becomes increasingly conspicuous, increasingly disabling. Moreover, my head with a headache is not a malfunctioning tool, but a way of being. My head as pain means that I experience my head as a region of pain, not as a malfunctioning brain. Such dysfunction also affects the entire way in which we inhabit the world. My head with a headache is experienced as the frustration of the attempt to read (Sartre 2003), as a darkening of my entire being, as a pressing demand on me to address the pain.

So although under a certain objective mode the body is a tool, it is also our medium for having a world. As Sartre observes: "when by means of universalizing thought I tried to think of my body emptily as a pure instrument in the midst of the world, the immediate result was the collapse of the world as such" (363–364). In other words, the body is not a tool in a crucial sense: it is the origin of our sense of

[11]The machinic model of the body is opposed to the phenomenological one and pushed to its logical conclusions by Cory Shores in Chap. 14.

being in the world and this feeling of inhabiting a world, although it is a tacit and normally unnoticed feeling, is anchored in the body and depends upon it (cf. Ratcliffe 2013).

Because of this fundamental dependence of the sense of reality (having a world that is familiar and feels real) on the body, a change to the body leads to a change in one's experience of the world. We experience the world not only empirically but also—and more fundamentally—existentially. So if a person goes blind, for example, she no longer experiences the world visually, and loses empirical data that comes from visual stimuli. But existence as a blind person will affect other senses, her sense of confidence, her projects and preferences, and so on. So the change in the case of bodily dysfunction runs much deeper than tool breakdown, despite the fact that a similar process of becoming conspicuous characterizes both tool and bodily breakdown. The possibility of bodily breakdown is foundational to our way of being and our experience of the world. Illness is a painful and violent way of revealing the intimately bodily nature of our being.

Bodily breakdown need not be dramatic in order to reveal our vulnerable nature to us. We have seen that even simple bodily disruptions, like a headache, may still reveal to us the contingency of our bodily being. The headache may be not severe and is transient. It is not life threatening. But even a simple headache disrupts whatever activity one is immersed it and thus reveals how our immersion in the everyday world is dependent upon bodily integrity. Vulnerability, limitation, and finitude are fundamental features of human life not only in its physiological objective mode, as knowledge in the abstract, but also in its experienced, subjective mode, as informing our ways of being in the world.

7 Conclusion

This chapter opened by examining Toombs' essential features of illness as five losses: loss of wholeness, certainty, control, freedom and loss of the familiar world. These were discussed and some problems with the view outlined. We then looked at the distinction between the objective body and the body as lived, that Husserl and Merleau-Ponty put forward as a fundamental phenomenology of the body. We saw how this distinction is useful for understanding the difference between disease and illness, as well as other issues in illness. This account was then supplanted by Sartre's three orders of the body: the body as objective and as subjective, but also the order of intersubjectivity, or of the body as I experience it as reflected in the experience of it by others.

We discussed the third order of the body as containing diverse experiences that make us conscious of how my body is perceived by others and how this affects my own understanding of my body. The three orders were then discussed in relation to interactions between health professionals and patients. I then presented the view that the healthy body is transparent, or absent, and discussed the limitations of this view, asking whether the healthy body really is transparent and offering examples of lost transparency in health. I suggested that a deep qualitative difference separates health and illness, and that this is not only a difference in the contents of experience but in one's entire being-in-the-world. I ended by examining the analogy between bodily and tool breakdown, using Heidegger's tool analysis, arguing that although the body is not a tool the analogy still holds.

These five phenomenological analyses cumulatively provide us with a general framework for understanding the experience of illness. This framework is underpinned by the understanding that the body has a central role in experience. So any substantial modification to the body must result in modification not only of the contents of experience, but also its structure and conditions of possibility. Because illness changes the body, and the body is so central to all experience, illness has such a tremendous impact. This framework makes that impact visible. On this view illness is not merely a suboptimal dysfunction of a body subsystem (cf. Boorse 1977) but a systematic transformation of the way the body experiences, reacts, and performs tasks as a whole. The change in illness is not local but global; it is not external but at the core of the self.

References

Angner, E., Ray, M. N., Saag, K. G., & Allison, J. J. (2009). Health and happiness among older adults. *Journal of Health Psychology, 14*(4), 503–512.

Bernet, R. (2013). The body as a 'legitimate naturalization of consciousness'. *Philosophy, 72*, 43–65.

Boorse, C. (1977). Health as a theoretical concept. *Philosophy of Science, 44*(4), 542–573.

Buber, M. (2010 [1923]). *I and thou*. Eastford CT: Martino Publishing.

Bury, M. (1982). Chronic illness as biographical disruption. *Sociology of Health and Illness, 4*(2), 167–182.

Canguilhem, G. (1991). *The normal and the pathological*. New York: Zone Books.

Carel, H. (2009). 'I Am well, apart from the fact that I have cancer': Explaining wellbeing within illness. In L. Bortolotti (Ed.), *Philosophy and Happiness* (pp. 82–99). Basingstoke: Palgrave.

Carel, H. (2012). Phenomenology as a resource for patients. *Journal of Medicine and Philosophy, 37*(2), 96–113. doi:10.1093/jmp/JHS008.

Carel, H. (2013a). *Illness*. London: Routledge.

Carel, H. (2013b). Bodily doubt. *Journal of Consciousness Studies* 20(7–8), 178–197.

Carel, H. & Kidd, I. J. (2014). Epistemic injustice in healthcare: a philosophical analysis. Medicine, Healthcare and Philosophy. doi:10.1007/s11019-014-9560-2.

Carel, H. & Macnaughton, J. (2012). How do you feel?: Oscillating perspectives in the clinic. *Lancet* 379(9834), 2334–2335 (23 June). doi:10.1016/S0140-6736(12)61007-1.

Carman, T. (1999). The body in Husserl and Merleau-Ponty. *Philosophical Topics, 27*(2), 205–226.

Chaung, H. T., Devins, G. M., Hunsley, J., & Gill, M. J. (1989). Psychosocial distress and wellbeing among gay and bisexual men with human immunodeficiency virus infection. *American Journal of Psychiatry, 146*(7), 876–880.

Chwalisz, K., Diener, E., & Gallagher, D. (1988). Autonomic arousal feedback and emotional experience: Evidence from the spinal cord injured. *Journal of Personality and Social Psychology, 54*(5), 820–828.

de Haes, J. C. J. M., & van Knippenberg, F. C. E. (1985). The quality of life of cancer patients: A review of the literature. *Social Science and Medicine, 20*(8), 809–817.

Frank, A. (1991). *At the will of the body*. New York: Mariner Books.

Gallagher, S., & Zahavi, D. (2008). *The phenomenological mind*. New York: Routledge.

Heiddeger, M. (1962 [1927]). *Being and time*. London: Blackwell.

Hoffman B. (2002). On the triad disease, illness and sickness. *Journal of Medicine and Philosophy 27*(6):651–673.

Leder, D. (1990). *The absent body*. Chicago: University of Chicago Press.

Levinas, E. (1969 [1961]). *Totality and infinity: An essay on exteriority* (A. Lingis, Trans.). Pittsburgh, PA: Duquesne University Press.

Merleau-Ponty, M. (2012 [1945]). Phenomenology of perception. New York: Routledge.

Mill, J. S. (1989). *Autobiography*. London: Penguin Books.

Moran, D. (2010). Husserl, Sartre and Merleau-Ponty on embodiment, touch, and the 'double sensation'. In K. Morris (Ed.), *Sartre on the body* (pp. 41–66). London: Palgrave Macmillan.

Ratcliffe, M. (2008). Touch and situatedness. *International Journal of Philosophical Studies, 16* (3), 99–322.

Ratcliffe, M. (2013). Phenomenology, naturalism and the sense of reality. *Philosophy, 72*, 67–88.

Riis, J., Baron, J., Loewenstein, G., & Jepson, C. (2005). Ignorance of hedonic adaptation to haemodialysis: A study using ecological momentary assessment. *Journal of Experimental Psychology, 134*(1), 3–9.

Sartre, J.-P. (2003 [1943]). *Being and nothingness*. London: Routledge.

Toombs, S. K. (1987). The meaning of illness: A phenomenological approach to the patient–physician relationship. *Journal of Medicine and Philosophy, 12*, 219–240.

Toombs, S. K. (1993). *The meaning of illness*. Amsterdam: Kluwer.

Twaddle A. (1968). *Influence and Illness*. PhD Thesis: Brown University.

Young, I. M. (2005). Pregnant embodiment: Subjectivity and alienation. In *On female body experience*, (pp. 46–61). Oxford: Oxford University Press.

Chapter 8
The Body Between Pathology and the Everyday

Eran Dorfman

1 Whose Body Is This?

"This body is mine!"—These words, accompanied by my finger pointing towards my chest, can be nothing but true. My body belongs to me; my body is mine. But when, or in what situation, might I find myself obliged to pronounce these words? Mostly when someone is trying to get hold of my body. It could be someone concrete who is harassing me and whom I try to push away, crying out "this is my body, not yours!"; or it could be someone or something more abstract, for instance, fashion magazines or TV commercials that dictate a certain model of the body and to whom I may silently reply: "This is my body, and it is for me, not you, to decide how to treat it."

The exclamation "this body is mine!" thus reveals the double face of the body: it is the most private and intimate thing that I have on earth, but it nevertheless remains a *thing*, which can consequently be treated as a mere object by others or even by myself. The body, my innermost everyday belonging, the house and shelter which I always carry with me and upon which everything I have is founded, constantly incarnates the risk of being appropriated by someone else.

The entire phenomenological enterprise of Maurice Merleau-Ponty (1908–1961) is aimed at extracting the personal dimension of the body from the impersonal one, showing the interactions and movements between the two. If in the work of Edmund Husserl we find the thinking-perceiving subject, and in Martin Heidegger the practical and engaged *Dasein* (the being-there), Merleau-Ponty develops the idea of an embodied subject. However, being embodied does not simply add another dimension to the subject, since the body, as Merleau-Ponty insists time and again, radically transforms the entire notion of subjectivity, being both inside and outside, both subject and object. If we wish to fully understand what it means to be

E. Dorfman (✉)
Tel Aviv University, Tel Aviv, Israel
e-mail: edorfm@post.tau.ac.il

D. Meacham (ed.), *Medicine and Society, New Perspectives in Continental Philosophy*, Philosophy and Medicine 120, DOI 10.1007/978-94-017-9870-9_8

an embodied subject and what everyday life this entails, we must therefore never neglect the double aspect of the body.

The body, according to Merleau-Ponty, is *ambiguous*. Yet ambiguity is not an accidental lack of clarity which can be fixed or got rid of by means of the right treatment. Ambiguity characterizes rather the human existence as such, that is, as embodied. However, ambiguity tends to hide itself in the everyday world, and therefore needs to be uncovered in order to gain a genuine understanding of what the body—my body—is. This is the task of Merleau-Ponty's phenomenological endeavor, which, by revealing ambiguity, aims not only at analyzing, but also at reviving and enriching human perception and existence. Accordingly, Merleau-Ponty's major work, *Phenomenology of Perception* (1945) goes through various aspects of existence such as space, time, sexuality, speech, otherness and freedom. For each of these Merleau-Ponty shows how it is based and constructed upon the ambiguity of the body, an ambiguity that is concealed in the everyday and needs to be exposed.

Merleau-Ponty delineates two extreme poles between which my attitude towards the body oscillates: total separation on the one hand, and total immersion on the other. In the first I feel my body itself as a thing in the world: an external and rather hostile object that I awkwardly move and which I am sadly doomed to carry until the end of my life. This attitude may come to the foreground due to illness, injury, depression or simply self-alienation. In the second extreme case objectivity disappears and I feel an inseparable and mutual belonging between myself and my body, as well as between my body and the world. When this feeling occurs, it is a powerful moment of inebriated joy and happiness, which I may feel when I dance, make love, engage in sport or am simply at peace with my body.

Merleau-Ponty calls this second realm of mutuality and intertwining *Flesh,* a notion he develops especially in his last two writings, *Eye and Mind* and the unfinished *The Visible and the Invisible.*[1] In the realm of the Flesh, which is more primordial than the realm of objectivity, only ontological ambiguity rules. In it I fully belong, through my body, to the carnal texture of the world, and the Flesh is defined precisely as this interdependence and mutual belonging:

> Once again, the flesh we are speaking of is not matter. It is the coiling over of the visible upon the seeing body, of the tangible upon the touching body, which is attested in particular when the body sees itself, touches itself seeing and touching the things, such that, simultaneously, *as* tangible it descends among them, *as* touching it dominates them all and draws this relationship and even this double relationship from itself, by dehiscence or fission of its own mass. (Merleau-Ponty 1968, p. 146)

We see here clearly how the different poles of the body and more generally of existence find their right balance: the touching and the touched, the seeing and the seen, the body as subject and the body as object. But where to locate the Flesh in

[1]For a classical analysis of Merleau-Ponty's notion of the Flesh see Dillon (1988).

relation to the everyday body, that is, the body in ordinary situations? Is ambiguity the ontological condition of the everyday body? Does it have different modes, and if so, how can one move between them?

2 The Mystery of the Phantom Limb

In reading *Phenomenology of Perception*, one is struck by the proportionally large number of pages dedicated to the analysis of pathological cases. The reason for this is simple: pathology shows what everyday normality conceals: the lack and finitude of the body. In order to illustrate this idea, Merleau-Ponty takes a case of pathology inspired by Heidegger. Indeed, Heidegger has often been criticized for having neglected the role of the body in Dasein's existence,[2] but this is not completely true, since there is one bodily organ that stands at the center of his phenomenology, namely the *hand*. The hand is the most useful organ for craft production, and as such it is emblematic of our practical attitude towards entities in the world. The worldly entities always need a hand to manipulate them actually and potentially, practically and theoretically. This is why Heidegger characterizes them as "ready-to-hand" (the practical tool) and "present-at-hand" (the reflected upon tool), and it is the movement between these two categories that guarantees a harmonious everyday practice (Heidegger 1962, pp. 98–107).[3] Merleau-Ponty aims to better understand the role of the hand in existence, which leads him to ask: what happens when one *loses* one's hand? This may seem at first to be a joke at the expense of Heidegger, but Merleau-Ponty is totally serious. In order to understand the function of the body in the creation of objects, he proposes to carefully examine the case of the loss of the hand. For it is this loss which requires one to confront the negativity of the body and find unusual ways to use it and the world.

Yet at this point there is another twist, since the negativity of the body is so difficult to support that one tends to resist it even when it is evident. Consequently, when a person loses a limb, one of the following related phenomena is often found to occur: either the person experiences the feeling of a *phantom limb*, that is to say a sensation of a real limb coming from the stump, or there is a refusal to admit the mutilation in the first place, a phenomenon called anosognosia, meaning in Greek "unawareness of the disease" (Merleau-Ponty 2012, pp. 78–79). Merleau-Ponty initially evokes these two phenomena in order to show that one cannot clearly distinguish between the body and the soul, the physiological and the psychological, since they act upon each other, and only their complicated interaction may explain the occurrence of the phantom limb and anosognosia. In other words, when I have a

[2]Heidegger himself evoked Sartre's critique on him and interpreted it as a misunderstanding of his ontology (Heidegger 2001, p. 231). See also Aho (2009), Haar (1993, pp. 34–35), Krell (1992, p. 52); Franck (1991, pp. 144–146). For interesting Heideggerian answers to these various critiques, see Cerbone (2000), Askay (1999).

[3]See Heidegger (1962, pp. 98–107); see also Carel, Chap. 6, this volume.

physiological problem it always has a psychological expression and vice versa, proving the unity—and ambiguity—of existence. But the phantom limb and anosognosia reveal much more than the mere interaction between the body and the soul. They also reveal my attitude to the *deficiency* of the body as what underlies my manner to live in the world and interact with it:

> To have a phantom limb is to remain open to all of the actions of which the arm alone is capable and to stay within the practical field which one had prior to the mutilation. The body is the vehicle of being in the world and, for a living being, having a body means being united with a definite milieu, merging with certain projects, and being perpetually engaged therein. In the evidentness of this complete world in which manipulable objects still figure, in the force of movement that goes toward it and where the project of writing or playing the piano still figures, the patient finds the certainty of his [bodily] integrity. But at the very moment that the world hides his deficiency from him, the world cannot help but to reveal it to him. [...] At the same moment that my customary world gives rise to habitual intentions in me, I can no longer, actually unite with it if I have lost a limb. Manipulable [*maniable*] objects, precisely insofar as they appear as manipulable, appeal to a hand [*main*] that I no longer have. Regions of silence are thus marked out in the totality of my body. The patient knows his disability [*déchéance*] precisely insofar as he is ignorant of it, and he ignores it precisely insofar as he knows of it. This is the paradox of all being in the world. (p. 84)

The mutilated patient can no longer get along with his or her habitual everyday movement, since the hand, responsible for so many projects and engagements, is suddenly gone. This could have opened him or her to new projects and engagements, inventing new ways of bodily gestures; but the patient cannot face the mutilation, negates it and sticks to the past world together with its no-longer-possible projects. In this way the patient is reassured of the stability of the world and the integrity of his or her body, but only at the price of ignoring and passing over in silence every project that would involve the missing hand. The patient's movement in and with the world is consequently degraded, not only because the body has been mutilated, but mostly because the mutilation is not admitted as such. Merleau-Ponty describes this situation as *déchéance*, his French translation of Heidegger's *Verfallen*, the Falling. According to Heidegger, the Falling does not concern lack or negativity as such, but rather the inability to acknowledge them and use them as an essential element in the movement of the everyday and the creation of new meanings (Heidegger 1962, pp. 210–24). This mechanism of degradation becomes more concrete with Merleau-Ponty, and, as he states at the end of the quotation, it does not stem from an accidental or hypothetical deficiency of the body, such as the case of the loss of the limb, but rather from the very condition of embodied being in the world.

Merleau-Ponty thus proposes an embodied version of Heidegger's theory, explaining how and why one moves from the presumably harmonious world of ready-to-hand "objects" to the inauthentic realm of the "they." In the same way that it is necessary to acknowledge the non-usability of the ready-to-hand in order to re-found and re-appropriate it by finding new ways to use it, so it is crucial to accept the essential insufficiency of the body in order to renew one's projects. Does this mean that the body is to be considered as an object or a tool? Yes and no. For the body, as we already know, is *both* subject and object, both the user of the tool and the tool itself. Yet the body tends to stick to its old habits and repeat them even when they are no longer possible:

> [I]t is as though our body comprises two distinct layers, that of the habitual body and that of the actual body. Gestures of manipulation that appear in the first have disappeared in the second, and the problem of how I can feel endowed with a limb that I no longer have in fact comes down to knowing how the habitual body can act as a guarantee for the actual body. How can I perceive objects as manipulable when I can no longer manipulate them? The manipulable must have ceased being something that I currently manipulate in order to become something *one* can manipulate; it must have ceased being something *manipulable for me* and have become something *manipulable in itself*. Correspondingly, my body must be grasped not merely in an instantaneous, singular and full experience, but moreover under an aspect of generality and as an impersonal being. (Merleau-Ponty 2012, pp. 84–85)

This passage gives a remarkable account of the bodily foundation of the everyday: on the one hand, the body stands as an apparently stable pole of habits, movements, functions and repetitive projects. On the other hand, it needs to dynamically adjust itself to present reality, looking for new things to manipulate and new work to be done. Ideally there is a continuous link between the habitual body and the actual body, the one permitting the other and vice versa. But in drastic cases of mutilation, such as the loss of one's arm, this link is severely damaged, so that past foundations no longer give place to new foundations. In fact, not only do handy tools become general objects but the body itself becomes an object too, as everyday language clearly shows. It hides the unpleasant and threatening bodily existence beneath reassuring impersonal and causal phrases like: "do not worry; *one* has a stomach-ache when *one* eats too much;" "try to do some jogging; *one* feels so good when *one* is doing sport," and so on. This is the language of the "they" or the "one" which does not regard the body as what ambiguously incorporates me in the world, but rather as a simple and isolated object that obeys physical and social rules. I therefore become alienated from my body, forgetting its double, ambiguous essence, being both inside and outside, constituting and constituted.

This, as I argued, is not an experience unique to illness; illness rather helps to show it more clearly, since its negativity (lack, deficiency, finitude of the body) is radical as opposed to the "small" and almost imperceptible negativity of everyday life. One should rather deduce the latter from the former and understand the negativity of the everyday by examining pathological cases of negativity. Merleau-Ponty does the same thing when he uses psychoanalytic terminology to connect the realm of pathology to the existential status of the body. He characterizes the body as an "inborn complex" that leads to its *repression* as an obstacle, and which one does not find the force either to overcome or to give it up (p. 86). One therefore remains blocked in "impersonal existence," which is equivalent to the inauthenticity described by Heidegger.[4] The easy external categories taken from the "they" and applied upon the self are thus a way of bypassing the obstacle that is the body.

---

[4]Merleau-Ponty distinguishes, though not systematically, between the "pre-personal" and the "impersonal" aspect of the body and existence. He tends to present the first as that from which one

The body reveals my constant disability, lack and finitude. In order to forget my unfulfilled needs, my not being whole, my situation as, so to speak, *always* lacking a hand, I must repress my bodily existence and isolate parts of my body, seeing them from now on as exterior, stable and eternal. My body, then, finally becomes a mere tool and a mere object, losing the movement which would connect it to my personal life.

To sum up, the description of the loss of the limb has helped us understand our existential loss, our essential negativity as bodily creatures. And yet, although Merleau-Ponty makes an analogy between the pathological body and the normal one, he does not further pursue it and does not mention how to embark upon the way that starts from the objectivist attitude and aims towards an integration of the body in our personal existence. In order to deepen our understanding of the normal and the pathological attitudes towards the body, I shall now examine the central case analyzed by Merleau-Ponty along many chapters of the *Phenomenology of Perception*, that is, the case of the brain-damaged Schneider.

3 Pathology and the Loss of Reflection

Schneider was a German solider who had suffered a brain injury in the First-World-War. His peculiar and multiple symptoms made a number of physiologists study his case in the 1920s, and in particular his personal doctor Kurt Goldstein.[5] Merleau-Ponty examines this case and proposes a re-interpretation of it, aiming to find the common existential denominator of Schneider's apparently unrelated symptoms, which affected his intellectual, emotional, motor, visual and sexual life.

At first sight, the symptom Merleau-Ponty chooses to focus on seems to be minor: Schneider is incapable, especially when his eyes are shut, of conducting movements outside a concrete everyday situation. For instance, when he is asked to make a military salute, he engages his entire body in the situation; he stands up straight and assumes a demeanor of respect and obedience, as if his commander were really there. In order to conduct an isolated or abstract movement Schneider thus needs to repeat the entire situation in which the movement normally takes place (pp. 106–07). This harmless symptom actually reveals in the eyes of Merleau-Ponty a most interesting psychological and philosophical phenomenon, namely the state of being imprisoned in the practical world without passive or active, intellectual or embodied reflection. When Schneider, his eyes shut, is told to touch a

(Footnote 4 continued)
emerges (the pre-objective) and the latter as that into which one falls (the objective). Interpreted in this manner, the impersonal can be related to Heidegger's inauthenticity.

[5]For the original case studies upon which Merleau-Ponty relied (available online), see Gelb and Goldstein (1918), Goldstein (1923). Goldstein and Gelb have been criticized in the following years for having relied on this single case that seemed to some "more like the platonic idea of a brain-injured patient than a patient himself" (Teuber 1966, p. 306). See also Goldenberg (2003).

specific part of his body, he cannot do so, but when a mosquito bites him he easily and spontaneously raises his hand and skillfully swats it (pp. 105–06). Practical and spontaneous situations are the only ones that Schneider can recognize and act upon, being deprived of the ability to detach parts from the whole, the necessary condition for reflection and theory. When his eyes are open, he can easily mask his disability,[6] but when he shuts them he cannot recognize, detach and reflect upon the objects, such that he must be totally immersed in the situation in order to act: "I experience movements as a result of the situation, as the sequence of events themselves; my movements and I, we are, so to speak, merely a link in the unfolding of the whole, and I am scarcely aware of any voluntary initiative [...] everything works by itself" (p. 107). This description reminds us of Dasein's everyday world, yet it is a world consisting of only ready-to-hand entities which can never be transformed or reflected upon. This everyday world moves as if by itself, so although it looks harmonious, it is soon revealed to be an oppressive prison.

We may thus conclude that reflection is not necessarily an intellectual activity, but can also be immersed in everyday life. Immersed or embodied reflection remains simultaneously distant from and close to the world, the body and oneself; it has the capacity to detach a specific element from the totality of experience, not in order to freeze it but, on the contrary, to create something new upon it. Immersed reflection thus permits one to be absorbed in the situation on the one hand, but able to slightly transform it on the other. This is the reason why Schneider's loss of reflection goes hand in hand with his inability to recreate the existing stock of objects and categories, for nothing new can be detached from the opaque mass of reality, and the only available objects are those which have already been founded before the mutilation. All Schneider can do now is mechanically repeat them. In this respect Schneider is not very different from the person suffering from a phantom limb, both being imprisoned in the past, unable in their present life to see any promise of the new.

Indeed, Merleau-Ponty does not call the capacity to renew the past and the present reflection but rather *projection*, an existential term borrowed from Heidegger and Sartre. But I would suggest that projection is in fact based upon reflection, provided that the latter is understood as immersed and embodied. Projection means throwing yourself from the past into the future; it is the ability to take one's past deeds and find in them the basis for future ones, a process which Heidegger named *repetition* (*Wiederholung*). This repetition, however, does much more than simply repeat, since it also re-appropriates and re-creates the past in the light of the present and the future (Heidegger 1962, p. 338). I propose to use the term "reflection" rather than "projection" since the former underlines the *circular* character of the movement: my past life is reflected upon the present environment and possibilities, which are simultaneously reflected by it in a two-way movement.

[6]In fact, Schneider also had numerous sight problems such that, for instance, he needed to touch and manipulate objects in order to recognize what they were. There is thus a strong interdependence between seeing and touching, as discussed by Gelb and Goldstein.

To return to Schneider and the person suffering from a phantom limb, we may say that both are "content" with what they have already acquired and cannot open themselves up to new projects, situations and significations. Both realize only one aspect of the ambiguity of the body—the constituted or founded pole—and are unable to activate their constituting or founding capacity. As a result, what Merleau-Ponty calls the "movement of existence" (projection/reflection) is slowed down in the case of the person suffering from a phantom limb, and is almost completely halted in the case of Schneider. Whereas the former may still retrieve his or her capacity of reflection by accepting the mutilation, Schneider is irreversibly deprived of this function, and he thus serves as an extreme example of its loss.

Now, taking a step from pathology back to the everyday, what may Schneider's radical loss of refection teach us about their role in everyday life? We may find a surprising answer to this if we examine Schneider's sex life. If sex is a "full" and self-enclosed experience which does not involve reflection, we would expect Schneider, who lacks this capacity, to have a normal or even enhanced sex life, free from unnecessary disturbing thoughts. Schneider, we might presume, would be able to get in touch with his "animal" or "instinctual" part and would spontaneously realize his desires. Yet curiously it is rather the opposite which turns out to be true:

> Obscene pictures, conversations on sexual topics, and the perception of a body fail to arouse any desire in him. The patient hardly ever kisses, and the kiss has no value of sexual stimulation for him. [...]. In the sexual act intromission is never spontaneous. If his partner reaches orgasm first and moves away, the half-fulfilled desire vanishes. Things happen at each moment as if the subject did not know what to do. (Merleau-Ponty 2012, p. 157)

Schneider's passivity and lack of interest in sex is moreover not only psychological, since he rarely has nocturnal emissions (p. 157), which are supposed to stem from a physiological mechanism. It is therefore the entire field of sexuality which is blocked for him.[7] Sexuality, for the human being, is revealed to be based upon something wider than a pure animal impulse. It involves imagination, virtuality and recognition of otherness. Schneider's lack of interest in sex shows how all these actually involve some form of reflection. In reflection one takes the given world and self, and, upon them, imagines something new, thus combining immersion and transcendence. Without this process I cannot make love, but neither can I dance or play

---

[7]Judith Butler severely criticizes Merleau-Ponty's analysis of Schneider's sexuality, claiming that it is based upon a heterosexual ideology of the male as supposedly active, dominant and objectifying the female body. I totally agree with Butler that Merleau-Ponty tends to set a "normal" ideal upon which he considers pathology, but I believe that rather than dismissing or deconstructing Merleau-Ponty, we should take his analyses of pathology as an integral part of normality. In this way we may arrive at a better understanding both of socially constructed ideals of the body and the empirical inability to achieve them, which leads to their transgression. The case of Schneider may describe a man who finds himself not "manly" enough, but the problem is that, exactly as the amputated patient, he is not able to benefit from his loss to change his ideas of sexuality. See Butler (1989).

football.[8] For all these situations require an attunement to the current environment (a partner, music, the field, the ball), connecting some of its elements to each other and to the self, and transforming something in them. This transformation is not necessarily active, as shows the case of hallucinatory drugs, when I just need to let the hallucination penetrate me and make me float over the different possibilities and variations of the given world which remain hidden in everyday perception. But in most cases we find a combination of passivity and activity, letting myself be absorbed in the situation while being active enough to respond, when I make love, to the gestures of my partner and myself, thus creating a new act of love making.

I thus suggest that every bodily gesture involves some degree of reflection. But does this mean that every reflection necessarily involves the body? Although reflection may be purely intellectual, most of the time it takes place within the everyday, with the body, even if one does not notice it playing a major role. A further illustration of this idea is given in another set of symptoms from which Schneider suffers: he has no ability or will to make new friends; he never spontaneously whistles or sings to himself; he does not have any opinion regarding politics, religion, or other abstract matters (pp. 159–60). All these attest again to a lack of reflection, and show how vast its influence upon practically every aspect of human life is. From a physical inability to locate a detached part of the body we finally arrive at a "mental" inability to reflect upon an abstract theme such as politics, and both cases are due to a lack of reflection as the ability to detach and reconnect elements in the world.

If this is so, what did Schneider's everyday life look like? The surprising answer is that it was apparently quite normal. He went to a wallet factory every day where he was employed as a simple worker, and despite his various symptoms his production rate was only a quarter less than the normal (p. 105). As long as he was not asked to go beyond his everyday mechanical routine, he mastered the situation almost perfectly, and yet it is reported that he had the feeling his life was not his; as if everything came from the outside and happened independently of himself. Pathology, I would suggest, has something important to tell us here about normal everyday life. It seems that Schneider is nothing but a very extreme case of the difficulty to found new meanings, and as such his behavior is not completely strange to us. We, too, find it very difficult to innovate our everyday routine; we, too, find ourselves repeating time and again the same movement; we, too, are afraid of shutting our eyes and remaining in the dark, striving to control the world with our eyes wide open, choosing between ready-made objects instead of creating new

[8]The opposite case of Schneider is that of Chuck Knoblauch, the baseball player who, due to an unexplained pathology, started to reflect upon his throwing the ball and consequently hit the crowd instead of the first base. This case has been debated by Hubert Dreyfus and John McDowell, the former deducing that reflection is not involved in coping skills, and any introduction of it would only disturb them (Dreyfus 2007, p. 354). McDowell, on the other hand, sees this case as proving that "when mindedness gets detached from immersion in activity, it can be the enemy of embodied coping" (McDowell 2009, p. 325). I tend to agree with McDowell here, putting the emphasis not on one of the poles (immersion/reflection) but rather on their relationship.

ones. The difference between Schneider and us lays rather in the *degree* of stagnation, as well as in the ability to act upon it, an ability which is closely connected to the function of reflection.

4 Body and Language

Although Merleau-Ponty hints at a link between the patient suffering from a phantom limb, Schneider, and finally everyday "normal" perception, he still maintains a clear distinction between "normality" and "pathology." The "normal" person, rather than sharing something with Schneider or other patients, is presented as opposed to them: "for the normal person, the subject's intentions are immediately reflected in the perceptual field: they polarize it, put their stamp on it, or finally, effortlessly give birth there to a wave of significations. For the patient, the perceptual field has lost this plasticity" (p. 133). Reflection and plasticity are the share of the normal person alone, who consequently possesses a full, vital and effortless perception, whereas the pathological patient is deprived of these, remaining prisoner in a frozen world: "The world no longer exists for these patients except as a ready-made or fixed world, whereas the normal person's projects polarize the world, causing a thousand signs to appear there, as if by magic, that guide action, as signs in a museum guide the visitor" (p. 115). But is it true that the "normal" always succeeds in maintaining this magic? Do we constantly give fresh sense to our everyday action?[9]

Merleau-Ponty tends to present the normal movement of existence as fully efficient but he must admit time and again that it is actually deficient. He says, for instance, that the normal person spontaneously creates his or her own linguistic categories, whereas Schneider uses only constituted language, that is, ready-made categories which structure and stabilize his perception (p. 130). But it soon appears that it is not only the pathological patient who finds it difficult to access living speech, but also every one of us in his or her everyday life: "We live in a world where speech is already *instituted*. We possess in ourselves ready-made significations for all these banal words [*paroles*]. They only give rise in us to second-order thoughts,

[9]In a radio broadcast from 1948 Merleau-Ponty claims himself that normality is only an ideal: "In the case of children, primitive people, the sick, or more so still, animals, the world which they occupy—insofar as we can reconstruct it from the way they behave—is certainly not a coherent system. By contrast, that of the healthy, civilised, adult human being strives for such coherence. Yet the crucial point here is that he does not attain this coherence: it remains an idea, or limit, which he never actually manages to reach. It follows that the 'normal' person must remain open to these abnormalities of which he is never entirely exempt himself; he must take the trouble to understand them. He is invited to look at himself without indulgence, to rediscover within himself the whole host of fantasies, dreams, patterns of magical behaviour and obscure phenomena which remain all-powerful in shaping both his private and public life and his relationships with other people" (Merleau-Ponty 2004, pp. 72–73). It is remarkable to note, however, that in the eyes of Merleau-Ponty, abnormality only inspires fantasy and magic and never rigidity and disenchantment.

which are in turn translated into other words that require no genuine effort of expression from us, and that will demand no effort of comprehension from our listeners" (p. 189).

The (normal) dynamic movement of existence is revealed to be an impossible ideal, since the everyday foundation has an inherent tendency to slow down. Whatever is founded soon takes the appearance of something stable which does not necessitate a further foundation. This is why "there is always a depersonalization at the heart of consciousness" (p. 139). In order to appropriate one's own foundation, in order to make it personal, one needs to constantly re-found it, that is, to repeat the movement and prevent it from becoming mechanical and external. As Heidegger claims too, a foundation that is not picked up time and again becomes alienated from its founder. Within myself I find a foreign body that is nonetheless familiar, something which I know well but which does not belong to me. Whereas this foreign body remains abstract in Heidegger, in Merleau-Ponty it really is a question of my concrete everyday body. The body is something into which I was born and which I did not choose: it is me and it is not me, and all life long I strive to appropriate and re-appropriate it.

Merleau-Ponty affirms that there is a constant struggle between personal and bodily existence: "most of the time personal existence represses the organism without being able either to go beyond it or to renounce itself" (p. 86). We saw earlier why the body, representing deficiency and finitude, needs to be repressed. This is where the "they" enters the scene, proposing to substitute the hard work of appropriation with easy categories which hide their bodily origin. Instead of the precarious foundation of the body, I then attain an illusion of a solid and objective basis, but the price I have to pay is alienation: from my body, from my language and finally from my entire perceptive field.

Both Heidegger and Merleau-Ponty propose ways to escape the suffocating yet comfortable realm of the "they," but their diagnosis and solution to the problem of the "they" is different. Whereas Heidegger sees Dasein as based upon nothingness and radical negativity, Merleau-Ponty locates the basis of existence in the body, which is not a pure nothingness but rather an ambiguous and fragile foundation. As a consequence, in order to get rid of the "they" I no longer need to annihilate my everyday world through anxiety, as was the case in Heidegger, but rather to re-attach myself to my body as the ambiguous vehicle of the movement of existence/foundation. But how, exactly, is one to do this?

We encountered pathology as standing for an extreme case of lack of reflection, such that the ambiguity of the body can be seen as *frozen*; but Merleau-Ponty also identifies several figures which possess an *enhanced* capacity of reflection or projection. These are the baby uttering its first word, the lover revealing his or her feelings, the writer, the artist, and, of course, the philosopher (p. 530n7; p. 203). All these use what Merleau-Ponty calls "speaking speech," in contrast to the everyday and common "spoken speech." They exploit the full potential of language and in this way overcome the tendency to remain only at its static and constituted pole.

But what role does the body play in the life of these figures? How do they combine the two apparently distinct realms of body and language? On the one hand, language goes well beyond the body: it enables me to bypass my physical situation and arrive at the realm of words which can invent imaginary times, places and creatures, having nothing to do with the limited and weak body of their author. But on the other hand, language has exactly the same structure as the body: I am born into it, I do not choose it, and yet through it I constitute my world. When I speak, I use ready-made words and yet I pronounce them in sentences which could only be mine. I am thus touched by language and am touching it at one and the same time, moving between its constituted and constituting poles. Touching and touched, founding and founded—this is the double and ambiguous structure of both the body and language. Is it a pure coincidence?

This question, which cannot be fully answered in principle, is one of the mysteries of human existence. What we can affirm is that through language I acquire a certain stability which would not be possible otherwise, in a purely bodily existence. Language enables rigid categories and this is why Husserl characterizes it as a *seduction* of which one should be vigilant.[10] Language supplies ready-made words which flatten the richness of their origin and hide their movement in time and the inability to fully grasp the object they point to. But this process of stabilization offered by language is not something to condemn or exorcize, since it allows one to bypass the purely corporal situation, to create new objects, new combinations, new connections between the body and the world. Reflection, projection and existence would not be possible without language, and the question is thus not how to attain a purely pre-objective realm, but rather how not to remain in a purely objective one.

5 Conclusion: Pathology at the Limits of Phenomenology

Merleau-Ponty, like Husserl and Heidegger, looks for the ideal essence of the body, perception, language, and time, and although he devotes many pages to various empirical figures he tends to classify them in the rubric of "pathology" rather than that of the everyday. *Phenomenology of Perception* was published in 1945, which explains why its unquestionable hero is Antoine de Saint-Exupéry, the famous author of *The Little Prince*, who was killed as a war-pilot during the Second-World-War. Merleau-Ponty cites Saint-Exupéry's *Flight to Arras* to illustrate the rich and full perception a war-pilot needs to adopt in his missions. He even closes *Phenomenology of Perception* with a declaration that "it is precisely here that we must remain silent, for only the hero fully lives his relation with men and with the world, and it is hardly fitting for another to speak in his name" (p. 483). The philosopher should thus clear the stage for the hero, but does Merleau-Ponty not forget that a war-pilot is, justly, a pilot of *war*, and that in moments of peace, when the sublime efforts taken in pursuit of a noble end are no longer necessary, the body tends again towards its own oblivion, the oblivion of its lack and finitude? Is there

[10] Husserl (2002, p. 100).

no everyday, peaceful manner of living in the world and in the body which is not condemned to inauthenticity?

In order to imagine a different everyday perception and action, we need first to understand the everyday not as the ordinary which is symmetrically opposed to the extraordinary and full, but rather as a positive phenomenon in its own right. Husserl, Heidegger and Merleau-Ponty describe various perceptive mechanisms involved in the everyday, but they secretly or openly wish to attain the full experience of the "things themselves," an experience in relation to which the everyday can be only an inauthentic shadow. We seem here to arrive at the limits of phenomenology, limits which stand between it and the historical, empirical and the objective world. Phenomenology looks for ideal essences, but after delineating them with care, it often deplores their "deterioration" in everyday life. It does not suppose, for instance, that the mechanical movement of the everyday is not only a stagnation of an allegedly "full" or "authentic" movement, but also a reaction to historical circumstances leading to new forms of experience. Neither does it suppose that technology has a potential not only to alienate one from the body, but also to open up new ways to access it.[11]

It is here that pathology may teach us a lesson about the reaction of the body to various circumstances, provided that we do not separate too sharply the pathological from the normal. The pathological body and the everyday body both try to find solutions to their inherent deficiency, but whereas these solutions "succeed" in the everyday body, and as such remain hidden, pathology stands as a striking "failure."[12] However, this failure is the share of each one of us as having an ephemeral body. I started this paper with the exclamation "this body is mine," and I shall thus conclude it with pathology's lesson: this body is always, to a certain degree, foreign to myself, and as such calls not only for a phenomenology which would take this aspect into account, but also for a corresponding ethics which is yet to be developed.

References

Aho, K. A. (2009). *Heidegger's neglect of the body*. Albany: SUNY Press.

Askay, R. R. (1999). Heidegger, the body, and the french philosophers. *Continental Philosophy Review, 32*, 29–35.

Butler, J. (1989). Sexual ideology and phenomenological description: A feminist critique of merleau-ponty's phenomenology of perception. In J. Allen & I. M. Young (Eds.), *The thinking muse* (pp. 85–100). Bloomington: Indiana University Press.

[11]For a discussion of contemporary technology in the context of Merleau-Ponty's phenomenology, see Ihde (2002).

[12]The idea of the body (or organism) finding solutions to problems posed by the environment is one that is developed with great nuance by Kurt Goldstein, a major influence on both Merleau-Ponty and Canguilhem, Dorfman's conclusion here brings his phenomenological analyses into some proximity with the work of Canguilhem, explored in the part III of this volume—the editor.

Cerbone, D. R. (2000). Heidegger and dasein's bodily nature: What is the hidden problematic? *International Journal of Philosophical Studies, 8*, 209–230.

Dillon, M. C. (1988). *Merleau-Ponty's ontology*. Bloomington: Indiana University Press.

Dreyfus, H. L. (2007). The return of the myth of the mental. *Inquiry, 50*, 352–365.

Franck, D. (1991). Being and the living. In E. Cadava, P. Connor, & J.-L. Nancy (Eds.), *Who comes after the subject?* (pp. 135–147). London: Routledge.

Gelb, A., & Goldstein, K. (1918). Psychologische analysen hirnpathologischer falle auf grund von untersuchungen hirnverletzer. *Zeitschrift für die gesamte Neurologie und Psychiatrie, 41*, 1–142.

Goldenberg, G. (2003). Goldstein and Gelb's case Schn: A classic case in neuropsychology? In C. Code, C. W. Wallesch, Y. Joanette, & A. R. Lecours (Eds.), *Classic cases in neuropsychology* (Vol. II, pp. 281–300). Hove: Psychology Press.

Goldstein, K. (1923). Über die Abhängigkeit der Bewegungen von optischen Vorgängen. *Monatsschrift für Psychiatrie und Neurologie, 54*, 141–194.

Haar, M. (1993). *The song of the earth: Heidegger and the grounds of the history of being* (R. Lilly, Trans.). Bloomington: Indiana University Press.

Heidegger, M. (1962). *Being and time* (J. Macquarrie & E. Robinson, Trans.). New York: Harper and Row.

Heidegger, M. (2001). *Zollikon seminars: protocol-conversations-letters* (F. K. Mayr & R. R. Askay, Trans.). Evanston: Northwestern University Press.

Husserl, E. (2002). The origin of geometry. In M. Merleau-Ponty (Ed.), *Husserl at the Limits of phenomenology* (pp. 93–116; L. Lawlor & B. Bergo, Trans.). Evanston: Northwestern University Press.

Ihde, D. (2002). *Bodies in technology*. Minneapolis: University of Minnesota.

Krell, D. F. (1992). *Daimon life: Heidegger and life-philosophy*. Bloomington: Indiana University Press.

McDowell, J. (2009). *The engaged intellect*. Cambridge, Mass.: Harvard University Press.

Merleau-Ponty, M. (1968). *The visible and the invisible* (A. Lingis, Trans.). Evanston: Northwestern University Press.

Merleau-Ponty, M. (2004). *The world of perception* (O. Davis, Trans.). London, New York: Routledge.

Merleau-Ponty, M. (2012). *Phenomenology of perception* (D. A. Landes, Trans.). London, New York: Routledge.

Teuber, H.-L. (1966). Kurt Goldstein's role in the development of neuropsychology. *Neuropsychologia, 4*, 299–310.

Part III
The Normal and the Pathological

Chapter 9
Towards a Critique of Normalization: Canguilhem and Boorse

Jonathan Sholl and Andreas De Block

> *[He] thought he was normal, like everyone else, when he imagined the crowd in abstract, a great, positive army united by the same feelings, the same ideas, the same aims; and it was comforting to be part of this. But as soon as individuals emerged out of that crowd, his illusion of normality shattered against the fact of diversity.*
>
> —*The Conformist*, Alberto Moravia

1 Introduction

In biomedical discussions, it is often the case that arguably the most crucial concept is taken for granted as being self-evident: normality. Yet the various meanings of the concept of normality undermine its self-evident application: e.g. the most frequent, the average, that which conforms to a type, that which occurs in healthy individuals, or an ideal to be attained (Vácha 1978). These various definitions have their roots in 19th century attempts to bring statistics into the biological and medical realms. While this statistical view of normality has been critiqued since its inception, a more recent formulation of it can be found in the biostatistical account of health and disease by Boorse (1975, 1977). What Boorse and these 19th century positions have in common is that they all assume an epistemological priority to normality such that it is in relation to what is deemed normal that we can determine the abnormal or the pathological: the normal is the standard by which divergences are measured. We shall label this view, also encountered in discussions on bioethics, disability and health care ethics (cf. Whitehouse et al. 2004; Daniels 1987; Amundson 2000), the normalization view.

J. Sholl (✉) · A. De Block
University of Leuven, Leuven, Belgium
e-mail: Jonathan.sholl@hiw.kuleuven.be

D. Meacham (ed.), *Medicine and Society, New Perspectives in Continental Philosophy*, Philosophy and Medicine 120, DOI 10.1007/978-94-017-9870-9_9

In this chapter, we will attempt to flesh out some recurring forms of the normalization view, ultimately claiming that those theories that aim to provide a statistical account of biomedical concepts, such as normality or abnormality, harbor problematic assumptions concerning the very concepts they seek to clarify. We will do so by first discussing one philosopher of biomedicine who was particularly attentive to such problems: Georges Canguilhem. His analyses of the relation between normality and disease will help to point out some of the common ways of thinking that this normalization view employs and some of the problems surrounding its formulation. Second, this will help us to question the very meanings of normality and abnormality that are found in a common naturalistic approach, such as Christopher Boorse's. We will show how, despite his appeals to biology to clarify biomedical concepts, normality is still viewed as both an average and an ideal, which ultimately undermines a coherent philosophical account of such concepts. Rather than concluding that such a problem renders the health/disease distinction illusory (Amundson 2000), we will argue that without a proper philosophical account of normality the ability to provide a more biologically accurate definition of health/disease will be hindered. Thirdly, we will briefly explore the insight from Canguilhem, corroborated by various findings in biology and medicine, that no organism or environment is normal in itself, but it is the historically changing relations between organisms and environments that make them normal or not. One interesting implication of this insight is that any naturalistic account of normality and abnormality would have to acknowledge that "normality" implies variation, both within and between environments. If there is no "normal" organism (Nesse 2001), no trait which is normal or pathological *in itself*, we seem led to define normality relative to the individual and its relation to its environment. We will end by posing some problems that arise with this "relativistic" account of disease.

2 Three Problems of Normalization

In order to elaborate this critique of the normalization view, we will first focus on three interrelated problems inherent to it: quantification, abstraction and exclusion. The next section will discuss these problems in relation to Christopher Boorse's theory of disease, as he allows us to test Canguilhem's insights against one of the most influential naturalist views.

In his central text, *Le normal et le pathologique* (1989[1]), Canguilhem provides both a critique of certain concepts within the history of the life sciences as well as a novel way to rethink these concepts. By tracing the historical alterations that these

[1]This text was published in two parts. The first part, *Essai sur quelques problèmes concernant le normal et le pathologique,* was published in 1943 and in 1966 a second part was added, *Nouvelle réflexions concernant le normal et le pathologique*, with the new title *Le normal et le pathologique*. We will refer to the English edition which contains both parts (1989), first translated in 1978, with an introduction by Michel Foucault.

scientific concepts have undergone and by acknowledging various scientific claims concerning the variability of biological norms he is able to uncover some philosophical and scientific problems inherent to what we have called the normalization view. For example, the normalization view understands the abnormal only in relation to the abstract statistical norm from which it deviates. However, this means that the normalization view runs into a problem precisely because it overlooks how the meaning of normality and pathology is actually derived from the individual's non-indifferent relation to its environment and not from a deviation from a statistical species norm. Thus, the relation of normality and pathology to individuality and the environment has to be reconsidered. This admittedly abstract sketch of the normalization view and its problems needs to be made more concrete: How did the statistical or quantitative view come about, what exactly does it amount to, and what are some examples of the recurring problems for such theories?

A quantitative approach was developed by various philosophers and scientists throughout the 19th Century who attempted to rethink the relation between physiology and pathology, as seen in Belgium with Quetelet, in France with Bernard and Comte, in Germany with Fechner and Rautmann, and in England with Galton and Pearson (Vácha 1985). Two historical factors were important for the development and scientific popularity of this view. First, there was a general aim to make physiology a more rigorous (nomological) experimental science that would approach the achievements of the physical sciences. Posed in this way, individual variations and pathologies became regrettable irregularities or "errors of measurement" whose underlying cause had to be explained so as to arrive at the supposed laws or regularities of physiology. Concomitantly, this understanding of "normality" became possible through the rise of statistics in the 19th century (particularly Gauss' normal distribution curve), as biologists and physiologists sought to speak more objectively about human beings. Moreover, from their inception these understandings of normality have been plagued by a possible conflation of facts with values: normality as not only what is average, but also as what is right or what *ought* to exist. Ian Hacking summarizes this view as follows: "The normal stands indifferently for what is typical, the unenthusiastic objective average, but it also stands for what has been, good health, and for what shall be, our chosen destiny" (Hacking 1990, p. 169).

The basic idea behind these quantitative theories, then, is that the statistical norm, as studied in physiology, takes precedence over the abnormalities and variations studied in pathology, entailing that the abnormal is merely a quantitatively determined lack or excess in relation to this norm. As mere quantitative deviations, or differences in degree, abnormalities can be derived from normality: they still refer to an underlying normal functioning, but with something added or lacking: "diseases are merely the effects of simple changes in intensity in the action of the stimulants which are indispensible for maintaining health" (Canguilhem 1989, p. 48).

Canguilhem challenges this by arguing that if there is no quality to quantitative variation,[2] then first, physiology has nothing new to learn from pathology, and second, biology and the life sciences more generally have nothing more to say concerning the nature of anomalies, sickness or death than physics or chemistry (Canguilhem 1988). If the difference between the normal and the pathological is merely quantitative, it becomes redundant and scientifically useless to distinguish between physiology and pathophysiology. By using the pathological to clarify the normal, the normalization view prevents the study of the pathological qua pathological.

This quantitative theory of disease also rests on the problem of abstraction whereby individuals are detached from their concrete circumstances by means of statistical analysis (Canguilhem 1989, p. 88). In order to determine pathological deviations, normality must first be established by abstracting from within individual (e.g. physiological fluctuations) and between individual (e.g. gender, geography, job differences, etc.) variations. The normalization view often assumes that there is a stable underlying type to which all organisms can be identified, with such variations being only accidental quantitative deviations. However, Canguilhem points out that from the very conception of this view in the 19th century, Claude Bernard already had his reservations since "the use of averages erases the essentially oscillatory and rhythmic character of the functional biological phenomenon" (Canguilhem 1989, p. 151).

Furthermore, this abstraction grounds the supposed epistemological and therapeutic implications of normality, with normality either serving as the goal of knowledge or the goal of medical intervention in its attempt to restore nature's order.[3] This reasoning is confronted with several problems. First, how do some variations result in disease in some individuals, whereas in others they pose no problem, as seen in multifactorially inherited diseases like cancer, hypertension or schizophrenia where environmental factors play a large role in how and whether the variation is expressed? Second, it seems obvious that there are variations that are not pathological even though they are deviations from this natural norm. Why is having green eyes not a pathology if only 2 % of humans have green eyes? Thirdly, even if such "oscillatory and rhythmic" characters are acknowledged, any judgment that a trait or individual is "normal" remains insufficient apart from the conditions in

[2]A certain reading of Canguilhem's focus on the quality of disease should be avoided. Canguilhem does not simply prefer quality over quantity, as if appealing to something intractable for scientific investigation, as is often implied (cf. Chimisso 2003; Roudinesco 2008), but argues that when dealing with living beings, quantitative changes always have a qualitative significance: quantification cannot erase quality, but neither does quality erase quantity: "The substitution of quantitative progression for qualitative contrast in no way annuls this opposition" (Canguilhem 1989, p. 111, 1988, p. 141).

[3]For Comte, "The identity of the normal and the pathological is asserted as a gain in *knowledge* of the normal" and for Bernard "The identity of the normal and the pathological is asserted as a gain in *remedying* the pathological." (Canguilhem 1989, pp. 43, 44, my italics). Canguilhem (1989, p. 45) points out that Nietzsche was also influenced by Bernard's view that pathology illuminates normality.

which it appears: tasks, length of time, previous state of the individual, environment, etc. As we will discuss later, the normality or pathology of a trait, e.g. being able to read, digest lactose or even to run quickly, depends on the environment in which the individual develops and its chosen or imposed tasks. Statistical abstractions would thus seem to offer no means *in themselves* for distinguishing between normal and abnormal variation (Canguilhem 1989, p. 155).

Finally, the problem of abstraction as the basis of knowledge of normality leads to the problem of the exclusion of differences. If diseases are explained by their relation to what is statistically normal, then that which would be different about them is regulated to that which contaminates or distorts normality: disease becomes an aberration which threatens our understanding of nature's regularity. "From this perspective, the singular—that is, the divergence, the variation—appears to be a failure, a defect, an impurity" (Canguilhem 2008, p. 123). It is the desire to establish how nature's lawful regularity can create ideal or normal individuals that explains why variations are seen as unnatural, deficient or excessive deviations: as the normal is the index for what *ought* to exist, the abnormal is unnatural, what *ought not* exist.

In all three instances, pathology is subordinated to physiology since disease is incapable of being a norm in itself apart from its relation to normality. It is because the abnormal is a quantitative deviation from a norm understood as an underlying essence that it can be considered unnatural. For the normalization view, the anomalous and the pathological are reduced to epistemological obstacles impeding the knowledge of normality and ontological obstacles to life's supposed goal of establishing or maintaining physiological constants.

3 Boorse's Naturalism as an Example of Normalization

A more recent attempt to uphold a similar line of argumentation can be seen in the work of Boorse (1975, 1997, 1997) who has argued for biostatistical, and value-free, concepts of health and disease. We will briefly outline the main arguments presented by Boorse and show how he exemplifies the problematic nature of normality discussed above.

Boorse develops his naturalistic theory in contrast to the normative view that health and disease imply value judgments, such as being desirable. Boorse claims that the "normativist" position is problematic when it comes to accounting for undesirable conditions that are not diseases. For example, infertility might be undesirable, but abstracted from the actual organism it is unclear whether it is related to disease. Moreover, many conditions that predispose people to immoral or even criminal behaviour are undesirable, but most people have the strong intuition that dispositions to immoral or criminal behaviour are not—or at least not necessarily—diseases. To better clarify disease, then, he aims to abstract from questions of desirability and to develop his own "naturalistic" account of disease. Boorse calls this account the biostatistical theory of disease as it combines evolutionary elements with statistical elements. In his view, the evolutionary elements neutralize the philosophically untenable implications of a purely statistical account, and the statistical elements neutralize the philosophically untenable or implausible implications of purely evolutionary account. For example, unlike a purely statistical account of disease, Boorse does not have to argue that bird flu stops being a disease as soon as everybody has bird flu (because having bird flu has then become statistically normal). According to Boorse, the bird flu would then still be a disease because the bird flu hampers the functioning of species typical processes that contribute to the survival and reproduction of organisms of that species.

In Boorse's biostatistical theory, "the normal is the natural" (1975, p. 57), in the sense that normality, which is the state of being free of disease and thus equated to health, entails a "mode of functioning [which] conforms to the natural design of that kind of organism" (57). As organisms are composed of a hierarchy of goal-directed functions, he posits the existence of a reference class of uniform functional design, such that "normal function" implies a statistically typical contribution to the goals of survival and reproduction (1976, p. 79). One can describe three aspects of this view of normality as that which is species-typical: quantitative, qualitative and dispositional normal function. Qualitative normal function refers to the causal contribution that a function gives to survival and reproduction, whereas quantitative normal function refers to the efficiency of that function (Kingma 2010). This can be seen in the distinction between whether an organ, such as the liver, performs its species-typical function of filtering toxins (qualitative), and whether it does so within the statistically typical level of efficiency (quantitative). Dispositional function (Kingma 2010) refers to the "readiness" that a given part has to perform "all its normal functions on typical occasions with at least typical efficiency" (Boorse 1977, p. 562). As such, a function can be considered normal, and thus healthy, even if it is not currently being used. This appeal to species-typical functions suggests a description of health and disease that makes no reference to the value of physiological functions, to whether an organism desires a certain goal—which would smell too much of "normativity"—but entails the objective empirical determinations of whether and to what degree a function contributes to physiological goals.[4]

As we have already mentioned, statistics are not sufficient to determine health or disease, since unusual conditions can be healthy and unhealthy conditions can be common (Boorse 1977, p. 546). Nevertheless, he maintains that "there is a persistent intuition that the average person—or at least the average heart, lung, kidney, thyroid, etc.—must be normal, or we would have no way of telling what the normal person or organ should be like" (546). Moreover, our "species and others are in fact highly uniform in structure and function; otherwise there would be no point to the extreme detail in textbooks of human physiology" (557). Thus, the claim that the normal is average, is retained because of the need for a standard, in the sense of the

[4]For another defense of "normal function" as that which is fixed by nature and thus allows for the objective determination of health care goals, see Normal Daniels (1987).

highly uniform species norms that have arisen and are maintained by natural selection. Since some of these norms that natural selection has established are not only relative to species, but also to sex and age, the reference class—the class that sets the standard or the norm—is not limited to the species but also includes age groups and sex groups (558). For instance, a condition that is species typical (e.g. the ability to control one's emotions), but not typical for pre-adolescent males of that species, would count as statistically abnormal for that individual, and could thus be a diseased process if it occurs in pre-adolescent males of that species. This latter relativity shows Boorse attempting to account for individual differences, but, as we will see below, he does not go far enough.

At first sight, there is much to praise in Boorse's view. His naturalistic view of disease has the advantages (1) of appealing to physiology and evolutionary biology so as to avoid the perils of pure normativism, (2) of being applicable across biological taxa (Nordenfelt 2007), and (3) of acknowledging that statistical deviations alone cannot account for how some deviations are abnormal and others are not (Boorse 1977). However, this view still falls prey to the three problems mentioned above. (1) Can empirical descriptions completely bracket their clinical significance?[5] What constitutes the difference between normal variation and abnormal variation? (2) Second, there is the assumption of some abstract identification of normality in the sense that underlying observed variations is the objective fixed design of the ideal organism that is established when the naturalist abstracts from "individual differences and from disease by averaging over a sufficiently large sample of the population" (557). This move is further sustained by arguing that these fixed designs are biological designs that are maintained in nature via "normalizing selection" (557). As such, Boorse's Platonism forces him to abstract from the actual individual for whom health is not merely the absence of disease or a statistical generality. (3) Finally, while he does acknowledge that variation is part of normality (563), the issue of exclusion remains when disease is seen as a failure that is "unnatural" and "foreign" to the species: "Diseases are, so to speak, failures to get as far as the rest of the species has been for millennia" (563). Despite a naturalistic approach, disease falls outside of nature, a mere derivation from naturally selected normality, and thus teaches us nothing about nature itself, except that it can, sometimes, go wrong.

We can see these three problems converging when Boorse discusses the controversial claim that homosexuality could be considered a disease since it is a deviation from one of the species-typical goals of sexuality, i.e. reproduction (1975, p. 63). Heterosexuality, by implication, is the normal, natural (and thus healthy) function of human sexuality since it conforms to this goal. David Hull (critically) summarizes such a view as follows:

[5]Méthot (2009) also argues that Canguilhem and Boorse diverge when it comes to the role of the clinic in conceptualizing disease.

> Heterosexuality is the normal state programmed into our genes. It needs no special explanation. Normal genes in a wide variety of normal environments lead most children quite naturally to prefer members of the opposite sex for sexual and emotional partners. Homosexuality, to the contrary, is an abnormal deviation which needs to be explained in terms of some combination of defective genes and/or undesirable environments. (1998, p. 390)

This captures what is at stake in the naturalistic view by explaining disease as either atypical or resulting from an environment gone wrong. Boorse adds that such an example shows how our desires might not conform to the species design and that in the case of homosexuality we would be better off asking what difference such a diagnosis would make. As biological normality is not a good in itself, but only instrumentally good in terms of contributions to the biological goals of survival and reproduction, then if one is happy with what he calls "a psyche full of deviant desires and unnatural acts" (Boorse 1975, p. 63), maybe it makes no difference on a practical level whether homosexuality would be a disease on the theoretical level. Is this not a prime example of normalization, whereby sexual variations are quantified (homosexuality as a deviation from the sex norms),[6] viewed abstractly (theoretically diseased), and excluded (as unnatural)? While it remains open for Boorse as to the value of sexual deviations and whether they should be medicalized, it is problematic at best to assume that such judgments about the variety of human sexuality in relation to ideal references classes, not to mention other forms of behavioural diversity, are free from being evaluative (Brown 1985; Kingma 2007).

Let us now focus on what might be the biggest problem of Boorse's account, the problem his account faces when it has to distinguish normal from abnormal variation. Boorse tries to solve this problem by invoking evolutionary elements ("contribution to survival and reproduction"). According to his view, deviations from statistical norms are not pathological as long as they do not undermine the trait's species-typical contribution to survival and reproduction. Furthermore, Boorse also thinks evolutionary theory supports his reliance on statistics in his biostatistical account. After all, natural selection tends to increase the frequency of adaptive and heritable traits in a population until these traits become the statistical norm. Having opposable thumbs is the statistical norm in our species because natural selection has resulted in the spread of that trait in our species. There are several problems with this reliance on evolutionary theory. First, it can be instructive to mention that some evolutionary theorists (and philosophers of biology) seem to call into question this stress on statistically determined norms by pointing out that variation is inherent to human populations such that

> [...] there is no one normal genome for the body. Likewise, there is no one perfect phenotype. There are just phenotypes that emerge from the products of genes interacting with environments. Thus, there is no ideal type to use as a benchmark for comparison to determine what is normal and what is not. (Nesse 2001, p. 44)

---

[6]Sexual desires for males are species typical: more than half of the population consists of individuals that have sexual desires for male individuals. However, such desires are not typical for males.

Yet, even Nesse seems to agree with Boorse that any deviation that negatively influences the ability of a bodily mechanism to perform its "normal function" in a given environment should be considered a disease: "Disease is a disadvantageous difference from normal" (Nesse 2001, p. 41). While this view claims to challenge the view that normality is an ideal that can be determined apart from the organism's, or the gene's, relation to a given environment, normality still refers to a supposedly "objective" standard in the form of what is "usual" for a given species (2001, p. 44).

This is where the second problem arises: why would evolutionary concerns be decisive for our judgment about health and disease? This problem can be formulated as follows: (a) trait T is not typical for an age group of a sex of our species whereas T' is typical, (b) individuals with T have on average lower reproductive success than individuals with T', and (c) it would be wrong to call T a disease (or people do not think of T as a disease or a disorder). Since there are plenty of examples of such traits, Boorse's account fails. For example, there seems to be a curvilinear effect of height on reproductive success in human males: average height men, compared to shorter and taller men, attain the highest reproductive success (Stulp et al. 2012). If one would apply Boorse's account to this example, one could conclude that only men of average height are normal and that all significant deviations from this norm are pathological. Yet, this conclusion is highly problematic. First, men of above average height are usually not seen as suffering from a disease. Secondly, the average that seems to matter here is not an average height of men in our species, but rather the average in a particular human population. In the US, males of average height have higher reproductive success than taller or shorter males. But the average that matters is the average height of males that live in the US. In the US, males of 178.2 cm have higher reproductive success than males of 184.8 cm. But in the Netherlands, males of 184.8 cm are of average height and they have more reproductive success than Dutch males of 178.2 cm. Would Boorse conclude that 184.2 cm is normal in the Netherlands but not in the US because Dutch men of that height have a higher than average reproductive success, whereas American men of that height have a lower than average reproductive success? In our view, this conclusion is absurd. The absurdity points out that adding another reference class (e.g. nationality) to the already existing reference classes in Boorse's account (age, sex and species) will not do. As such, the problematic nature of the concept of normality remains, as do the limitations of a biostatistical approach, with disease still being conceived as a deviation from supposedly objective biological norms.

While Boorse and other naturalists are right to critique normative theories for viewing biological norms solely in terms of social ideals or subjective evaluations, the claim that these norms are better understood in relation to a species-typical design is to overlook an important problem with species-typicality or types more generally. By claiming to simply describe nature's norms, Boorse makes the unfounded assumption that his reference class is sufficiently uniform (Hull 1998). Moreover, he ignores the fact that biological organisms tend to adapt to changes in their environments. As long as these adaptive changes result (on average) in more reproductive success, Boorse would not call them diseases. Yet, he would have to conclude that individuals that are unable to adapt to new environmental circumstances but that do conform to a statistical species-typical (and age and sex-typical) average are not suffering from a disease, even though this "common" phenotype would turn out to be fatal for that organism. It seems that one should take the evolutionary challenge more seriously than Boorse does[7]: there are no ideal genotypes or phenotypes, but simply gene-environment interactions that produce a variety of functions and behaviours (Pigliucci 2001).

4 The Problem of the Abnormal and the Anomalous

As was discussed in the previous section, Boorse himself acknowledges that statistical deviations are not sufficient conditions to determine whether a given phenomenon is a disease. We believe that one of the main problems with Boorse's account is that statistical abnormality is not a necessary condition either. Rather than just accepting this as a difficulty inherent to statistics, however, our intent is to show why this difficulty arises. If we begin with the view that normal and abnormal variation are two kinds of natural variability, rather than with the view that abnormality is "foreign" to an underlying species design, then we can mitigate the problems of normalization. To do so, we will further explore the insights of Canguilhem.

We first need to clarify Canguilhem's distinction between "anomaly" and "abnormality" because there is a tendency to conflate these terms and thereby prevent the ability to understand the difference between mutations and diseases (cf. Blumberg 2009). For example, if deviation from the species design is retained as one basis for disease, some problems emerge. Insofar as a genetic mutation expressed in the phenotype deviates from the typical species design and entails the possibility of a new variety, or insofar as an organism whose physiological mutation prevents adaptation in one environment and forces it into a new environment that allows it to flourish there, the normalization view would be led into the paradox of calling such mutations both pathological, insofar as they are deviations, and normal, insofar as they maintain their form via reproduction (Canguilhem 1989, p. 144). For Canguilhem, however, the pathology of such anomalies would be based on their inability to establish a new norm, not merely their deviation from the species ideal. Conversely, the "normality" of such anomalies would be based on their ability to survive in the new environment, thereby establishing a new norm:

[7]See also van der Steen and Thung (1988, p. 90) for a similar critique that Boorse's view, while relative to age and sex, does not adequately account for how environmental changes produce physiological changes. The reference values used to establish "normal" function cannot be separated from the environment in which they occur, thereby undermining Boorse's idealized account of normality. Van der Steen and Thung accuse Boorse of appealing to hypothetical "non-biological" environments and thus of doing "bad biology." This issue is further discussed in Ananth (2008, pp. 159–161) who argues that despite his attempts Boorse has not provided a convincing reply.

"biological normality is determined by the interaction between structures and behaviours, on the one hand, and environmental conditions, on the other" (Canguilhem 1994, p. 352). Some recent findings in the field of developmental plasticity suggest that a "non-typical but viable phenotype is not *broken* by its failure to comply with some imagined blueprint for its species. It will function anyhow, in spite of its a typicality" (Amundson 2000, p. 39). The usual example given is that of the goat born without forelegs but which, through various morphological alterations, was able to adapt to living as a biped (West-Eberhard 2005). Such examples suggest that while biological processes do contribute to the goals of survival and reproduction, these processes often have no inherent aim at reproducing identical functioning, but are flexible so as to produce a variety of adaptations depending on the environmental conditions (Amundson 2000, p. 43). It is thus not relative to a species ideal, but to how the individual organism or function finds its own way to live and operate in relation to various environmental demands that the distinction between anomaly and disease is to be determined.

It seems plausible to argue that as mutations are not pathological simply because they are anomalous or atypical, then biological norms are not normal or pathological in themselves, but only in relation to the individual and its environment: "These two [anomaly and mutation] express other possible norms of life. If these norms are inferior to specific earlier norms in terms of stability, fecundity, variability of life, they will be called pathological" (Canguilhem 1989, p. 144). New variations or mutations involve spatial considerations, describing facts of individual variation in structure and function, whereas pathologies involve temporal considerations, referring to a disruption, actual or possible, of an organism's actions or course of life.[8] Of course, one can object that this distinction is rarely contested, but the point is that within the normalization view, this distinction can become obscured, and possibly conflated, if it does not fully account for the individual-environment relation.

To address such a possible problem, Boorse does say (1977, p. 566) that structural deformities are only diseases when they disrupt normal functioning. However, the point that we wish to make is that it is not merely by a divergence from species-typical functioning that the anomalous becomes abnormal, but *relative to the individual for whom the deformity may or may not inhibit some function in a given environment*. The example of the anomaly thus seems to be the exception that proves the rule regarding the relativity of health judgments (Canguilhem 2008, p. 129). Boorse is correct to argue that statistical divergence is insufficient, but he

[8]"An anomaly is a fact of individual variation which prevents two beings from being able to take the place of each other completely. [...] But diversity is not a disease; the *anomalous* is not the pathological. Pathological implies *pathos*, the direct and concrete feeling of suffering and impotence, the feeling of life gone wrong" (Canguilhem 1989, p. 137). However, as deterioration and impotence with regards to biological normativity are equivalent to the suffering of the organism, this implies, as has been pointed out with regards to mental disorders, that calling diseases "harmful dysfunctions" (Wakefield 1992) is redundant (De Block 2008).

does not follow through with the implications of this. As such, naturalism could be both extended and limited: extended so as to include the particular environment in which a function or individual lives, but limited by making the individual the crucial reference class.[9] This is not to deny physiological regularities, but rather to acknowledge that such norms result from historically and geographically contingent behaviours whose individuality goes beyond sex and age to include the specific demands of everyday life:

> Instead of considering a specific type as being really stable because it presents characteristics devoid of any incompatibility, it could be considered as being apparently stable because it has temporarily succeeded in reconciling opposing demands by means of a set of compensations. A normal specific form would be the product of a normalization between functions and organs whose synthetic harmony is obtained in defined conditions and is not given. (Canguilhem 1989, p. 162)

Normality is thus the *effect* of the competing demands of the organism and its environment. Rather than abstracting from such specific conditions, a theory of health and disease would do better to embrace them.

A few examples can help to illustrate this point and show the limitations of the naturalistic approach. First, it can be argued that dyslexia need only be considered a dysfunction within an environment where the behaviour of reading is widespread and important. It seems, at the least, very awkward to say that people in illiterate societies can have dyslexia. Canguilhem provides similar examples: "With a disability like astigmatism or myopia, one would be normal in an agricultural or a pastoral society but abnormal for sailing or flying" (1989, p. 201). Also, whether seasonal affective disorder (SAD) is considered a dysfunction can change depending on an individual's country of origin and their current environment. Someone from Africa diagnosed with SAD can be said to have a dysfunction while in Africa, but upon moving to a northern climate the changed environment can render the condition liveable, thus negating the diagnosis of having a dysfunction *in that environment* (De Block 2008). This view helps to account for the role that social norms, cultural practices, and the physical environment play in shaping diagnoses, and exemplifies Canguilhem's claim that there is no normal or pathological phenomenon in itself but only through its relation to a particular environment.

The example of intercultural differences regarding the ability to digest the lactose found in cows' milk (Canguilhem 1989, p. 168) and how this ability is based on differing social norms further shows the environmental and individual relativity of health judgments. More recently, this example of culturally relative differences in the presence of genes for lactose absorption has been described from the perspectives of niche construction and gene-culture co-evolution (Laland et al. 2010). These theories argue that it was not because there were such genes, established in

---

[9]In fact, Kingma (2010, p. 247) claims that the "situation-specificity" of functions seems to be implicit in Boorse. However, she admits that by making such an element explicit, she could be modifying the theory. It is our contention that even if such an element is implicit in his theory, the implications of making it explicit require some changes that Boorse would likely object to, such as the individual relativity of health judgments.

relation to some underlying species ideals, that the practice of dairy farming emerged, but rather that the activity of dairy farming itself created the selection pressures for such genes to spread (Laland et al. 2007, p. 55). Here what becomes biologically normal is based on different ways of life, not vice versa, thus showing how physiology is shaped by historically changing behaviours of niche construction. Furthermore, whether or not a given trait or mutation, such as the inability to digest lactose, needs to be diagnosed as a disease depends on whether a given individual is in an environment where dairy is consumed. It does not depend on the average impact of dairy consumption on the reproductive success and longevity of the average human (or the average adult woman). Gluckman et al. point out the difficulty in defining disease in such an example:

> Can we really say that the majority of humans have a disease because they do not carry a single nucleotide polymorphism that causes lactase to persist into adulthood, a deficiency that is of no consequence for their health or fitness in the context of an environment free from cows' milk? Rather, should we label the species-atypical state of lactase persistence in people of northern European origin as the *abnormal* condition and then reflect on the context-sensitive dichotomy between abnormality and ill-health? (2009, p. 5)

Rather than shy away from the context-sensitivity of medical judgments, Canguilhem's individual and environmental relativity of health and disease help to explain such examples. What these examples suggest is that as physiological changes take place within and because of human norms, it is not the average that determines norms of life, but norms of life that determine what will be considered average (Canguilhem 1989, p. 178). The point is not to deny that some conditions such as lactose persistence can become statistically average in a given population, but to stress the fact that such averages are the result of historically changing human activities and environments and thus medical judgments concerning the nature of such conditions would be more accurate if kept relative to such norms.

Given this environmental and individual relativity regarding disease, Canguilhem's view seems to ameliorate the naturalist position by defining disease as a "positive, innovative experience in the living being" (1989, p. 186) that cannot be accounted for if disease is *merely* quantitative or subordinated to normality. More completely, disease is a "behaviour (*comportement*) of negative value for a concrete individual living being in a relation of polarized activity with [its] environment" (223). In this view, disease is not unnatural as it "is still a norm of life but it is an inferior norm in the sense that it tolerates no deviation from the conditions in which it is valid, incapable as it is of changing itself into another norm" (183). This definition describes three aspects of disease.

First, rather than being merely the violation of a norm, it entails the *presence* of new physiological or structural norms that have a negative value as they involve a limitation on an individual's range of behaviours. Disease is not viewed as a privation or lack of organization, but a new organization which obliges the individual to behave differently (Canguilhem 2008, p. 132). Oliver Sacks has similarly captured the problem of reducing disease to mere deviations when he argues that "disease is never a mere loss or excess—that there is always a reaction, on the part of the affected organism or individual, to restore, to replace, to compensate for and to preserve its identity, however strange the means may be" (1998, p. 6). Disease is lived as an inferior norm since it entails a hindrance or limitation on the comportment of the individual in relation to its environment, but it also expresses the organism's ability to find new ways of meeting environmental demands. As disease reveals new physiological possibilities it expresses the organism's non-indifference to its life and as such is in no way unnatural.[10]

Second, the qualification of disease rests on *individual* norms, implying that the individual should be compared to itself, at different times and in different environments and that because each individual is different, even if only slightly, what is abnormal for one need not apply to others depending on their unique physiology and their environment. "It is the individual who is the judge of this transformation [from normal to pathological] because it is he who suffers from it from the very moment he feels inferior to the tasks which the new situation imposes upon him" (Canguilhem 1989, p. 182). He thus starts from the claim that the value or viability of an individual (or a function), i.e. whether or not it will survive (or contribute to survival), is not determined a priori by its relation to some transcendent Platonic ideal or statistical norm, but according to the individual's contingent ability to establish its own norms in a particular environment (2008, p. 125). While this individual relativity seems to erase the boundary between health and disease, Canguilhem argues that even if we accept that "from one individual to the next the relativity of the normal is the rule" (2008, p. 130), this does not erase the absolute difference between these states for the individual. For the individual, disease is *qualitatively* different than health.[11]

Third, these first two aspects are understood in relation to the individual's *mode of life*, i.e. its actions, needs and preferences as expressed in a changing environment.[12] This claim that disease is experienced as a negative value in a given environment can help to address the possible objection that this would imply a normative definition of health and disease in terms of desirability. While Canguilhem stresses the role that the conscious experience of disease has played in the historical development of medicine as a human practice, which is what ultimately forces him to appeal to the "subjective" elements of disease (1989, p. 229),

---

[10]The "sick man is not abnormal because of the absence of a norm but because of his incapacity to be normative" (Canguilhem 1989, p. 186). In other words, "for the individual, disease is a new life, characterized by new physiological constants and new mechanisms for obtaining apparently unchanged results" (ibid, p. 188).

[11]For a thorough description of the concept of individuality in Canguilhem, see Gayon (1998).

[12]Giroux (2008, 2010) criticizes this aspect of Canguilhem's theory by claiming that it cannot account for more recent advances in biology regarding multi-level selection and it inhibits an understanding of epidemiology. These critiques, while interesting, tend to miss one main point: individual differences matter because organisms actively shape their environments, whether singularly or in groups, thereby demanding that norms be considered relative to this organism-environment relation. Giroux also misrepresents the current state of biology, overlooking how the organism, or at least the level of phenotypes, still plays a crucial role in natural selection (Bateson 2005; Huneman 2010).

what is implied is not necessarily a psychological or phenomenological evaluation, such as referring to one's subjective description of what it means to be diseased, e.g. what disease means *for me* as I experience it or as I form a conscious representation of it. Rather, what is at stake is describing how disease affects the activities, the modes of living of individuals, which as we saw in the above examples, are thoroughly influenced by social norms. As such, irrespective of one's desires, the judgment of the distinction between health and disease can still be made relative to an individual's activity in a particular milieu. For example, even the diagnosis of sterility as a disease cannot be based solely on physiological determinations, since it need only be considered a dysfunction for an individual who is trying to reproduce (irrespective of whether they value such reproduction). Regardless of the supposed "demands" of our genes, reproduction is a luxury, not a necessity. Similarly, while celiac disease prevents one from eating foods containing gluten, the judgment that the lack of certain enzymes entails a dysfunction seems unwarranted in a gluten-free environment, i.e. where the *practice* of eating gluten is absent. In both cases, the judgment that such conditions are pathological would be more accurate by incorporating the individual's environment and behaviours.

Disease is thus a disruption of one's actions, regardless of whether these actions are based on desires. Mirroring Spinoza's critique of teleology (*Ethics*, Book 1, trans. Parkinson, 2000), we could argue that disease is not devalued in relation to what is objectively good (as an ideal), but its (negative) value is based on the organism's activity amidst the changing conditions of its life. Thus, it is not the normalizing scientist who dictates which values are positive or negative to the living being based on quantification, abstraction and exclusion,[13] making the line between health and disease decidedly not a mere academic affair (Boorse 1977, p. 559): it is relative to the concrete living individual, in its particular environment, that such judgements should be made.

5 From Environmental to Social Relativity?

According to Canguilhem, normality cannot be established a priori, or deduced from physiological regularities, but is relative to the individual and to the environment the individual is living in. It is this relativity that leads him to argue that the "normal is not a static or peaceful, but a dynamic and polemical concept" (Canguilhem, 1989, p. 239). We presented evidence and arguments in favour of this view. Moreover, we also argued that this view solves many of the problems that Boorse's biostatistical account of disease is confronted with. We conclude this paper with a short discussion of the role of social norms for disease judgments and the problems this issue might or might not raise for Canguilhem.

---

[13] "One does not scientifically dictate norms to life" (Canguilhem 1989, p. 226).

Many species are social species, our species being one of them. This means that we rely on other human beings for teaching us what to eat and what not, for healing us when we are sick and for consoling us when we are feeling sad or lonely. An interesting consequence is that the human environment is—to a large extent—a social environment, both because it was constructed in part by other individuals of our species, and because other people are part of the environment. Now, if health and disease are relative to the environment, as Canguilhem claims, then one can expect that health and disease in a social species like ours are, in part, relative to the social environment.

To some extent, this point was already underscored by our example of dyslexia: in environments where reading and writing are expected and important for the well-being and overall functioning of an individual, dyslexia can be a disorder, whereas the condition is not pathological in illiterate societies. Yet, it seems that there are examples of "social relativity" that challenge Canguilhem's account. Take for instance homosexuality. Individuals who prefer to have sex with individuals of their own sex have been treated differently by different cultures. In Western Europe prejudice against homosexuality and homosexuals was almost endemic for much of the last millennium. Even worse, during that period many homosexuals were incarcerated for their homosexuality and it was not uncommon to execute so-called "sodomites" (Gerard and Hekma 1989). Luckily, Western Europe has witnessed a dramatic change in sexual values to such a degree that discrimination based on sexual orientation or preference has become illegal in many countries. In this case, the emphasis on the environmental relativity of disease may seem to lead to the judgment that homosexuality is a disease in some social environments and normal/healthy in other environments. But wouldn't this conclusion be too close to the normativist view that defines health and disease in terms of desirability?

In our view, Canguilhem's position leads to the conclusion that homosexuality was a disease during the era that it was heavily stigmatized, and stopped being a disease after it was (widely) accepted. Yet, for several reasons this might be easier to accept than many would expect. For instance, it is clear that calling homosexuality a disease (or a sin) may convince some homosexual individuals that they are suffering from a disease, especially if they cannot adapt their desires and behaviours to the very strict sexual norms of the society they grew up in. Furthermore, the social nature of humans also implies that humans are very good at internalizing social norms. If the homosexual individual has internalized the anti-gay norms, he is bound to feel extremely guilty for his desires, or he may feel extremely disgusted about himself every time he acts upon his desires. You do not have to be a Freudian to see that this intra-psychic conflict can lead to serious psychiatric problems. These first two points might serve as a lubricant for accepting the view that homosexuality is a disease in some societies (and not in others!). However, they are far from compelling since the real problem seems to be that Canguilhem has to claim that homosexuality is a disease in some homophobic societies *even when the homosexual individual does not see his sexual orientation as a disease and even if there is no intra-psychic conflict within the homosexual individual*. In such a context the threat of being ostracized, the continual policing of one's behaviour, or the general social pressures to conform would be sufficient.

Why could that be an acceptable view? First, saying that homosexuality is a disease in some environments does not necessary reflect a moral condemnation of homosexuality. To be perfectly clear about this, we condemn homophobia while still arguing that a homophobic environment could make homosexuality a diseased condition. Secondly, emphasizing the environmental relativity of normality and disease also entails that therapeutic interventions and prophylactic measures can focus on the interaction between individual and environment, but also *solely* on the environment or on the individual. The case of homosexuality seems to be an example where the best results are to be expected from changes in the social environment.

References

Amundson, R. (2000). Against normal function. *Studies in History and Philosophy of Biological and Biomedical Sciences, 31*(1), 33–53.

Ananth, M. (2008). *In defence of an evolutionary concept of health: Nature, norms, and human biology*. Hampshire: Ashgate Publishing.

Bateson, P. (2005). The return of the whole organism. *Journal of Biosciences, 30*(1), 31–39.

Blumberg, M. S. (2009). *Freaks of nature: And what they tell us about development and evolution*. Oxford: Oxford University Press.

Boorse, C. (1975). On the distinction between disease and illness. *Philosophy and Public Affairs, 5* (1), 49–68.

Boorse, C. (1976). Wright on functions. *The Philosophical Review, 85*(1), 70–86.

Boorse, C. (1977). Health as a theoretical concept. *Philosophy of Science, 44*(4), 542–573.

Boorse, C. (1997). A Rebuttal on Health. In J. M. Humber & R. F. Almeder (Eds.), *What is disease?* (pp. 3–134). Totowa: Humana Press.

Brown, W. M. (1985). On defining "disease". *The Journal of Medicine and Philosophy, 10*, 311–328.

Canguilhem, G. (1988). *Ideology and rationality in the history of the life sciences* (A. Goldhammertrans, Trans.). Cambridge: MIT Press.

Canguilhem, G. (1989). *The normal and the pathological* (C. R. Fawcett & R. S. Cohen, Trans.). New York: Zone Books.

Canguilhem, G. (1994). Normality and normativity. In F. Delaporte (Ed.), *A vital rationalist: Selected writings from Georges Canguilhem* (A. Goldhammer, Trans.). New York: Zone Books.

Canguilhem, G. (2008). *Knowledge of life* (S. Geroulanos & D. Ginsberg, Trans.). New York: Fordham University Press.

Chimisso, C. (2003). The tribunal of philosophy and its norms: History and philosophy in George Canguilhem's historical epistemology. *Studies in History and Philosophy of Biological and Biomedical Sciences, 34*, 297–327.

Daniels, J. (1987). Justice and health care. In D. Van deVeer & T. Regan (Eds.), *Health care ethics* (pp. 290–325). Philadelphia: Temple University Press.

De Block, A. (2008). Why mental disorders are just mental dysfunctions (and nothing more): some Darwinian arguments. *Studies in History and Philosophy of Science, 39*(3), 338–346.

Gayon, J. (1998). The concept of individuality in Canguilhem's philosophy of Biology. *Journal of the History of Biology, 31*, 305–325.

Giroux, É. (2008). N'y a-t-il de santé que de l'individu ? Un point de vue épidémiologique sur les thèses de Canguilhem. In Hee-Jin Han (Ed.), *Philosophie et Médecine: En hommage à Georges Canguilhem* (pp. 171–193). Paris: Vrin.

Giroux, É. (2010). *Après Canguilhem: définir la santé et la maladie*. Paris: Presses Universitaires de France.

Gluckman, P., Beedle, A., & Hanson, M. (2009). *Principles of evolutionary medicine*. Oxford: Oxford University Press.

Hacking, I. (1990). *The taming of chance*. Cambridge: Cambridge University Press.

Gerard, K., & Hekma, G. (Eds.). (1989). *The pursuit of sodomy: Male homosexuality in renaissance and enlightenment Europe*. Binghampton: Harrington Park Press.

Hull, D. (1998). On human nature. In D. L. Hull & M. Ruse (Eds.), *The philosophy of biology* (pp. 383–397). Oxford: Oxford University Press.

Huneman, P. (2010). Assessing the prospects for a return of organisms in evolutionary biology. *History and Philosophy of the Life Sciences, 32*, 341–372.

Kingma, E. (2007). What is it to be healthy? *Analysis, 67*, 128–133.

Kingma, E. (2010). Paracetamol, poison, and polio: Why Boorse's account of function fails to distinguish health and disease. *British Journal for the Philosophy of Science, 61*, 241–264.

Laland, K. N., Kendal, J. R., & Brown, G. R. (2007). The Niche construction perspective: Implications for evolution and human behaviour. *Journal of Evolutionary Psychology, 5*(1-4), 51–66.

Laland, K. N., Odling-Smee, J., & Myles, S. (2010). How culture shaped the human genome: Bringing genetics and the human sciences together. *Nature Reviews, 11*, 137–148.

Méthot, P.-O. (2009). French epistemology overseas: Analyzing the influence of Georges Canguilhem in Québec. *Humana Menta, 9*, 39–58.

Nesse, R. M. (2001). On the difficulty of defining disease: A Darwinian perspective. *Medicine, Health Care and Philosophy, 4*, 37–46.

Nordenfelt, L. (2007). The concepts of health and illness revisited. *Medicine, Health Care and Philosophy, 10*, 5–10.

Pigliucci, M. (2001). *Phenotypic plasticity: Beyond nature and nurture*. Baltimore: The Johns Hopkins University Press.

Roudinesco, E. (2008). *Philosophy in turbulent times: Canguilhem, Sartre, Foucault, Althusser, Deleuze, Derrida* (W. McCuaig, Trans.). New York: Columbia University Press.

Sacks, O. (1998). *The man who mistook his wife for a hat: And other clinical tales*. New York: Touchstone.

Spinoza, B. (2000). *Ethics* (G. H. R. Parkinson, Trans.). Oxford: Oxford University Press.

Stulp, G., Pollet, T. V., Verhulst, S., & Buunk, A. P. (2012). A curvilinear effect of height on reproductive success in human males. *Behavioral Ecology and Sociobiology, 66*(3), 375–384.

Vácha, J. (1978). Biology and the problem of normality. *Scientia, 113*, 823–846.

Vácha, J. (1985). German constitutional doctrine in the 1920s and 1930s and pitfalls of the contemporary conception of normality in biology and medicine. *The Journal of Medicine and Philosophy, 10*, 339–367.

van der Steen, W. J., & Thung, P. J. (1988). *Faces of medicine: A philosophical study*. Dordrecht: Kluwer Academic Publishers.

Wakefield, J. (1992). The concept of mental disorder: On the boundary between biological facts and social values. *American Psychologist, 47*(3), 373–388.

West-Eberhard, M. J. (2005). Developmental plasticity and the origin of species differences. *Proceedings of the National Academy of Sciences, 102*(suppl. 1), 6543–6549.

Whitehouse, P. J., Juengst, E. T., Mehlman, M., & Murray, T. H. (2004). From "enhancing cognition in the intellectually intact". In A. L. Caplan, J. J. McCartney, & D. A. Sisti (Eds.), *Health, illness, and disease: Concepts in medicine* (pp. 263–267). Washington, D.C.: Georgetown University Press.

Chapter 10
Are Paraphilias Mental Disorders? The Case of the DSM

Pieter R. Adriaens

1 Introduction

Throughout history, many unusual[1] sexual behaviors and desires have been considered problematic. First of all, they have often been seen as criminal offenses. Numerous books of the Old Testament already stipulated that transvestism and bestiality, among many other things, should be punished harshly (Aggrawal 2009). Having sex with animals, for example, was described in *Leviticus* (20:16) as a capital offence for all parties involved: "And if a woman approach unto any beast, and lie down thereto, thou shalt kill the woman, and the beast: they shall surely be put to death; their blood shall be upon them." More recently, since 1871, the infamous "paragraph 175" of the German penal code made some homosexual acts punishable by imprisonment. The law remained on the books, at least in West Germany, until 1994 (Whisnant 2012). Secondly, unusual sexual behaviors and desires have also been condemned as vices. The moral condemnation of such behaviors and desires can be inferred from the wide range of depreciatory adjectives that have been used in the canon of Western literature to describe them: "inappropriate", "unfortunate", "depraved", "regrettable", "unnatural" and even "monstrous" (Bagemihl 1999). In this context, animals (again) often met with the same fate as humans. For example: when a nineteenth-century entomologist observed repeated copulations between male soldier beetles and male fireflies, he charged them with blatant immorality ("*une immoralité flagrante*") and guilty complicity ("*une complaisance coupable*") (Peragallo 1863, p. 663). Thirdly and finally, since

[1]The word "unusual" is used here to refer to both the (relative) statistical rarity of certain sexual behaviours and desires, *and* their salience, i.e. their being able to generate heated debates and extreme emotions.

P.R. Adriaens (✉)
Institute of Philosophy, University of Leuven, Leuven, Belgium
e-mail: Pieter.adriaens@hiw.kuleuven.be

D. Meacham (ed.), *Medicine and Society, New Perspectives in Continental Philosophy*, Philosophy and Medicine 120, DOI 10.1007/978-94-017-9870-9_10

the mid-nineteenth century, unusual sexual behaviors and desires have also been conceptualized as disorders (or symptoms of disorders). Variously labeled as "sexual perversions", "sexual deviations" or, in recent years, "paraphilias" (Bullough 2003), they came to be seen as "aberrant", "abnormal", "defective" and "disordered".[2] Early psychiatrists and psychologists indeed interpreted these behaviors and desires as pathological modifications of the sexual instinct, rather than crimes or moral lapses (Oosterhuis 2000). They also devised new names for (some of) them, and constructed a list of "usual suspects"—a list of disease categories that included homosexuality, sadism, pedophilia, fetishism, exhibitionism, voyeurism, masochism, zoophilia, frotteurism, necrophilia and transvestism.

The above three attitudes towards unusual sexual behaviors and desires—criminalizing, moralizing, and pathologizing—peacefully coexisted throughout the past two centuries, and in fact they still do in many parts of the world. The main aim of this chapter is to contribute to a burgeoning literature that questions the legitimacy and usefulness of the third and most recent attitude towards sexual deviance, i.e. pathologizing (see, e.g. Davidson 2001; Roughgarden 2004; Moser and Kleinplatz 2005). Why are certain sexual behaviors and desires still conceptualized as (symptoms of) mental disorders? In other words: what reasons are there to believe that these conditions are *disorders* rather than, for example, instances of ordinary criminality, immorality, or eccentricity (social deviance)?

Here I will answer this question by focusing on the American Psychiatric Association's dealings with sexual deviance, as laid out in the consecutive editions of its famous manual, the *Diagnostic and Statistical Manual of Mental Disorders* (DSM). There are three reasons for choosing this particular focus. First, the DSM is the leading clinical manual of contemporary psychiatry. It is used worldwide for diagnostic and administrative purposes, and it provides the backbone of much of today's psychiatric research. Even though the manual has attracted vehement criticism in the past decades, and even though it certainly does not represent the opinions of all psychiatrists all over the world, it is unmistakably an authoritative document, compiled by the world's most powerful professional organization of psychiatrists. As such, it deserves our attention. Secondly, focusing on the DSM is timely. Its long-anticipated fifth edition (DSM-5) was published just recently, in May 2013, and the working group devoted to revising the subclass of the paraphilias in this edition announced some important changes vis-à-vis earlier editions. Ever since its first edition in 1952, the DSM has listed the sexual deviations as mental disorders. Will this tradition be continued, and perhaps legitimated, in DSM-5?

A third and final reason to focus on the DSM relates to the fact that it is based on an explicit definition of the concept of mental disorder. The question whether paraphilias are mental disorders inevitably leads us back to an underlying

[2]Note that, for reasons of readability, I will use such expressions and terms as "unusual sexual behaviours and desires," "sexual perversion," "sexual deviation," and "paraphilia" interchangeably. "Sexual deviance" refers to the set of unusual sexual behaviours and desires available to a particular society at a particular time.

conceptual question: what is mental disorder? What necessary and sufficient conditions, if any, does a set of behaviors and desires have to fulfill in order to be a mental disorder? Since 1980, the DSM provides, in its general introduction, an answer to this question. I will argue, however, that the manual fails to provide an exhaustive and coherent analysis of the concept of mental disorder. Moreover, it also fails to design a classification of mental disorders that is consistent with whatever analysis it does provide. In other words: given the manual's messy definition of mental disorder, advocates of the DSM cannot convincingly continue to claim that all paraphilias are mental disorders.

In the present chapter, I will start by explaining briefly how psychiatry got involved in studying sexual deviance in the first place. Then I will move on to a discussion of the DSM's conceptualization of sexual deviance, starting with the first two editions. These set the stage for one of the most intriguing chapters in the history of the American Psychiatric Association: the controversy over homosexuality. I will argue that this controversy has been vital in the introduction and formulation of a general definition of mental disorder in DSM-III, published in 1980. Further, in discussing the later editions of DSM, including the recent fifth edition, it will become clear that the paraphilias provide an excellent example of the manual's constant struggle to be consistent with its own definition of mental disorder. I conclude with a general critique of the DSM approach of sexual deviance.

2 Revolutionizing Sexual Deviance

In retrospect, one may wonder why sexual deviance became a medical and psychiatric issue in the first place. Since time immemorial, sexual deviations had been repudiated by philosophers, physicians and naturalists, either as crimes or as vices. So how did they "suddenly"[3] come to be seen as disorders? Here I list two important reasons that help explain the nineteenth-century pathologising of sexual deviance.

First of all, the eighteenth and nineteenth century witnessed a growing political concern about the vitality and health of nations and peoples (Gerard and Hekma 1989); the birth of what French historian and philosopher Michel Foucault would later call "biopolitics". To address the spectre of depopulation and degeneration, politicians enlisted the help of physicians and psychiatrists, as they were held in high regard by both the public opinion and the authorities. Thus originated the eighteenth-century medical literature about the health hazards of masturbation and various other kinds of non-reproductive sexual behavior—a literature that continued to be popular

[3]Some historians of sexuality have argued that sexual deviance had in fact been pathologized before the nineteenth century. Commenting on Avicenna's work, for example, the fifteenth-century French physician Jacques Despars interpreted same-sex sexuality as a disorder that is not amenable to medical treatment (Neal 2008).

until well into the first half of the twentieth century. The nineteenth-century pathologizing of sexual deviance probably reflected (and certainly fed) a similar anxiety.[4] Much like the other two attitudes vis-à-vis unusual behaviors and desires, i.e. criminalizing and moralizing, pathologizing acted as a powerful deterrent to engage in such practices, and it provided the extra bonus of possible therapeutic interventions.

Secondly, nineteenth-century psychiatrists were able to set themselves up as experts in the domain of sexual deviance because they succeeded in *psychologizing* such deviance (Oosterhuis 2000). Unusual sexual behaviors and desires, they argued, should be understood at the level of an individual's psychology, rather than his or her behavior or anatomy. One of the landmarks in this process of psychologizing is the work of Richard von Krafft-Ebing—an Austrian forensic psychiatrist who authored the famous *Psychopathia Sexualis* in 1886. Krafft-Ebing drew an important distinction between sexual perversions and sexual perversities, equating the former with "diseases" and the latter with "vices" (Krafft-Ebing 1965 [1886], p. 54). In his view, *perversities* are occasional unusual sexual behaviors. It is only when the individual's personality as a whole becomes involved in producing such perversities that one is entitled to speak of a sexual *perversion*. The different perversions, then, are in fact different ways of being a person. As such, they cannot be diagnosed on the basis of behaviors alone; mental states, such as feelings and beliefs, need to be taken into account too. When discussing homosexuality, for example, Michel Foucault accurately captured Krafft-Ebing's "revolution" when he observed that "homosexuality appeared as one of the forms of sexuality when it was transposed from the practice of sodomy into a kind of interior androgyny, a hermaphroditism of the soul. The sodomite had been a temporary aberration; the homosexual was now a species" (Foucault 1978, p. 43). If psychiatrists are any good in dealing with the troubled mind, and if homosexuality is a "hermaphroditism of the soul" (43), then psychiatrists are indeed entitled to deal with homosexuality and, by extension, with all kinds of sexual deviations.

3 The Early DSM and the Paraphilias (1952–1980)

Many of Krafft-Ebing's ideas on sexual deviance have been immensely influential in twentieth-century psychiatry. His nomenclature and general biomedical perspective, for example, still pervade many contemporary psychiatric classifications of sexual deviations, including the *Diagnostic and Statistical Manual of Mental Disorders* (DSM). In this section, I will briefly discuss the origins and early editions of this manual, while focusing on their dealings with sexual deviance.

---

[4]In fact both episodes in the history of sexuality are connected, to the extent that many nineteenth-century psychiatrists emphasised the role of masturbation in the aetiology of sexual deviations and various other kinds of insanity (Rimke and Hunt 2002).

The DSM originated from the need for a uniform reporting of statistics of the many mental hospitals in early twentieth-century America (Grob 1991). Its predecessor, the *Statistical Manual for the Use of Hospitals for Mental Diseases*, first published in 1918, reflected the then population of these hospitals, as it concentrated mostly on severe brain disorders, often with an organic etiology (National Committee for Mental Hygiene [NCMH] 1918). One of the manual's clinical groups was given the enigmatic name "Not Insane", and included a disease category called "constitutional psychopathic personality (without psychosis)," which in its turn referred to "criminal traits, moral deficiency, tramp life, sexual perversions and various temperamental peculiarities" (27). In a way, then, DSM's predecessor did not consider the sexual perversions as mental disorders. The message was more ambiguous, however, since "perverts" and tramps and criminals were also referred to as "pathological" and even "abnormal personalities" (27).

The origin of the *Statistical Manual* as an instrument to collect mental hospital data was predictive of the difficulties it was about to encounter. The strains and rigors at the fronts of World War II brought back shipments of American soldiers whose illnesses were nowhere to be found in the manual. Combat fatigue and shell shock produced relatively mild mental disorders, at least when compared to the grave afflictions found in mental hospitals. Faced with an enormous new patient population, the American Psychiatric Association quickly understood the need to expand its stock of disease categories. In 1952, it published the first edition of the *Diagnostic and Statistical Manual: Mental Disorders* (DSM-I; APA 1952). Among its novelties was an extensive category of *Transient Situational Personality Disorders*.

DSM-I had very little to say about the sexual deviations. They were catalogued as one of the "sociopathic personality disturbances" that, in their turn, were part of the general category of "personality disorders." Interestingly, the description of "sociopathic personality disturbance" reads: "Individuals to be placed in this category are ill primarily in terms of society and of conformity with the prevailing cultural milieu, and not only in terms of personal discomfort and relations with other individuals" (APA 1952, p. 38). It is one of the rare occasions where the editors of DSM-I hint at a definition of mental disorder. Unlike later editions of the manual, the first DSM did not provide an explicit definition of mental disorder (and neither did DSM-II), but its general outlook suggested that mental illness be understood either in terms of some organic defect, as in the case of the many brain disorders listed, and/or in terms of personal distress, as in the case of the neuroses. Somehow (some of) the perversions fell outside this implicit definition of mental illness, as they were seen primarily as instances of social deviance, rather than mental illness.

Like any psychiatric classification, DSM-I was a child of its time. Its descriptions of disease categories were riddled with psychoanalytic terms and concepts, such as "unconscious affects", "projection mechanisms" and "regressive reactions". Contrary to what some historians of psychiatry (e.g. Shorter 1997) and also some biological psychiatrists (e.g. Maxmen 1985) have claimed, the second edition of DSM, first published in 1968, did not really continue this tradition. Its descriptions were shorter, and speculations as to the causes and mechanisms of disorders were kept to a minimum. The pursuit of a theory-neutral or "atheoretical" nomenclature would become ever more important in later editions of DSM.

As to the perversions, one of the minor novelties of DSM-II was the introduction of an extensive list of eight sexual deviations: homosexuality, fetishism, pedophilia, transvestism, exhibitionism, voyeurism, sadism and masochism. Also, while DSM-I and its precursor considered the perversions as a kind of personality disturbances, DSM-II listed them under the rather vague heading of "certain non-psychotic mental disorders." More importantly, however, all references to the pathogenic power of social norms in the general description of the sexual deviations were omitted. Whereas DSM-I had noted that "perverts" "are ill *primarily* in terms of society and of conformity with the prevailing cultural milieu, and *not only in terms of personal discomfort*" (APA 1952, p. 38; italics mine), DSM-II resolutely focused on the personal distress accompanying these deviations: "Even though many find their practices distasteful, they remain unable to substitute normal sexual behavior for them" (APA 1968 p. 44). Much like the concern of theory-neutrality, the increasing emphasis on the criterion of personal distress was an early announcement of the looming landslide created by the appearance of DSM-III.

4 Homosexuality: A Crucial Controversy

The 1970s were turbulent times for the American Psychiatric Association. Since World War II, the majority of its members had been practicing psychoanalysts, but now the powers of psychoanalysis were waning (Decker 2007). This decline of psychoanalysis set the stage for a new wave of research psychiatrists, thus revealing a power struggle within the APA—a struggle that culminated in one of the most pressing, and perhaps even embarrassing problems in the build-up to the creation of DSM-III: the problem of homosexuality.

Perhaps more than DSM-I, DSM-II unambiguously qualified homosexuality as a mental disorder. Many commentators have coordinated this view with the predominance of psychoanalysis in the early post-war intellectual climate (e.g. Friedman and Downey 1998). Apparently many of the then psychoanalysts disagreed with Freud on the topic since Freud did *not* unambiguously consider all homosexuals to be mentally ill. In his famous letter to the mother of a homosexual man, he stated that "homosexuality is assuredly no advantage, but it is nothing to be ashamed of, no vice, no degradation; it cannot be classified as an illness" (Freud 1960 [1935], p. 423).[5] Another important difference between Freud and mid-twentieth-century psychoanalysts related to their views on the need for, and the prospects of, therapeutic interventions. Freud was remarkably clear on this topic:

---

[5]Elsewhere, however, he spoke of it as an "aberration" and an "abnormality" (Freud 1960 [1905]).

"In general to undertake to convert a fully developed homosexual into a heterosexual is not much more promising than to do the reverse, only that for good practical reasons the latter is never attempted" (Freud 1955 [1920], p. 32). For some reason, the therapeutic optimism of post-war psychoanalytic psychiatrists was markedly greater than Freud's, and many of them were actively engaged in so-called "conversion therapy" when the controversy over homosexuality erupted in the early 1970s (see, e.g. Bieber et al. 1962).

So why was it fashionable for psychoanalysts to consider homosexuality as a pathological condition? In fact many of them firmly believed that heterosexuality is a natural norm—again disagreeing with Freud. In the words of one of them, Irving Bieber: "humans are biologically programmed for heterosexuality" (Bieber 1987, p. 425). Traumatizing experiences and disturbed parent-child or peer relationships were thought to dislocate this "natural urge", thus resulting in abnormal sexual behavior. Psychoanalysts like Bieber indeed defined illness by its antecedents, and since their research supposedly showed these antecedents to be pathological, psychoanalysts could not but conclude that homosexuality was an illness. Coincidentally, the claim that heterosexuality is a natural norm was also defended by non-psychoanalysts in the 1970s. As Scholl and De Block relate, in this volume, the philosopher Christopher Boorse thought it reasonable to consider homosexuality as a disease, even though he was quick to add that such a claim would not have much practical significance (Boorse 1975, p. 63). In his view, homosexuality could be conceptualized as a disease because it conflicts with "one normal function of sexual desire," which is "to promote reproduction" (63). We will take a close look at this last claim in the final section of this chapter.

Throughout the 1960s, the illness view came under increasing attack from a variety of actors, including gay activists and public intellectuals. Judd Marmor, for example, an outspoken opponent of the psychoanalytic view, put it this way: "It is our task as psychiatrists to be healers of the *distressed*, not watchdogs of our social mores" (Marmor 1973, p. 1209). Critics of the illness theory of homosexuality put forward a number of arguments—some of which were reminiscent of the work of early European sexologists, including Magnus Hirschfeld and Havelock Ellis. First of all, they claimed that homosexuality was biologically natural. Marmor, for example, paraphrased "an eminent biologist" saying "human homosexuality reflects the essential bisexual character of our mammalian inheritance" (1209).[6] Secondly,

---

[6]Marmor obviously referred to the work of the American ethologist Frank A. Beach, who co-authored the classic *Patterns of Sexual Behavior* in 1951. Here the authors indeed made reference to "the bisexuality of the physiological mechanisms for mammalian mating behaviour" and a "fundamental mammalian heritage of general sexual responsiveness" (Ford and Beach 1951, pp. 258–9). By summarising evidence of same-sex sexual behaviour in humans and other animals, they also hoped to strengthen the view later defended by Marmor, i.e. that homosexuality should not be seen as some kind of physical abnormality, nor as a perversion of the sexual instinct. In the glossary of the book, the authors define "perversion" as "[a] term without scientific meaning. It refers to any form of sexual activity which a given social group regards as unnatural and abnormal. Activities that are classified as perversions by one society may be considered normal in another" (283).

they argued that even if heterosexuality would be a natural norm, then it would not follow that homosexuality is an illness. Celibacy and vegetarianism can also be considered as "violations" of a natural norm, Marmor argued, and yet we do not generally see them as illnesses. Thirdly, history and daily experience teach us that not all homosexuals are, or were, ill. Most of the evidence brought forward by psychoanalysts came from clinical practice, and to their critics it was obvious that such evidence could not be representative for the whole population of homosexuals (Torrey 1974). Fourthly and finally, even if the overwhelming majority of contemporary homosexuals would turn out to have psychological problems, then the question would be whether they do so because of some inherent pathology, as psychoanalysts maintained, or because of the oppressive power of a homophobic society (Gold 1973). The latter position was defended, at least implicitly, by the editors of DSM-I, and it matches the view that Scholl and De Block attribute, in this volume, to the French philosopher Georges Canguilhem. Basically, these authors take Canguilhem's analysis of the concept of normality to imply that some conditions, such as homosexuality, are diseases in some social environments, while they are normal in other environments. A homophobic society, then, is what transforms homosexuality into a disease.

By setting up arguments to show that homosexuality was neither abnormal nor an illness, Marmor provided fuel to the work of a variety of gay activist groups. From 1970 onward, some of these groups started protesting at the annual meetings of the American Psychiatric Association, where leading psychoanalysts presented their evidence to show that homosexuality was a truly pathological condition (Bayer 1981). In the midst of this dispute between activists and psychoanalysts, a young psychiatrist, Robert Spitzer, stepped up as a go-between. Spitzer was originally convinced that homosexuality did belong in DSM. Various events, however, including his attending an informal meeting of the "Gay-PA"—a secret group of homosexual APA members later known as the Association of Gay and Lesbian Psychiatrists—made him realize that many homosexuals were actually healthy and high-functioning individuals, who were often satisfied with their sexuality (Bayer 1987). Soon afterward he drafted a first compromise: homosexuality as such was to be removed from DSM, and to be replaced by "sexual orientation disturbance," which included those individuals troubled by their own sexual orientation (later rebranded as "ego-dystonic homosexuality," only to be removed altogether from DSM-III-R in 1987).

One of the important mainsprings behind this proposal was an attempt to define the concept of mental disorder. In Spitzer's view, such definition should entail two elements: "[I]t must either regularly cause subjective distress, or regularly be associated with some generalized impairment in social effectiveness or functioning" (Spitzer 1973, p. 1215). Many homosexuals did not fulfill either of these criteria, and therefore they should not be considered mentally ill. Importantly, Spitzer did not consider homosexuality as normal either: "No doubt, homosexual activist groups will claim that psychiatry has at last recognized that homosexuality is as 'normal' as heterosexuality. They will be wrong" (1216). To meet the expected objections of the psychoanalysts, he suggested to describe homosexuality as "an Irregular Form of Sexual Development" that is "suboptimal" when compared to heterosexuality. Yet suboptimal behavior, he argued, need not necessarily constitute disorder, as was shown in the examples of celibacy, racism, religious fanaticism, or vegetarianism, which he jokingly describes as "unnatural avoidance of carnivorous behavior" (1215; see also Spitzer 1981).

Despite its obvious diplomatic qualities, Spitzer's proposal met with fierce protest, and for different reasons. Activists expressed anger about the contention that homosexuality would not be as "valuable" as heterosexuality, while psychoanalysts, in their turn, repeatedly called on the APA officials not to capitulate to political pressure. Nevertheless, the proposal to eliminate homosexuality from DSM (and replace it with "sexual orientation disturbance") was unanimously accepted by the APA's board of trustees in December 1973. Following further protest from a number of leading psychoanalysts, the APA then organized a referendum: Should homosexuality be in the APA nomenclature or not? Spitzer's proposal was accepted by 58 % of the APA membership, and consequently homosexuality as such was deleted from the seventh printing of DSM-II in 1974. According to some commentators, the referendum was a public relations disaster for the APA. Devising a psychiatric nomenclature turned out to be a matter of politics rather than science (Shorter 1997; Kirk and Kutchins 1992).

Despite this sobering history, many of the then architects of DSM continued (and continue) to claim that the manual, and certainly its third edition, was the first real evidence-based and scientifically sound psychiatric classification. Until recently, Robert Spitzer stood by such views (see, e.g. Spitzer 2001). For some reason, however, he seems to have changed his mind. In an interview from early 2007, he conceded that the DSM-III task force did not always rely on research evidence. When asked about how new disease categories were included in the nomenclature, the following conversation ensued:

> Spitzer: You have to have a lobby, that's how. You have to have troops.
> Fink [one of the interviewers]: So it's not a matter of…
> Spitzer: Having the data? No.
> Fink: It's nothing to do with science then, and nothing to do with evidence?
> Spitzer nodded (Shorter 2008, p. 168).

The interviewers seem to have been shocked at this "confession," but in a sense Spitzer's honesty should not really surprise us. Immediately after the APA board's decision to delete homosexuality from their manual, the psychoanalyst Irving Bieber publicly asked Spitzer whether he would consider deleting other sexual deviations from DSM, too. Spitzer answered: "I haven't given much thought to [these problems] and perhaps that is because the voyeurs and the fetishists [unlike the homosexuals] have not yet organized themselves and forced us to do that" (quoted in Bayer 1987, p. 397; see also Bieber 1987, p. 433).

5 On Being Consistent: Defining the Paraphilias in DSM-III and DSM-IV (1980–2012)

In May 1974, immediately after the controversy over homosexuality, the American Psychiatric Association appointed Spitzer chair of the new Task Force on Nomenclature and Statistics, and his first decision was to assemble a completely new core committee. Unlike the task force of DSM-II, all members of Spitzer's group were in favor of biological psychiatry, rather than psychoanalysis, and a symptom-based rather than etiologic approach to diagnosis (Shorter 1997).

As a consequence, DSM-III, first published in 1980, differed in many ways from its predecessor (Mayes and Horwitz 2005). One novelty was the introduction of diagnostic criteria—in order to be eligible for a particular diagnosis, the patient had to fulfill a specific number of such criteria. Together with a significant increase in the number of disease categories,[7] the inclusion of these criteria more than doubled the size of the manual's previous edition. Another interesting novelty was an attempt, on the very first pages of the manual, to define the concept of mental disorder:

> In DSM-III each of the mental disorders is conceptualized as a clinically significant behavioral or psychological syndrome or pattern that occurs in an individual and that is typically associated with either a painful symptom (distress) or impairment in one or more important areas of functioning (disability). In addition, there is an inference that there is a behavioral, psychological, or biological dysfunction, and that the disturbance is not only in the relationship between the individual and society. (APA 1980, p. 6)

As I explained earlier, homosexuality was deleted from DSM-II mainly because it did not fit in with this definition of mental disorder that, according to Spitzer (1981), was also employed, though implicitly, when constructing the first two editions of the manual. This implicit definition was based on two criteria: distress and disability (or functional impairment). Because many homosexuals were not in any way distressed by their sexual orientation, and since most of them appeared to function very well, both socially and professionally, it was clear that homosexuality per se should be excluded from the manual.

But what about the other sexual deviations, such as voyeurism or sexual sadism? What evidence was there to believe that these conditions, unlike homosexuality, did cause significant distress or disability? Spitzer himself believed that the status of some of the perversions, particularly voyeurism and fetishism, as mental disorders was "questionable," and he was aware that many expected him, following the APA decision about homosexuality, to delete these conditions from the manual (Spitzer 1981, p. 406). It is possible that these reservations led him to conclude the manual's definition of mental disorder with the following caveat: "When the disturbance is limited to a conflict between an individual and society [which, according to DSM-I,

---

[7]The total number of diagnostic categories increased from 106 in DSM-I to 182 in DSM-II, and again to 265 in DSM-III. The penultimate edition, DSM-IV (APA 1994), contained no less than 297 different categories (Mayes and Horwitz 2005, p. 251).

was certainly the case for many sexual deviations], this may represent social deviance, which may or may not be commendable, but is not by itself a mental disorder" (APA 1980, p. 6); the very same statement was repeated more or less verbatim in all subsequent editions of DSM.

Still, all of DSM-II's sexual deviations simply reappeared in DSM-III, if only under a different name ("paraphilias"), and in a different diagnostic class ("psychosexual disorders"). The term "paraphilias" was preferred to the old "sexual deviations" "in that it correctly emphasizes that the deviation (para) is in that to which the individual is attracted (philia)" (APA 1980, p. 267). The new name was not just more accurate, however; it also sounded more scientific and less moralistic or judgmental (Bullough 2003). The manual went on with a list of the usual suspects: fetishism, transvestism, zoophilia, pedophilia, exhibitionism, voyeurism, sexual masochism, sexual sadism, and some "atypical" paraphilias (e.g. frotteurism and necrophilia). According to DSM-III, the common denominator of all paraphilias is "that unusual or bizarre imagery or acts are necessary for sexual excitement," involving "sexual objects or situations that are not part of normative arousal-activity patterns and that in varying degrees may interfere with the capacity for reciprocal affectionate sexual activity" (261).

It is noteworthy that the general description accompanying this class of disorders again reflected Spitzer's reservations to include them in the manual. First of all, and contrary to his aversion to all things related to theory and tradition, he noted that "the Paraphilias included here are, by and large, conditions that *traditionally* have been specifically identified by previous classifications" (APA 1980, p. 267; italics mine). Secondly, Spitzer seemed to be doubtful about how to fit in the paraphilias with DSM-III's general definition of mental disorder. He himself noted that "these individuals [with a paraphilia] assert that the[ir] behavior causes them no distress" (267) (the first criterion in the definition). Moreover, he could not but concede that at least some of them appeared to function well, both socially and professionally (the second criterion in the definition). So why did DSM-III continue to present sexual deviations as mental disorders?

DSM-III explicitly acknowledged that there may well be a continuum between sexual health and sexual deviance (APA 1980, p. 6), and that paraphilic fantasies or acts could be part of a normal sexual repertoire and a healthy sexual relationship. It recognized, for example, that "women's undergarments and imagery of sexual coercion are sexually exciting for many men" and that "masochistic fantasies of being bound, beaten, raped or otherwise humiliated may facilitate sexual excitement in some [normal] individuals" (267 and 273–274). Diagnostic criterion A stipulated, for all paraphilias, that it was only when such imagery or fantasies became "insistently and involuntarily repetitive," "repeatedly preferred or exclusive," or even "necessary" in order to achieve sexual gratification, that it was to be considered part of a proper paraphilia. In sum, what made an unusual sexual behavior or desire (or fantasy) a mental disorder, according to DSM-III, was its exclusivity and its repetitivity in arousing sexual excitement. Curiously, DSM-III seemed to follow a Freudian characterization of the paraphilias here,[8] thereby *ignoring* its very own definition of mental disorder, which it did use to legitimate the removal of homosexuality[9] (Primoratz 1997; Silverstein 1984). The general definition of mental disorder in DSM-III did not mention a word about repetitivity.

In a paper published shortly after DSM-III, Spitzer (1981) provided an alternative account of the decision to keep the paraphilias listed as mental disorders. His account focused on the importance of impairment, rather than distress or repetitivity. As Spitzer said: "we decided that even in those cases where there was no distress, the behavior represented impairment [...] in the important area of *sexual* functioning" (Spitzer 1981, p. 406, italics in original). Fetishists, zoophiliacs, and voyeurs were considered mentally ill because their behaviors and desires impaired them to engage in affectionate and reciprocal relationships; and somehow such relationships were valued more highly than a relationship between a human being and an animal, or between a human being and an inanimate object. As Spitzer concluded his paper: "I guess that deep in our bones we [psychiatrists] must believe that sex is more fulfilling when it is between human beings" (414). This argument was then and remains debatable, as I will argue later on, but it was at least compatible with the DSM's own definition of mental disorder. For some reason, however, later editions of the manual tended to ignore this specific argument, as they focused more or less exclusively on the role of distress, and introduced new disorder conditions that were not part of the general definition.

Spitzer and his colleagues were quick to spot some of the inconsistencies of DSM-III in dealing with the sexual deviations, and partly corrected them in a major revision, which was published in 1987 as DSM-III-R. One of the important novelties in DSM-III-R was that considerations of exclusivity and repetitivity were no longer deemed essential in diagnosing the paraphilias. Such considerations were replaced by two basic diagnostic criteria that applied to all paraphilias listed.

---

[8]In his early work, Freud indeed focused on the exclusivity of particular sexual behaviors and desires to distinguish between normal sexuality and pathological sexuality. Thus he claimed, in his *Three Essays on the Theory of Sexuality*: "In the majority of cases we are able to find the morbid character of the perversion not in the content of the new sexual aim but in its relation to the normal. It is morbid if the perversion does not appear beside the normal (sexual aim and sexual object), where favourable circumstances promote it and unfavourable impede the normal, or if it has under all circumstances repressed and supplanted the normal; the *exclusiveness* and *fixation* of the perversion justifies us in considering it a morbid symptom" (Freud 1960 [1905], p. 22; italics in original). .

[9]In the annotated listing of the differences between DSM-II and DSM-III (Appendix C; APA 1980, p. 380), Spitzer cited some evidence to warrant the exclusion of homosexuality: "The crucial issue in determining whether or not homosexuality per se should be regarded as a mental disorder is not the etiology of the condition, but its consequences and the definition of mental disorder. A significant proportion of homosexuals are apparently satisfied with their sexual orientation, show no significant signs of manifest psychopathology [...], and are able to function socially and occupationally with no impairment. If one uses the criteria of distress or disability, homosexuality per se is not a mental disorder."

Criterion A required the presence of "recurrent intense sexual urges and sexually arousing fantasies, over a period of at least six months," while Criterion B stipulated that "the person has acted on these urges, *or* is markedly distressed by them" (APA 1987, pp. 282–90; italics mine). There was no mention of impairment or disability in the criteria. The latter part of Criterion B, about distress, could be seen as an attempt to fit the paraphilias into the manual's general definition of mental disorder. Surprisingly, however, and contrary to this definition, distress was considered as sufficient but not necessary for a condition to qualify as a paraphilia. According to DSM-III-R, some urges and fantasies needed only be acted on to indicate disorder, even if they did not cause any distress to the individual. Repeated sexual behaviors, then, or even a single sexual behavior, could constitute a mental disorder. This conclusion was rather counter-intuitive, and it was certainly at odds with an intellectual heritage that dates back to the work of Krafft-Ebing, and his distinction between sexual perversities and sexual perversions. Krafft-Ebing once noted that "[t]he nature of the act can never, in itself, determine a decision as to whether it lies within the limits of mental pathology [...]. The perverse act does not per se indicate perversion of instinct" (Krafft-Ebing 1965 [1886], p. 501).

In DSM-IV, published in 1994, the above inconsistency was resolved by omitting the first part of criterion B. This criterion now required, for all paraphilias, only that "the fantasies, sexual urges, or behaviors cause clinically significant distress or impairment in social, occupational, or other important areas of functioning" (APA 1994, p. 523). Failing distress or impairment, unusual sexual fantasies, urges or behaviors were considered non-pathological. They may well be seen as instances of criminality or eccentricity, but not as disorders.

Even though the DSM-IV's wording of the diagnostic criteria of paraphilia was by far the most consistent with the DSM's own definition of mental disorder, its amendment was short-lived. In a later editorial, the editors of DSM-IV-TR (APA 2000), Michael First and Allen Frances, related how they were attacked by "conservative religious groups" who "*mistakenly* worried that the change meant DSM-IV did not recognize pedophilia as a mental disorder unless it caused distress" (First and Frances 2008, p. 1240; italics mine). In the view of First and Frances, the editors of DSM-IV *did* think pedophilia was a mental disorder even if it caused no distress—a statement that is obviously incorrect. As I just explained, DSM-IV stipulated that child offenders should not be considered mentally ill unless their offenses caused them distress or impairment in functioning. Yet the editors of DSM-IV-TR explicitly speak of a "misinterpretation" of DSM-IV (1240). In the end, DSM-IV-TR simply reverted to the (inconsistent) diagnostic criteria for paraphilia in DSM-III-R. For those paraphilias that may involve non-consenting victims (e.g. pedophilia) the authors simply reintroduced the old Criterion B, which required either acting on unusual urges or fantasies, *or* experiencing distress about these urges or fantasies (APA 2000, p. 566). For the remaining paraphilias (e.g. fetishism) the diagnosis is made if the urges, fantasies, or behaviors cause distress or impairment in functioning.

Elsewhere, and adding to the confusion, the editors of DSM-IV-TR also emphasized that sexual offenders should not be considered mentally ill simply because they have committed sexual offenses. They concluded: "Defining paraphilia based on acts alone blurs the distinction between mental disorder and ordinary criminality" (First and Frances, 2008, p. 1240). More recently, First has argued that, in order to avoid such confusion, it is absolutely essential to take into account the nature of the fantasies and urges preceding or accompanying the acts. Thus he remarked: "A paraphilia is [...] fundamentally a disturbed internal mental process (i.e., a deviant focus of sexual arousal) which is conceptually distinguishable from its various clinical manifestations" (First 2010, p. 1240). First's recommendation to DSM-5 is to revive a forgotten aspect of the DSM's general definition of mental disorder. Ever since DSM-III, this definition indeed specifies that a condition can only qualify as a disorder if it causes distress or impairment *and* if it is considered "a manifestation of a behavioral, psychological, or biological dysfunction in the individual" (APA 2000, p. xxiv). Unfortunately neither First nor any of the editions of DSM tell us how to define such underlying dysfunction, or how it is to be ascertained. What part of the mind would be dysfunctioning in the case of the paraphilias, for example? The answer to that question depends on how one defines the concept of function, and how one understands the function of sexuality. I will return to this issue in the final section of this chapter.

6 DSM-5, Paraphilias, and Paraphilic Disorders

Looking back, the first four editions of the *Diagnostic and Statistical Manual of Mental Disorders*, perhaps excluding DSM-II, at least allowed for the possibility that some paraphilias were not mental disorders. Both in the manual and elsewhere, editors reminded us that not all unusual sexual behaviors and desires should be considered as pathological. This view is in line with a growing literature suggesting that many paraphilias are actually harmless and hence do not necessitate any kind of intervention, whether legal or psychiatric. Studies have shown that people with paraphilias are often of above-average intelligence and social status (McConaghy 1997); that they enjoy their sexual behaviors and desires; and that actually such fantasies etc. are reported by a significant number of healthy subjects (Hinderliter 2010). On the other hand, there is also a sizable literature about putative genetic or hormonal defects and anomalous brain development in people with paraphilia (Blanchard et al. 2006); and about comorbidity with other mental disorders and various medical conditions (Kafka and Hennen 2002; Gijs 2008).

The fifth edition of DSM seems keen on making this distinction between "harmless" and "harmful" paraphilias more explicit. Early on in the revision process, the work group devoted to revising the subclass of the paraphilias in DSM-5 announced a consensus that paraphilias are not "*ipso facto* mental disorders" and that by themselves they would "not automatically justify or require clinical intervention" (APA 2012; italics in original). Therefore, the work group proposed to differentiate between paraphilias and paraphilic disorders: "A Paraphilic Disorder is a paraphilia that is currently causing distress and impairment to the individual or a paraphilia whose satisfaction has entailed personal harm, or risk of harm, to others in the past. A paraphilia is a necessary but not a sufficient condition for having a Paraphilic Disorder" (APA 2012).

Even though DSM-5 explicitly distinguishes between deviance and disorder, it makes the very same mistake it has often made in the past. Like all past editions of the manual, excluding DSM-IV, the proposal of the work group suggests indeed that acting on unusual sexual urges is relevant for psychiatric diagnosis: "[A] paraphilia whose satisfaction has entailed personal harm, or risk of harm, to others in the past" is considered as a paraphilic disorder (APA 2012). In this view, acting on unusual sexual urges determines the difference between a (harmless) paraphilia and a (harmful) paraphilic disorder. Hence, in some cases of pedophilia, sadism, voyeurism, exhibitionism, and frotteurism, the only difference between a non-disordered individual with a paraphilia and an individual with a paraphilic disorder is that the latter has had victims. The work group fails to explain, however, why and how harming others would amount to more than merely immoral or criminal behavior. Why would sexual offenses be mental disorders?

7 Arguing Against the DSM

Are paraphilias mental disorders, or are they not? To answer this question, I have scrutinized the presentation and discussion of unusual sexual behaviors and desires in the consecutive editions of the *Diagnostic and Statistical Manual of Mental Disorders*, from its very first edition in 1952 up until the freshly printed DSM-5. Since 1980, the manual boasts an elaborate definition of the concept of mental disorder—a definition it can fall back on to decide whether specific (sets of) mental or behavioral states are to be considered as mental disorders. At first glance, the DSM definition of mental disorder includes three basic conditions: distress, impairment (or disability), and dysfunction. It would seem relatively easy, then, to answer the question whether paraphilias are mental disorders or not. We just need to check whether they fulfill the relevant conditions.

Unfortunately there are a number of difficulties in following this strategy. First of all, many editions of the manual have smuggled in new disorder conditions while discussing the paraphilias—conditions that are nowhere to be found in the definition of mental disorder in the manual's general introduction. In this chapter I provided two examples of such ad hoc conditions: the condition of repetitivity in DSM-III, and the condition of acting in DSM-III-R, DSM-IV-TR, and DSM-5. The presence of these conditions conveys the impression that some juggling was needed to keep the paraphilias listed as mental disorders.[10] Secondly, some of the conditions in question are rather vague. I explained earlier, for example, that it is unclear what it means for a mental or behavioral state to be a manifestation of an underlying dysfunction. What is a dysfunction anyway? And how does it differ from impairment ? The manual itself remains utterly silent on this issue. In the remainder of this section, I will focus on this condition of dysfunction, which has been taken up by some of the past editors of DSM (Spitzer 2005; First 2010), and I will argue that in at least some of the interpretations of this condition, paraphilias need not be dysfunctions.

Ever since its third edition, the DSM has stipulated that in order for a "behavioral or psychological syndrome or pattern" to be a mental disorder, it must not only be associated with distress or impairment, but also with "a behavioral, psychological, or biological dysfunction" (APA 1980, p. 6). The latter condition is extremely important, as it allows us, still according to DSM-III, to differentiate deviance from disorder: "Neither deviant behavior (e.g., political, religious, or sexual) nor conflicts that are primarily between the individual and society are mental disorders unless the deviance or conflict is a symptom of a dysfunction in the individual" (APA 1994, p. xxxi). As explained earlier, none of the editions of DSM provides any definition of the concept of dysfunction. Spitzer (1999) acknowledged this lacuna and suggested adoption of Jerome Wakefield's evolutionary interpretation of the concept of dysfunction in the construction of DSM-5. In Wakefield's view, the concept of mental disorder is intrinsically hybrid, in that a disorder judgment requires both a value judgment that there is harm (more or less equivalent to the notion of distress in DSM) and a scientific judgment that there is a dysfunction. Wakefield (1992, p. 384) then defined dysfunction as "the inability of some internal mechanism to perform its naturally selected function." Depression, for example, can be seen as a mental disorder because it is a harmful dysfunction of our capacity to experience low mood—a mental mechanism that evolved to allow us to deal with various adverse life events (see, e.g. Price et al. 2007).

Spitzer attempted to apply this concept of dysfunction to the paraphilias in a book devoted to a critique of the sexual and gender diagnoses of DSM-IV-TR (Karasic and Drescher 2005). There he argued that sexual arousal has a specific evolutionary function, which consisted of "facilitating pair bonding which is facilitated by reciprocal affectionate relationships" (Spitzer 2005, p. 114). In Wakefield's terminology, the paraphilias represent a failure of sexual arousal to perform its naturally selected function, because people with a paraphilia are unable to be sexually aroused by

[10]Moreover, I have already explained that the ad hoc condition of acting cannot, in itself, be considered a sufficient condition for an unusual sexual desire or urge to be a disorder. The editors of DSM-IV-TR indeed admitted as much themselves, when they claimed that "[d]efining paraphilia based on acts alone blurs the distinction between mental disorder and ordinary criminality" (First and Frances 2008, p. 1240). Some would probably go one step further to argue that, for most paraphilias, the condition of acting cannot even qualify as a *necessary* condition. In Krafft-Ebing's view, for example, one can be a paraphiliac without ever realizing any of one's unusual sexual desires or fantasies (Oosterhuis 2000).

another human being or are unable to engage in a mutual loving relationship. Curiously, Spitzer's wording reminds us of an argument that he already put forward in 1981, when defending the decision of the DSM-III core committee to keep the paraphilias in the manual. At that time, he said: "we decided that even in those cases [of paraphilias] where there was no distress, the behavior represented impairment [...] in the important area of *sexual* functioning" (Spitzer 1981, p. 406, italics in original). If impairment and dysfunction are indeed identical disorder conditions, why are they systematically and explicitly distinguished in all editions of DSM since 1980?

More importantly, however, one wonders what to think of Spitzer's evolutionary argument that the sole function of sexual arousal is to facilitate pair bonding. In my view, his argument is questionable, and for two reasons. First, pair bonding can be facilitated in many ways, including, but most certainly not limited to "reciprocal affectionate relationships" (Spitzer 2005, p. 114). Sexual arousal can indeed serve to form and maintain pair bonds, but human history and the animal sciences teach us that this connection can be established via many intermediaries, including various paraphilias such as pedophilia, sadism, masochism, and transvestism. Secondly, Spitzer's argument ignores the extensive literature on the many different functions of sexuality and sexual arousal (see, e.g. Symons 1981; Roughgarden 2004). According to evolutionary biologists, any one organismal trait can have several evolutionary functions, and it is very likely that the same is true for sexual arousal. Recent work in behavioral ecology, for example, distinguishes at least half a dozen potential evolutionary functions of animal homosexuality, some of which are not directly related to pair bonding. Thus it would serve to communicate one's rank within a so-called dominance hierarchy, i.e. a ranking system which determines access to resources and mates (Vasey 1995); or it would help to reduce tension and facilitate reconciliation among group members (Bailey and Zuk 2009), and even to control population size (discussed in Vasey and Sommer 2006). Unfortunately, there is very little research on the potential function(s) of unusual sexual behaviors and desires other than homosexuality,[11] but it is possible that at least some of them may turn out to be functional, rather than dysfunctional. If so, then they cannot be considered as disorders, at least when "disorder" is defined as dysfunction, and "dysfunction" in its turn is defined as the failure of an evolved mental mechanism.

8 Conclusion

Are paraphilias mental disorders, then, or are they not? The cautious answer to this question is that it depends on what conditions we associate with the concept of mental disorder. In the end, the DSM definition of mental disorder stands on two relevant conditions: distress and dysfunction. I have argued that it is at least unclear

[11]Aronsson (2011) is an intriguing exception, but it is based on the assumption that paraphilias are biologically dysfunctional sexual preferences.

whether all unusual sexual behaviors and desires fulfill both of these conditions. By distinguishing between (non-disordered) paraphilias and paraphilic disorders, DSM-5 acknowledges this argument. Like most previous editions of the manual, however, it fails to explain where and how we should draw the line between both. Why are we to regard some unusual sexual behaviors and desires as disorders, and others as normal variations of human sexuality?

References

Aggrawal, A. (2009). References to the paraphilias and sexual crimes in the Bible. *Journal of Forensic and Legal Medicine, 16*, 109–114.

American Psychiatric Association. (1952). *Diagnostic and statistical manual: Mental disorders* (1st ed.; DSM-I). Washington, DC: Author.

American Psychiatric Association. (1968). *Diagnostic and statistical manual of mental disorders* (2nd ed.; DSM-II). Washington, DC: Author.

American Psychiatric Association. (1980). *Diagnostic and statistical manual of mental disorders* (3rd ed.; DSM-III). Washington, DC: American Psychiatric Press.

American Psychiatric Association. (1987). *Diagnostic and statistical manual of mental disorders* (3rd ed., rev.; DSM-III-R). Washington, DC: American Psychiatric Press.

American Psychiatric Association. (1994). *Diagnostic and statistical manual of mental disorders* (4th ed.; DSM-IV). Washington, DC: American Psychiatric Press.

American Psychiatric Association. (2000). *Diagnostic and statistical manual of mental disorders* (4th ed., text rev.; DSM-IV-TR). Washington, DC: American Psychiatric Press.

American Psychiatric Association. (2012). Changes affecting the diagnostic criteria for all paraphilic disorders. Retrieved from http://www.dsm5.org/ProposedRevision/Pages/proposed-revision.aspv?rid=62#.

Aronsson, H. (2011). Sexual imprinting and fetishism: An evolutionary hypothesis. In P. Adriaens & A. De Block (Eds.), *Maladapting minds: Philosophy, psychiatry, and evolutionary theory* (pp. 65–90). Oxford: Oxford University Press.

Bagemihl, B. (1999). *Biological exuberance: Animal homosexuality and natural diversity*. New York: St. Martin's Press.

Bailey, N. W., & Zuk, M. (2009). Same-sex sexual behavior and evolution. *Trends in Ecology and Evolution, 24*, 439–446.

Bayer, R. (1981). *Homosexuality and American psychiatry: The politics of diagnosis*. Princeton, NJ: Princeton University Press.

Bayer, R. (1987). Politics, science, and the problem of psychiatric nomenclature: A case study of the American Psychiatric Association referendum on homosexuality. In T. Engelhardt & A. Caplan (Eds.), *Scientific controversies: Case-studies in the resolution and closure in science and technology* (pp. 381–400). New York: Cambridge University Press.

Bieber, I. (1987). On arriving at the American Psychiatric Association decision on homosexuality. In H. Engelhardt & A. Caplan (Eds.), *Scientific controversies: Case studies in the resolution and closure of disputes in science and technology* (pp. 417–436). New York: Cambridge University Press.

Bieber, I., Dain, H., Dince, P. R., Drellich, M., Grand, H., & Gundlach, R. (1962). *Homosexuality: A psychoanalytic study of male homosexuals*. New York: Basic Books.

Blanchard, R., Cantor, J. M., & Robichaud, L. K. (2006). Biological factors in the development of sexual deviance and aggression in males. In H. Barbaree & W. Marshall (Eds.), *The juvenile sex offender* (pp. 77–104). New York: Guilford Press.

Boorse, C. (1975). On the distinction between disease and illness. *Philosophy and Public Affairs, 5*, 49–68.
Bullough, V. L. (2003). The contributions of John Money: A personal view. *Journal of Sex Research, 40*, 230–236.
Davidson, A. (2001). *The emergence of sexuality: Historical epistemology and the formation of concepts*. Cambridge, MA: Harvard University Press.
Decker, H. S. (2007). How Kraepelinian was Kraepelin? How Kraepelinian were the neo-Kraepelinians? From Emil Kraepelin to DSM-III. *History of Psychiatry, 18*, 337–360.
First, M. (2010). DSM-5 proposals for paraphilias: Suggestions for reducing false positives related to use of behavioral manifestations. *Archives of Sexual Behavior, 39*, 1239–1244.
First, M., & Frances, A. (2008). Issues for DSM-V: Unintended consequences of small changes: The case of paraphilias. *American Journal of Psychiatry, 165*, 1240–1241.
Ford, C. S., & Beach, F. A. (1951). *Patterns of sexual behavior*. New York: Harper & Brothers.
Foucault, M. (1978). *The history of sexuality: An introduction* (Vol. 1). New York: Pantheon Books.
Freud, S. (1955 [1920]). The psychogenesis of a case of homosexuality in a woman. In J. Strachey (Ed., Trans.), *The standard edition of the complete psychological works of sigmund freud* (Vol. 18, pp. 145–172). London: Hogarth Press.
Freud, S. (1960 [1905]). Three essays on the theory of sexuality. In J. Strachey (Ed., Trans.), *The standard edition of the complete psychological works of sigmund freud* (Vol. 7, pp. 123–246). London: Hogarth Press.
Freud, S. (1960 [1935]). Anonymous (Letter to an American mother). In E. Freud (Ed.), *The letters of sigmund freud* (pp. 423–424). London: Hogarth Press.
Friedman, R. C., & Downey, J. I. (1998). Psychoanalysis and the model of homosexuality as psychopathology: A historical overview. *American Journal of Psychoanalysis, 58*, 249–270.
Gerard, K., & Hekma, G. (1989). *The pursuit of sodomy: Male homosexuality in renaissance and enlightenment Europe*. Binghamton, NY: Harrington Park Press.
Gijs, L. (2008). Paraphilia and paraphilia-related disorders: An introduction. In D. Rowland & L. Incrocci (Eds.), *Handbook of sexual and gender identity disorders* (pp. 491–528). Hoboken, NJ: Wiley.
Gold, R. (1973). Stop it, you're making me sick! *American Journal of Psychiatry, 130*, 1211–1212.
Grob, G. N. (1991). Origins of DSM-I: A study in appearance and reality. *American Journal of Psychiatry, 148*, 421–431.
Hinderliter, A. (2010). Disregarding science, clinical utility, and the DSM's definition of mental disorder: The case of exhibitionism, voyeurism, and frotteurism. *Archives of Sexual Behavior, 39*, 1235–1237.
Kafka, M., & Hennen, J. (2002). A DSM-IV Axis I comorbidity study of males (n = 120) with paraphilias and paraphilia-related disorders. *Sexual Abuse: A Journal of Research and Treatment, 14*, 349–366.
Karasic, D., & Drescher, J. (2005). *Sexual and Gender Diagnoses of the Diagnostic and Statistical Manual (DSM): A reevaluation*. Binghampton: The Haworth Press.
Kirk, S. A., & Kutchins, H. (1992). *The selling of the DSM: The rhetoric of science in psychiatry*. New York: Aldine De Gruyter.
Krafft-Ebing, R. (1965 [1886]). *Psychopathia sexualis with special reference to the antipathic sexual instinct: A medico-forensic study*. New York: Paperback Library.
Marmor, J. (1973). Homosexuality and cultural value systems. *American Journal of Psychiatry, 130*, 1208–1209.
Maxmen, J. (1985). *The new psychiatry*. New York: Morrow.
Mayes, R., & Horwitz, A. V. (2005). DSM-III and the revolution in the classification of mental illness. *Journal of the History of the Behavioral Sciences, 41*, 249–267.
McConaghy, N. (1997). Sexual and gender identity disorders. In S. Turner & M. Hersen (Eds.), *Adult psychopathology and diagnosis* (pp. 409–464). New York: Wiley.

Moser, C., & Kleinplatz, P. (2005). DSM-IV-TR and the paraphilias: An argument for removal. *Journal of Psychology and Human Sexuality, 17*, 91–109.

National Committee for Mental Hygiene. (1918). *Statistical manual for the use of hospitals for mental diseases*. New York: Author.

Neal, D. (2008). Disorder of the body, mind or soul: Male sexual deviance in Jacques Despars's commentary on Avicenna. In K. Borris & G. Rousseau (Eds.), *The sciences of homosexuality in early modern Europe*. New York: Routledge.

Oosterhuis, H. (2000). *Stepchildren of nature: Krafft-Ebing, psychiatry, and the making of sexual identity*. Chicago: University of Chicago Press.

Peragallo, M. (1863). Seconde note pour servir à l'histoire des Lucioles. *Annales de la Société Entomologique de France, 21*, 661–665.

Price, J., Gardner, R., Wilson, D. R., Sloman, L., Rohde, P., & Erickson, M. (2007). Territory, rank and mental health: The history of an idea. *Evolutionary Psychology, 5*, 531–554.

Primoratz, I. (1997). Sexual perversion. *American Philosophical Quarterly, 34*, 245–258.

Rimke, H., & Hunt, A. (2002). From sinners to degenerates: The medicalization of morality in the 19th century. *History of the Human Sciences, 15*, 59–88.

Roughgarden, J. (2004). *Evolution's rainbow: Diversity, gender, and sexuality in nature and people*. Los Angeles: University of California Press.

Shorter, E. (1997). *A history of psychiatry: From the era of the asylum to the age of prozac*. New York: Wiley.

Shorter, E. (2008). *Before prozac: The troubled history of mood disorders in psychiatry*. New York: Oxford University Press.

Silverstein, C. (1984). The ethical and moral implications of sexual classification: A commentary. *Journal of Homosexuality, 9*, 29–38.

Spitzer, R. (1973). A proposal about homosexuality and the APA nomenclature: Homosexuality as an irregular form of sexual behavior and sexual orientation disturbance as a psychiatric disorder. *American Journal of Psychiatry, 130*, 1214–1216.

Spitzer, R. (1981). The diagnostic status of homosexuality in DSM-III: A reformulation of the issues. *American Journal of Psychiatry, 138*, 210–215.

Spitzer, R. (1999). Harmful dysfunction and the DSM definition of mental disorder. *Journal of Abnormal Psychology, 108*, 430–432.

Spitzer, R. (2001). Values and assumptions in the development of DSM-III and DSM-III-R: An insider's perspective and a belated response to Sadler, Hulgus, and Agich's "On values in recent American psychiatric classification". *Journal of Nervous and Mental Disease, 189*, 351–359.

Spitzer, R. (2005). Sexual and gender disorders: Discussions of questions for DSM-V. In D. Karasic & J. Drescher (Eds.), *Sexual and gender diagnoses of the diagnostic and statistical manual (DSM): A re-evaluation* (pp. 111–116). Binghamton, NY: Haworth Press.

Symons, D. (1981). *The evolution of human sexuality*. Oxford: Oxford University Press.

Torrey, E. F. (1974). *The death of psychiatry*. Radnor, PA: Chilton.

Vasey, P. L. (1995). Homosexual behavior in primates: A review of evidence and theory. *International Journal of Primatology, 16*, 173–204.

Vasey, P. L., & Sommer, V. (2006). Homosexual behavior in animals: Topics, hypotheses and research trajectories. In V. Sommer & P. Vasey (Eds.), *Homosexual behavior in animals: An evolutionary perspective* (pp. 3–42). Cambridge: Cambridge University Press.

Wakefield, J. (1992). The concept of mental disorder: On the boundary between biological facts and social values. *American Psychologist, 47*, 373–388.

Whisnant, C. J. (2012). *Male homosexuality in West Germany: Between persecution and freedom, 1945–1969*. Basingstoke: Palgrave Macmillan.

Chapter 11
Liberal Eugenics, Human Enhancement and the Concept of the Normal

Catherine Mills

> *We no longer ask, in all seriousness, what is human nature? Instead we talk about normal people.*
>
> (Hacking 1990, p. 161).

1 Introduction

The development of technologies such as preimplantation genetic diagnosis, reproductive cloning, and genetic therapy and enhancement have prompted considerable public and scholarly concern about a return to the eugenic projects of the early Twentieth century. But while there has been much disagreement on whether new genetic technologies are eugenic or not, with the implication being that their moral acceptability rests on this designation, some contributors to this debate have taken a different approach. They argue that while new genetic technologies may well be eugenic, they constitute a new form of "liberal" or "*laissez faire*" eugenics, which are morally distinct from the totalitarian eugenics of the twentieth century. The core idea driving the formulation of this notion is that even if genetic practices are considered eugenic, this is not necessarily an indication that they are morally indefensible, since a certain form of eugenic intervention may be compatible with the key moral principles of liberal democratic societies. In apparent opposition to the more familiar form of eugenics, it is argued that this form of eugenic intervention extends individual freedom in reproductive choices and insists upon state neutrality and value pluralism.

Preserving value pluralism is thus central to maintaining the liberalness of liberal eugenics over and against the older, indefensible, counterpart of totalitarian eugenics. One of the concerns that arises in relation to this is what role the idea of the "normal" person should play in debates about genetic interventions. The point of

C. Mills (✉)
Monash University, Melbourne, Australia
e-mail: catherine.mills@monash.edu

D. Meacham (ed.), *Medicine and Society, New Perspectives in Continental Philosophy*, Philosophy and Medicine 120, DOI 10.1007/978-94-017-9870-9_11

contention is whether the standard of normality provides a way of dissecting morally acceptable and unacceptable practices in a way that maintains liberal value pluralism without ceding to relativistic libertarianism. But the concept of the normal is slippery, and the relationship between notions of biological normality and normative judgements is far from clear. To tease out some of this complexity, I consider various approaches to the question of whether the standard of normality can ground ethical limitations on the use of genetic technologies within bioethical debates about liberal eugenics. Through the lens of the controversy over the distinction, or lack thereof, between therapy and enhancement, I briefly consider three different approaches to human nature and normality. These are: Jürgen Habermas's emphasis on human nature as a normative concept that grounds the distinction between therapy and enhancement; the use of the "normal species functioning" model of normality by Allen Buchanan and his co-authors in *From Chance to Choice*; and finally, John Harris's rejection of normality and consequent embrace of enhancement. Following this discussion, I begin to develop an outline of a conception of the normal that would both avoid the worries that hound Habermas's strong attachment to a normative conception of human nature, while still allowing for a distinction between therapy and enhancement. To do this, I draw on the work of Georges Canguilhem, especially his influential book, *The Normal and the Pathological*.

2 Shaping People: Human Enhancement and Normality

If the addition of the word liberal transforms a morally evil practice into a morally acceptable one as Nicholas Agar (2004, p. 135) suggests, then there is considerable pressure to establish the liberality of the new eugenics.[1] In order to do this, those arguing for a liberal eugenics attempt to distinguish themselves from previous generations of eugenicists by insisting upon several important points of difference. The most central of these derive from two fundamental principles of liberalism, specifically the related tenets of value pluralism in relation to the good and the priority of individual liberty. These principles give rise to an insistence on state neutrality alongside the minimisation of state intervention in decision-making processes relating to reproduction (Agar 1998). In this view, the key moral wrong of the earlier eugenics was the coercive and highly interventionist role the state played in shaping reproductive choices of citizens (e.g. see, Kitcher 1996). The totalitarian characteristics of coercive intervention curtail individual autonomy by enforcing a particular conception of the good, and restrict freedom by narrowing the scope of choices available to prospective parents. In contrast, a liberal eugenics actually enlarges the scope of reproductive liberty by minimising state regulation and coercion of reproductive choices.

[1] For a strong critique of Agar, see Fox (2007).

There are two aspects to this claim. First, libertarian advocates of technological enhancements emphasise the necessity of restrictions on state intervention per se, such that free or unrestricted parental choice is the final arbiter of moral acceptability. A second, more complex, idea is that the liberal state must maintain a neutral stance in relation to conceptions of the good to be sought through genetic interventions. This means that even if the state plays a regulatory function in relation to reproductive technology, it should not positively intervene to enforce a particular conception of individual wellbeing or population health since it is constrained by the liberal commitment to value pluralism. It is argued that if the state maintains neutrality in this way, then rather than reinvigorating the spectre of Nazism, the new eugenics or liberal eugenics will reinforce and enhance the freedoms associated with reproduction and parenting. It will do so by giving parents more choice in and control over the genetic profile of the child that is born to them, and by reinforcing reproductive rights, such as the right to found a family established in the United Nations Declaration of Human Rights.[2]

While this construal of state neutrality and non-intervention seems to lead away from a totalitarian eugenics and thereby helps to establish the liberality of the new eugenics, value pluralism is more complicated than this supposes. For one, Buchanan et al. (2000, p. 51) in *From Chance to Choice* point out that it is overly simplistic to think that statism itself establishes the immorality of totalitarian eugenics: a strong interventionist state is neither essential to eugenics nor the core wrong of early eugenics.[3] Indeed, the founder of eugenics in Britain, Francis Galton, rejected coercive decision-making and instead favoured an educational approach predicated on informed voluntarism. Additionally, Buchanan et al. point out that the requirements of pluralism differ for the state than for parents (170–175). The former requires non-interference in parental reproductive decision-making, and ensures a domain of individual liberty within which parents are free to make their own decisions about reproduction without the imposition of state sanctioned reproductive goals. However, the standards required by pluralism within parental decision-making may be better understood through the principle of harm and the notion of a "right to an open future" (167–172).[4] Value pluralism therefore pertains not only to states, but also to the nature of the choices made by individuals.

Seen from the perspective of the necessity of maintaining value pluralism, a central issue in liberal eugenics is the (individual or collective) prerogative to shape the lives of others. The key questions are: what are the limits of state intervention, and conversely, what duties does the state have in relation to maintaining and promoting population health? What are the limits of the prerogative of parents to shape the lives of their children according to their own values? To what extent do

---

[2]The right to found a family is especially important in defences of reproductive cloning such as Harris (2004).

[3]For further discussion of the relation of contemporary genetics to eugenics, see in particular, Burdett and Richardson (2007), Lemke (2005), Paul (1994).

[4]For more on the notion of a "right to an open future," see Feinberg (1980).

parental decisions concerning new genetics foster or restrict the prospective freedoms and rights of their future child? That is, does parental control legitimately extend so far as to allow interventions in the genetic profile of the child born to them? Or, should it be limited to interventions for which it is possible to conceive that the future child would give consent? And if consent is withheld, for which it is then possible for them to reject the choices of their parents in morally significant ways? The extent to which new reproductive technologies have become controversial is indicative of the significance of these questions for the moral and ethical inflection of liberal democratic societies.

In addressing questions such as these, those in favour of liberal eugenics tend to reject two "conventional distinctions in shaping people" (Agar 1998, p. 139). The first of these is the distinction between biological and social influences on childhood development. As Agar outlines, intervention by parents upon the genetic profile of their future child differs from totalitarian eugenics in a number of ways, but is not in itself radically different from other choices and influences that parents have over the lives of their children. While intervention in the genetic profile of an embryo may well be novel, this kind of influence is not qualitatively different from the manipulation of environmental factors in order to enhance a child's natural skill, talent or ability. Thus, genetic enhancement is akin to private education, additional tutoring or experimental diets (139–40). This means that certain forms of genetic intervention may be no more morally problematic than practices that are routinely accepted as part of parenting and may in fact, "preserve our children's capacity to fully participate in society" (Agar 2006, p. 5). By the same token, it also means that certain exercises of social control by parents over children may be as morally problematic as some genetic interventions (5). By this light then, the distinction between the natural and the social is morally insignificant; instead, the point of moral arbitration is simply the *degree* of control a parent may have over the "life plan" of their child. That is, the measure of parental control is merely quantitative, not qualitative (5; Agar 2004). One consequence of this construal of the social and biological is that it rejects the idea that the "natural" has any normative force in itself; thus, recourse to the "natural foundations" of the human being cannot ground moral opposition to genetic interventions.

The second, related, distinction that liberal eugenicists tend to reject is the oft-made moral differentiation between genetic interventions for therapeutic reasons and interventions for reasons of enhancement (Agar 1998, pp. 141–142). In broad terms, this distinction attempts to capture the intuitive difference between addressing deficiencies therapeutically to restore the human body to health on the one hand, and on the other, boosting capacities beyond what is normal. But while that intuitive distinction may seem relatively straightforward at a descriptive level, it becomes more complicated in the context of the moral permissibility or otherwise of genetic inventions. For while therapeutic practices are usually seen as uncontroversial interventions to improve the wellbeing of an individual, enhancements are often seen as a step beyond the rightful limits of human control over others. However, the problem with this characterisation lies in the fact that it proves difficult to identify and isolate therapeutic practices over and against enhancements:

in short, one person's therapy is another person's enhancement and vice versa (Harris 2007).

Central to the task of disambiguating therapy and enhancement is the standard of "the normal," whether understood as normal biological functioning or more speculatively (and controversially) as normal "human nature." For it is often reference to a concept of normality that allows the identification of therapeutic restoration of a biological function (to its "normal" level), as opposed to the illegitimate enhancement of a function (that is otherwise "normal"). But while the idea of the normal is commonplace, it is both more philosophically interesting and more complicated than its everyday usage might suggest. For the concept of the normal incorporates both descriptive and normative implications, with the consequence that it cannot be simply an objective standard from which abnormalities deviate. Thus, it is not clear how, or whether, it helps to distinguish enhancement from therapy. Three broad types of responses to this conceptual ambiguity can be identified in debates on genetics and eugenics: (1) a restrictive approach to genetic enhancement that maintains the distinction on the basis of a moral conception of human nature; (2) a moderately restrictive approach that attempts to base the distinction upon a non-moral conception of normal human functioning; and (3) those who reject the standard of normality and the correlative distinction between therapy and enhancement altogether and adopt a more *laissez faire* approach. I will briefly discuss each of these in turn.

Perhaps the most popularly resonant argument against dissolving the distinction between therapy and enhancement draws on the trope of "transforming human nature," to argue that a moral conception of human nature should place limits on the technological intervention into and transformation of the human genome. In this approach, a normative conception of human nature grounds a distinction between acceptable therapeutic interventions and unacceptable enhancements. More grandly, some claim that a normative conception of human nature is required to stave off the threat to liberal democratic values that the project of a liberal eugenics is seen to augur. These arguments take several forms, including the strongly Aristotelian approach of Frances Fukuyama (2003), who posits that a substantive idea of human nature is intrinsic to our conceptions of justice, rights and morality. More Kantian approaches move away from this teleological perspective and argue that the distinctive and essential human feature of autonomous individuality is threatened by technological instrumentalization. Similar in ways to both these arguments, the most philosophically elaborate intervention in the "moralisation of human nature" position has been the post-metaphysical arguments of Jürgen Habermas.

The overall thrust of Habermas's argument in *The Future of Human Nature* (2003) is that new genetic technologies transform our "ethical self-understanding" by undermining the Aristotelian distinction between the "given" and the "made," which he sees as having a constitutive effect within our lifeworld. To the extent that this distinction underpins our ethical self-understanding and correlative moral and political principles, the "dedifferentiation" of the given and the made threatens to undermine those principles. In particular, Habermas worries that the dedifferentiation of the given and the made introduces a novel asymmetric relation between the "designer and the designed" that is contrary to the value of universal egalitarianism. Further, this may prevent the designed from establishing an ethically autonomous or self-defined life for themselves. Because of these worries, he argues that difficult as a distinction between therapy and enhancement may be to maintain at a conceptual level, it is nevertheless practically crucial.

Notably, Habermas's emphasis on ethical self-understanding distinguishes his position from the more straightforward Aristotelianism of Fukuyama. For Habermas, the notion of human nature has an importance within our "lifeworld," but it is not tied to ontological claims about human nature per se, whether understood in the form of "Factor X" or species-typical characteristics (Fukuyama 2003, p. 149). But, regardless of the nuances of Habermas's view, or its virtues and vices, the project of developing a species ethic founded on a normative conception of human nature worries some commentators. Their concern is that if substantive content is given to a notion of human nature, then it may be mobilised as a means of political exclusion and, further, appears to contradict the central liberal virtue of value pluralism (Mendieta 2003, pp. 135–138; Rabinow 2008, p. 24). And a move away from liberal pluralism threatens to collapse the new eugenics back into the old totalitarian eugenics (Agar 1998, p. 137).

A second, more moderate, position on genetic interventions including enhancements also draws on a notion of human nature, but one that is understood as non-normative, since it refers only to an empirical ideal of species-typical functioning. Developed by Boorse (1977), the notion of "normal species functioning" has been imported into bioethics by Daniels (1985), Brock (1993), and Buchanan et al. (2000). Boorse proposes this notion in the context of developing a functional definition of health and disease, in which diseases are "internal states that depress a functional ability below species-typical levels," and "health as freedom from disease is statistical normality of function, i.e. the ability to perform all physiological functions with at least typical efficiency" (Boorse 1977, p. 542). Boorse's naturalistic and functional conceptions of health and disease rely upon the identification of statistically ideal characteristics of species or populations. He argues that these ideal-types are neither aesthetic nor moral, but simply non-normative descriptors of typical species characteristics, from which any and all individuals might vary in some way or another, but which provide an abstracted empirical ideal to which judgements about health and disease can refer (557). This means then that health is essentially non-evaluative: for Boorse, because it refers to an empirical ideal, the concept is value free. Further, this leads to the view that "the normal is the natural" and disease is consequently "foreign to the nature of the species" (554).

Buchanan et al. take up this conception of health as a way of parsing therapy and enhancement without having to posit a substantive view of human nature. Countering the "shadow" of eugenics, they argue that eugenics may be acceptable if it is driven by concerns with justice. This raises the significant question of the extent to which genetic resources allocated by the "natural lottery" can be subjected to the requirements of distributive justice. Addressing the resulting "colonisation of the natural by the just," they adopt the notion of "normal species function" to differentiate between the restoration of normal functioning versus attempts to extend the capacities allocated to a person in the natural lottery beyond the statistically normal range. Within this, disease is defined as any "adverse departures from normal species functioning" (Buchanan et al. 2000, p. 72), and therapeutic interventions would entail re-establishing normal species functioning. Importantly, the limited defence of the therapy/enhancement distinction that they develop is not supposed to derive moral force from the empirical ideal of the normal per se (the normal is statistically descriptive, not normative), but from a broader argument for a "social structural" conception of just health care.

That is, genetic therapies provide a means of curing or preventing disease in accordance with Rawlsian principles of justice as fairness, aimed at ensuring equality of opportunity. Hence, it is not the normal per se that acts as a "regulative ideal," but rather, the imperative of equality of opportunity; normal species functioning is only important to the extent that it contributes to that, by allowing for fair competition in social cooperation. Normal species functioning thus provides one abstract indicator in establishing the "level playing field" required for equality of opportunity. The implication of this is that interventions may be undertaken that help to establish that measure, particularly by eliminating disease conditions,[5] but genetic interventions should not undermine it by raising some above the bar of the normal. That said, it is worth noting that the equality of opportunity view of genetic interventions offered by Buchanan et al. does not require an absolute equality of genetic resources, since, for one, this fails to appreciate "the limitations imposed by the fact of value pluralism" (80).[6] Instead, they suggest that it may aim at something akin to a "genetic decent minimum" that promotes the prevention or amelioration of the most serious disabilities that negatively impact on an individual's equality of opportunity (82).

In developing this view, Buchanan et al. adopt and defend the model of just health care proposed by Norman Daniels, in which normal species functioning anchors the obligations of health care. That is, his "normal function" model of fair equality of opportunity entails for health care the "relatively modest and limited task of keeping people functioning as close to normal as possible," in order to preserve their "capacity to participate in political, social and economic life" (127; 22). Such participation is not, however, guaranteed on the basis of being "equal competitors" but rather, of being "normal competitors." Buchanan et al. thus draw on the conception of normal species functioning posed by Boorse; but they also move away from his strong claim that this conception of health and disease is entirely non-evaluative. Instead, they concede that the social context in which adverse departures from

[5]Though, it should be noted that acceptable interventions are not strictly limited to the treatment of disease, but may also include conditions that do not count as disease. Nevertheless, the treatment of disease conditions provides the primary rationale of just health care. See Buchanan et al. (2000, p. 74).

[6]In this, it is less expansive than the 'brute luck' view. See the discussion at Buchanan et.al. 2000, pp. 66–84.

normal functioning are manifest will impact upon their specification as disease conditions or not. Further, they note that "sometimes values, including prejudices, as well as errors, intrude" into the relatively "objective and non-evaluative context provided by the biomedical sciences" (122).

However, several difficulties can be seen in this view. For one, the conception of biomedical sciences indicated here is naïve; as science and technology scholars have shown, (biomedical) science is not a value-free activity, in which values, prejudices and errors intrude only occasionally. Instead, values are intrinsic to the practice of science in a number of ways, from the personal values of individual scientists, the social norms that shape scientific practice through funding priorities and economic and political agendas for example, and the norms that legitimate and support scientific epistemology itself.[7] More importantly for my purposes here, though, Buchanan et al. forget that the concept of the normal is itself a confusion of fact and value: the term "normal" derives from the Latin term "*norma*," meaning to set right or to straighten, such that the norm (understood as the typical) and the right are etymologically intertwined. As Ian Hacking pithily writes, "[f]rom the beginning of our language the word 'normal' has been dancing and prancing all over" the fact/value distinction (Hacking 1990, p. 163). This means that a purely descriptive conception of the normal will be difficult to achieve, and it is not at all clear that Buchanan et al. do achieve such a conception.

Additionally, disability theorists point to the significant ambiguities embedded in notion of "normal species functioning" that underpins the aim of ensuring "normal competitors." For instance, Ron Amundson argues that the notion of biological normality is itself part of social prejudices against individuals with certain functional modes or styles. He draws the conclusion that disadvantages and limitations on opportunity cannot be causally linked to biological characteristics but instead, always derive from the environments in which individuals operate and live (Amundson 2000, p. 51). Extending on this, Shelley Tremain argues that while the notion of normal species functioning seems to imply a statistical conception of "the typical" or most common—the statistical mode—it actually operates to indicate something more like the mean or average. Moreover, deviations from this average are negatively evaluated such that the guiding presumption is that "the more an organism diverges from the species average, the worse it will function" (Tremain 2006, p. 43). The worry underlying this critique relates to the interaction of the ostensibly biologically derived "species-typical" norms and the "normal" understood as a regulative ideal that is externally applied as a means of delimiting the socially accepted standards of bodily capacities. What is embedded within the critique of the mobilisation of the statistically typical as an evaluative tool, then, is the concern that the "normal" is no longer taken as a normatively neutral indicator but instead is conflated with a social ideal, such that the formula of "species typical

[7]This insight is commonplace in science and technology studies, but for especially interesting examples see Latour (1986), Rabinow (1999), Fox Keller (2003).

characteristics" actually operates as a normative conception of human nature, rather than a "purely" statistically descriptive one.

Whether Buchanan et al. fall foul of this critique or not would be a question worth exploring in more detail, though I cannot attempt such an exploration here. The question that would have to be asked is whether the notion of statistical normality can do the work that they wish it to do without recalling the fact/value confusion that Hacking suggests is intrinsic to the concept of the normal. Further, does the emphasis on intervening therapeutically to ensure that an individual attains a condition akin to, or at least in the vicinity of, normal species functioning as a matter of justice mean that the normal is implicitly taken as the right or even the ideal? Does this view presuppose that to be "normal" is better than being "abnormal," such that deviation from the normal is itself negatively evaluated? And if so, what are the implications of this for an understanding of just health care in the context of a new eugenics? Their limited defence of the therapy/enhancement distinction through the notion of normal species functioning, and elaboration of a "normal function" model of just health care, thus raises complex questions for anyone interested in the political implications of the concept of the normal.

Buchanan et al.'s primary concern is to establish a social and political obligation to provide therapeutic measures that restore normal functioning as a matter of justice, while avoiding claims for a comparable obligation to undertake enhancements (apart from in exceptional cases). The third approach I wish to consider here takes a stronger line, to argue for an obligation to enhance. One of the key proponents of this approach is John Harris, who has recently attempted an extensive justification of human genetic enhancement. In this, he argues that references to the normal should play no role in establishing the moral permissibility of either therapy or enhancement. Harris emphasises the indistinction between therapy and enhancement, and, moreover, argues that enhancement technologies have long played a fundamental part in human life. Vaccinations, for instance, are not simply therapeutic, since they provide an ability to resist disease that humans would not otherwise have, and yet they are generally seen as not only beneficial but also morally acceptable. By extension, he also implies that all other enhancements are similarly morally acceptable. But Harris's argument is not only for the freedom but the obligation to undertake enhancements. He contends that insofar as enhancements are beneficial—which they are by definition—then individuals and governments should pursue them, since there is a similar obligation to confer benefit as there is to avoid harm. For him, "the moral imperative is the safety of the people and the duty to compare risks with benefits, not on the basis of the normality of the risks or of the benefits, or of their contribution to equality of opportunity, but on the basis of their magnitude and probability" (Harris 2007, p. 54). Harris's use of the principle of harm, drawn from John Stuart Mill, eschews any conception of the normal, whether understood as descriptive or normative, and instead simply emphasises the calculation of likely harms and benefits. Thus, he adopts a libertarian position in which the only potential limit on an individual's freedom to enhance is the likelihood and magnitude of harm.

However, while Harris explicitly rejects any reference to normality, it may be that he nevertheless implicitly relies upon some conception of the normal. For one, this is because the designation of interventions as beneficial or harmful seems to require some standard against which to judge whether they are in fact benefits or harms. While Harris avers that, "normalcy plays no part in the definition of harm and therefore no part in the way the distinction between therapy and enhancement is drawn" (46) it is difficult to see that he provides a compelling alternative standard by which harms can be identified. What he does offer as a way of identifying a harmed condition is the "emergency room" test. He elaborates the test: "if a patient was brought unconscious into the ER department of a hospital in such a condition and it could be reversed or removed, the medical staff would be negligent if they failed to reverse or remove it" (54). Even so, while this test suggests that the failure to reverse a condition would indicate negligence (because the condition is deemed harmful), it does not clarify why the condition is thought of as harmful in the first instance, such that the failure to reverse or remove it would be negligent.

There is, then, a significant circularity in this test—a condition is considered harmful if the failure to remove or reverse it is negligent. But that failure is only negligent because the condition is intuitively understood as harmful in the first place. This circularity appears again when Harris writes, "a harmed condition is defined relative both to one's rational preferences and to conditions which might be described as harmful" (92). It is surely truistic that a harmed condition refers to conditions that might be described as harmful. But even if this definition is granted, a question remains about the work that the idea of harmed conditions referring to rational preferences does for Harris. The emergency room test is, for Harris, a way of determining that disabilities are and should be treated as harmed conditions. While it might seem that the rejection of a notion of biological normality might lead Harris to an extreme position of abjuring the very idea of disability—since ostensibly he has no criteria against which to identify some bodily capacities as diminished in relation to others—this is not the case. Instead, the reference to rational preferences is central to his definition of disability and provides him with that criterion.

While rejecting reference to biological functionality for defining disability, Harris does not therefore take up the opposing social model of disability either. In this model, disability is the social condition of discrimination that attaches to biological conditions of impairment. Thus, disability is to impairment what gender (understood as socially constructed) is to sex (understood as an irreducible biological substrate). But as such, the identification of impairment still seems to require reference to biological functionality. In rejecting such reference, Harris instead proposes to define disability as "a condition that someone has a strong rational preference not to be in and one that is moreover in some sense a harmed condition" (91).[8] In this "harmed condition" model of disability, the important point of

[8]See Harris (2001). Also see the alternative formulation of this definition in Bortolotti and Harris (2006, p. 32), where it is argued that, "conditions are disabling if they are physical or mental conditions that constitute a harm to the individual which a rational person would wish to be without."

reference for identifying disability is "alternative possibilities" of bodily capacities, where harm is established through the above mentioned emergency room test. A bodily capacity is considered a disability if it is conceivable that someone could have a strong rational preference not to be in that condition, where that condition can in some sense fail the emergency room test such that it would be negligent to fail to remove or reverse the condition.

Apart from the fact that some disabilities are neither reversible nor removable, this construal of the emergency room test as a way of identifying harmed conditions reveals several points about it. For one, it highlights the significantly counterfactual nature of this model: that is, a given condition is identified as a disability because it is seen as undesirable or harmful in relation to a counterfactual alternative existence without the condition. Further, when this is combined with the standard of rational preferences, it becomes clear that Harris's approach to disability is, for want of a better term, "able-centric." That is, it is from the perspective of a rational, *able-bodied* person, and in relation to such a counterfactual alternative person, that a condition is seen as rationally desirable or not. Hence, while Harris rejects recourse to the "subjective experience" of a disabled person as a relevant factor in reproductive ethics, he nevertheless implicitly relies on the (notional) subjective experience of an able-bodied, rational person as the measure against which disability is considered harmful. That is, he implicitly relies on a conception of a "normal" person.

In more general terms, the problem with Harris's approach is that he fails to grasp the ways in which social norms shape the very desirability of a condition as compared with counterfactual alternatives. That is, he fails to see that what might be rationally desirable is itself normatively framed. Clearly, the sense in which I use the term "normative" here does not simply refer to more or less explicit formulations of moral principles or declarations of what ought to be distinct from what is. Instead, I refer to an understanding of social life itself as fundamentally normative. One characteristic of this view is that it insists on the pervasive and ineluctable power of norms in shaping what bodies appear within the social field as desirable possibilities for living. Judith Butler poses this claim most forcefully, when she argues that the materiality of the body is fundamentally shaped by the reiteration and enactment of regulatory social norms. She writes that "bodies only appear, only endure, only live within the productive constraints of […] regulatory schemas" (Butler 1993, p. xi) such that the appearance of the body within the social sphere is simultaneous with the attribution of value or worth. For Butler, norms impose "a grid of intelligibility" on the social and, in doing so, delineate possible modes of bodily life. One consequence of this is a blurring of the distinction between the descriptive and the normative—bodies that appear within the social field embody the norms that productively constrain their own intelligibility and recognisability. Additionally, norms are embedded within the practical exercise of power across various institutions such as law and medicine, and as such, they can be mobilised—explicitly or implicitly—as standards of evaluation and exclusion. Hence, this perspective makes it clear that his abstraction from the social condition of norms in shaping the desirability of bodily forms hides a deeper attachment to normality than Harris acknowledges.

3 Rethinking Normality

Given the apparent difficulty in avoiding use of the concept of normality altogether, even if it is only appealed to implicitly, it may serve those involved in debates on enhancement well to attempt to address the concept of the normal more explicitly. Further, though, the critiques of the "normal species functioning" model of the normal suggest that it does not stand up to scrutiny and may well mire its advocates in bioethics in problematic assumptions about idealised "normal" bodies that work to denigrate bodies that differ from "species typical" bodies, but are nevertheless functionally sound (see esp. Kingma 2007). To address these issues, I want here to briefly discuss the conception of the normal proposed by French historian and epistemologist of science, Georges Canguilhem, who extends the work of the neuropsychologist, Kurt Goldstein (2000). Canguilhem's approach to the normal is distinguished by his insistence on a normativity inherent to living itself, whereby the "normal" only emerges in the relationship between an organism and its environment. I argue that this approach to the normal can allow for bodily variation without falling into a relativism that would undermine all grounds for a distinction between therapy and enhancement.

In his "holistic" approach to understanding conditions of health and pathology in the organism, Goldstein argues that neither statistical nor idealistic conceptions of the norm and normal are sufficient, since neither can do justice to the individual. Instead, he argues that only a norm that "permits taking the entire concrete individuality into consideration, a norm that takes the individual himself [sic] as a measure" (329) can be adequate to understanding conditions of health, disease and abnormality. From the point of view of the whole individual organism, then, health amounts to a situation of "ordered behaviour" which allows the organism to meet the demands made upon it by the environment in which it exists. Disease arises as a "catastrophic reaction" to changes within an organism such that it is no longer able to meet the demands placed upon it in its "proper, 'normal' milieu" (329), and which thereby threatens the very existence of the organism itself. As this implies, Goldstein makes a distinction between disease and variation from the norm as abnormality: he writes, "any disease is an abnormality but not ... every abnormality is a disease" (326), since not every deviation from the normal will threaten the organism in an existential way. Further, rehabilitation from disease is not simply the eradication of a catastrophe, but may come about through the development of a new state of health, understood as a previously non-existent set of ordered relations between the organism and its environment; that is, health is not an ideal condition to which the organism is restored, but an active interaction and "negotiation" between the organism and its environment.

This insight that health describes functional relations between an individual and its environment is central to Canguilhem's extension of Goldstein's understanding of norms and health in his study of the concepts of the normal and the pathological in medicine. Canguilhem argues that life itself is inherently normative, insofar as it aims at the restoration of functional or "normal" relations between an individual organism and its environment. He writes:

> Taken separately, the living being and his [sic] environment are not normal: it is their relationship that makes them such. For any given form of life the environment is normal to the extent that it allows it fertility and a corresponding variety of forms such that, should changes in the environment occur, life will be able to find the solution to the problem of adaptation… in one of these forms. A living being is normal in any given environment insofar as it is the morphological and functional solution found by life as a response to the demands of the environment. Even if it is relatively rare, this living being is normal in terms of every other form from which it diverges, because in terms of those other forms it is *normative*, that is, it devalues them before eliminating them. (Canguilhem 1991, p. 143–144)

For Canguilhem, health amounts to a "normal" situation, one in which the organism is normatively attuned to its environment and is thus able to meet the demands of it. Conversely, pathology or disease is the incapacity to meet those demands; but while it amounts to a deviation from the normal state, it is not strictly speaking, a situation of disorder or normlessness. Rather, "the pathological is not the absence of a biological norm: it is another norm but one which is, comparatively speaking, pushed aside by life" (144). Thus, norms are not only internally specific to the organism but vary across the conditions of its existence, either when its normal condition is disrupted by physiological changes or changes in the demands that an environment places upon it such that it can no longer meet those demands.

But while placing emphasis on the normal as the normative relation between an organism and its environment, this does not mean that Canguilhem privileges stasis or stability at the expense of diversity, divergence and mutation. In fact, he argues that life includes within itself a capacity for errancy that ensures that no state of being is ever entirely fixed. Moreover, even if it is logically second, the abnormal is existentially prior to the norm. Related to this, Canguilhem is careful to distinguish the anomalous from the abnormal, suggesting that the former is a descriptive concept while the latter is evaluative and normative. That is, the anomalous refers to the statistically infrequent, but the abnormal refers to that which is against the normal. However, the relation of the abnormal and normal is not simply one of "contradiction and externality." It is instead one of "inversion and polarity": the abnormal does not exist outside the extension of the norm as such, but indicates a less preferable possibility in relation to the norm (239–240). That is, abnormality indicates that all possible modes of living are not normatively equivalent for an organism, since some (and only some) divergences from a norm will be experienced as an obstacle or hindrance in living. As François Ewald writes, "if all possible forms are not normal, it is not because some forms are naturally impossible but because the various possible forms of existence are not all equivalent for those who must exist in them" (Ewald 1990, p. 157). Thus, the importance of the designation of the normal and abnormal is not that it indicates simple variation from an *a priori* model or type, but instead evaluates the ways that such divergences affect the modes of living of an organism in a specific environment.

To return to the debate on liberal eugenics, this characterisation of norms and the conceptions of health, disease and diversity that it gives rise to may provide important leverage in discussions of therapy and enhancement. For one, it provides a way of differentiating between disease and divergence, abnormality and anomaly.

In doing so, it may help to recuperate a sense of therapeutic practice aimed at the restoration of health. Of prime importance for this view of health are not "species-typical" characteristics or functions but the essentially normative relation between an individual organism and the environment in which it exists. Within this view, to attain a normal state for an individual is not to regularise that individual in relation to others or in reference to an abstract empirical ideal, but to attain a condition under which the individual themselves can flourish, even if that condition appears as statistically anomalous or atypical. Perhaps one controversial example of such a therapeutic practice would be self-demand amputation for "Body Integrity Identity Disorder," in which sufferers are psychologically debilitated by living with a body that is otherwise considered morphologically normal. Or, conversely, the provision of cochlear ear implants to restore hearing may be an important therapeutic practice for some individuals, and not simply a "normalising" measure that destroys the distinctive identity of Deafness (though it may also be that for others).

This is not to say that the immanent approach to norms that Canguilhem proposes eliminates reference to species-typical traits altogether; but these traits are not the standard from which divergences are therapeutically assessed. In effect, the evaluation of the health of an individual in relation to species-typical functioning confuses statistical norms and therapeutic norms. That is, while the notion of species-typical functioning attempts to describe a non-normative statistical regularity across numerous individuals, the therapeutic question addresses variation in relation to the individual's own trajectory and existential milieu. In other words, while the statistical norm is synchronic insofar as it indicates divergences across individuals in space, therapeutic norms are diachronic in that they allow for the comparison of states within the lifespan of an individual and their assessment as more or less successful forms of living for that individual. Variation and disease, then, are normative in the sense that they require consideration of the value for the living organism of divergences from its normal state of health. No doubt, the opposition between statistical norms and therapeutic norms as synchronic or diachronic is too simplistic on its own; but the basic point is that "diversity is not disease; the *anomalous* is not the pathological" (Canguilhem 1991, p. 137). The reduction of one of these categories to the other entails collapsing different conceptions of norms that should be kept analytically distinct.

While restoring sense to ideas of therapy, the perspective that I propose also allows for a more differentiated approach to the question of human enhancement. As we saw in the first section of this paper, the idea of the normal has been mobilised in various ways in debates on therapy and enhancement, often appearing as the point of descriptive and moral differentiation between them. In response to this, other commentators have rejected the notion altogether, claiming that it cannot do the work of distinguishing therapeutic interventions from enhancements. Indeed, they reason that as it is not possible to distinguish between therapy and enhancement, the latter must be as morally acceptable (if not obligatory) as the former. I argued, though, that even these theorists unwittingly relied upon an idea of the normal. The question, then, is whether the normal can be recuperated in such a way that it does not commit one to either a strong conception of human nature or of species-typical functioning and their attendant problems. I have argued that it can be; moreover, it can be in such a way that does not lead to an overly simplistic *tout court* rejection or endorsement of enhancement technologies. As Joanna Zylinska has argued, being "for" or "against" enhancement is an "impossible position to sustain"; instead, then, the ethical task in relation to enhancement is "*knowing how to differentiate*" and "*how to use our prostheses well*" (Zylinska 2010, 155, 158). The kind of internally differentiated conception of the normal that I am proposing here, which focuses on the flourishing of an individual as living being in its always already social environment, may be one of the tools we need in order to take up this task.

References

Agar, N. (1998). Liberal eugenics. *Public Affairs Quarterly, 12*, 137–156.
Agar, N. (2004). *Liberal eugenics: In defence of human enhancement.* Oxford: Blackwell.
Agar, N. (2006). The debate over liberal eugenics. *Hastings Center Report, 36*, 4–5.
Amundson, R. (2000). Against normal function. *Studies in the History and Philosophy of Biology and Biomedical Sciences, 31*, 33–53.
Boorse, C. (1977). Health as a theoretical concept. *Philosophy of Science, 44*, 542–573.
Bortolotti, L., & Harris, J. (2006). Disability, enhancement and the harm-benefit continuum. In J. R. Spencer & A. Du Bois-Pedain (Eds.), *Freedom and responsibility in reproductive choice* (pp. 31–49). Oxford: Hart Publishing.
Brock, D. W. (1993). *Life and death: Philosophical essays in biomedical ethics.* Cambridge, New York: Cambridge University Press.
Buchanan, A., Brock, D. W., Daniels, N., & Wikler, D. (2000). *From chance to choice: Genetics and justice.* Cambridge: Cambridge University Press.
Burdett, C., & Richardson, A. (2007) Eugenics, old and new. Special Edition of *New formations: A journal of culture/theory/politics*, 60.
Butler, J. (1993). *Bodies that matter: On the discursive limits of 'sex'.* New York: Routledge.
Canguilhem, G. (1991). *The normal and the pathological* (C. Fawcett, Trans.). New York: Zone Books.
Daniels, N. (1985). *Just health care.* Cambridge, New York: Cambridge University Press.
Ewald, F. (1990). Norms, discipline and the law. *Representation, 30*, 138–161.
Feinberg, J. (1980). The child's right to an open future. In W. Aiken & H. LaFollette (Eds.), *Whose child? Children's rights, parental authority, and state power* (pp.124–153). Totawa, NJ: Rowman and Littlefield.
Fox, D. (2007). The illiberality of liberal eugenics. *Ratio 20*, 1–25.
Fox Keller, E. (2003). *Making sense of life: Explaining biological development with models, metaphors and machines.* Cambridge, MA: Harvard University Press.
Fukuyama, F. (2003). *Our posthuman future: Consequences of the biotechnology revolution.* London: Profile Books.
Goldstein, K. (2000). *The organism: A holistic approach to biology derived from pathological data in man.* New York: Zone Books.
Habermas, J. (2003). *The future of human nature.* Cambridge, MA: Polity.
Hacking, I. (1990). *The taming of chance.* Cambridge: Cambridge University Press.
Harris, J. (2001). One principle and three fallacies of disability studies. *Journal of Medical Ethics, 27*, 383–387.
Harris, J. (2004). *On cloning.* London, New York: Routledge.

Harris, J. (2007). *Enhancing evolution: The ethical case for making better people*. Princeton, Oxford: Princeton University Press.
Kingma, E. (2007) What is it to be healthy? *Analysis*, *67*(2), 128–133.
Kitcher, P. (1996). *The lives to come: The genetic revolution and human possibilities*. London: Penguin Press.
Latour, B. (1986). *Laboratory life: The construction of scientific facts* (2nd ed.). Princeton: Princeton University Press.
Lemke, T. (2005) From eugenics to the government of genetic risks. In R. Bunton & A. Petersen (Eds.), *Genetic governance: Health, risk and ethics in the biotech Eera* (pp. 95–106). Abingdon: Routledge.
Mendieta, E. (2003). Communicative freedom and genetic engineering. *Logos, 2*(1), 124–140.
Paul, D. B. (1994) Is human genetics disguised eugenics? In R. F. Weir, S. C. Lawrence & E. Fales (Eds.), *Genes and human self-knowledge: Historical and philosophical reflections on modern genetics* (pp. 67–83). Iowa City: University of Iowa Press.
Rabinow, P. (1999). *French DNA: Trouble in purgatory*. Chicago: Chicago University Press.
Rabinow, P. (2008). *Marking time: On the anthropology of the contemporary*. Princeton: Princeton University Press.
Tremain, S. (2006) Reproductive freedom, self-regulation and the government of impairment in Utero. *Hypatia, 21*(1), 35–53.
Zylinska, J. (2010). Playing god, playing Adam: The politics and ethics of enhancement. *Journal of Bioethical Inquiry, 7*(2), 149–161.

Part IV
Life Itself: From Bio to Political

Chapter 12
Was Canguilhem a Biochauvinist? Goldstein, Canguilhem and the Project of Biophilosophy

Charles T. Wolfe

> *Nous n'avons pas l'outrecuidance de prétendre rénover la médecine en lui incorporant une métaphysique*
> Canguilhem (1972, p. 9).

> *la vie déconcerte la logique*
> Canguilhem (1977, p. 1)

1 Introduction

In what follows I reflect on the possible contribution of Georges Canguilhem (1904–1995) to a discourse in the philosophy of the life sciences which would not be content to locate itself squarely within either of two classic and enduring orthodoxies: reductionism or holism. Granted, these two extremes often coexist, if not very happily, and the different subdisciplines approach them in a very different way. As Gayon has noted (Gayon 2010), the philosophy of biology as a professional discipline, which primarily focuses on a kind of specialized conceptual analysis aiming at clarifying the implications and consequences of biological claims in mainstream science, has kept a safe distance from what it perceives as "vitalism" throughout its existence as an Anglophone genre. This is less true of the philosophy of medicine, inasmuch as it focuses more on "whole person" analyses, subjectivity, qualitative dimensions of suffering and well-being, and so on (see Giroux (2010) for a useful contrast between Canguilhem and analytic philosophy of medicine).

C.T. Wolfe (✉)
Sarton Centre for History of Science, Department of Philosophy and Moral Science, Ghent University, Ghent, Belgium
e-mail: charles.wolfe@ugent.be

D. Meacham (ed.), *Medicine and Society, New Perspectives in Continental Philosophy*, Philosophy and Medicine 120, DOI 10.1007/978-94-017-9870-9_12

Canguilhem was a prominent figure in these disciplines, particularly in the rather short-lived intellectual formation known as "biophilosophy" (along with Raymond Ruyer and Gilbert Simondon; Ruyer's early works are contemporary with Canguilhem's, in the 1940s, while Simondon shares with Canguilhem a 'heyday' in the 1960s). The latter precisely was the project to understand Life, living beings, the concept of organism, and so on, in terms not exclusively dictated either by mechanistic science or by the philosophical fellow-travellers of such science. The question of whether such a project is necessarily "vitalistic" or "biochauvinist" [to use a recent coinage by the biological theorist and embodied-cognition researcher Ezequiel Di Paolo, in Di Paolo (2009)], and of course, what these terms mean in the present context, shall be part of my concern in this essay.

Canguilhem sometimes described himself as a vitalist—playfully, but perhaps not ironically (Canguilhem 1965 and 1977, Preface), and one should not forget that in the decades he did so, particularly the 1950s–1960s, it was at the very least provocative (Geroulanos 2009); there was after all no scholarship either on eighteenth-century vitalism (like that of the Montpellier School) or on early nineteenth-century German biology (like Blumenbach's embryology), nor of course was there such a thing as "theory" and its invocations of vitalism (such as Bennett 2010b). Canguilhem returned to the theme several times, and of course in a broader sense if we reflect on some of the core arguments of his classic, *The Normal and the Pathological*, we find an implicit presupposition that normativity is a power or capacity proper to *living* beings. This may not be full-blown "vitalism" [whatever that is; see Wolfe (2011a, b); Normandin and Wolfe (2013)], but it is an insistence that there is something unique about living entities that makes them creators of a certain world which they inhabit.

This should not be taken so much in the sense of classical idealism, for which "nothing whatsoever can have a positive relation to the living being if the latter is not in its own self the possibility of this relation, i.e. if the relation is not determined by the Notion and hence not directly immanent in the subject" (Hegel 1817/1970, § 359R, p. 385); it is closer for instance to von Uexküll's sense of *Umwelt*, according to which "[e]very subject spins out, like the spider's threads, its relations to certain qualities of things and weaves them into a solid web, which carries its existence" (von Uexküll 2010, p. 53). But we can also detect in this idea of living beings as creators, some Nietzschean overtones or *arrière-pensées* [and of course Foucault pointed to this aspect in his mentor's work, emphasizing that "forming concepts is a way of living, not of killing life, of living in complete mobility and not immobilizing life" (Foucault 1985/1989, p. 21)]: the idea that values, norms and other higher-level constructs are in fact products of our vital instincts. For Canguilhem, who was interested in such illustrations of the unpredictability of life as monsters:

> Man is only truly healthy when he is capable of multiple norms, when he is more than normal. The measure of health is a certain capacity to overcome organic crises in order to

> establish a new physiological order, different from the initial order. In all seriousness, health is the ability [*le luxe*] to fall ill and then get over it. On the contrary, illness is the reduction of the power to overcome other illnesses.[1]

Closer to the present topic, we can also recognize in this idea the influence of Kurt Goldstein, who elaborated, in his lengthy and difficult work on "the structure of the organism" (Goldstein 1934/1995), a conception of organisms as interpretive and indeed *meaning-creating* beings; beings for whom being alive, acting, is, aside from other metabolic processes, also a process of the production of meaning. Or, in a more recent restatement of the same core idea: "organisms are subjects having purposes according to values encountered in the making of their living" (Weber and Varela 2002, p. 102). Differently put, the kind of vitalism at work in Goldstein and Canguilhem is explicitly *not* like the vitalism of those people who contemplate little squiggly bundles of life (from Trembley's polyp to Driesch's sea urchin blastomeres, via Réaumur's frogs which he made to wear little taffetas shorts to catch their sperm) and then assert that they have witnessed the difference between Life and non-Life: "A vitalist, I would suggest, is someone who is led to reflect on the nature of life more because of the contemplation of an egg than because she has handled a hoist or a bellows" (Canguilhem 1965a, p. 88). Rather, it is a vitalism of meaning and projection.

Yet Canguilhem (unlike, say, Hans Jonas) is genuinely concerned with the nature of *biological* life, not with some secret way of defending human uniqueness over and against the rest of the physical universe. In his major collection of essays on the topic, *The Phenomenon of Life*, Jonas opposes the world of conscious organisms to the "dead" world of mechanical Nature and insists that "the point of life itself" is "its self-centered individuality," which he insists must be an "ontological concept" (Jonas 1966, p. 79); from the outset, he explains that he is interested in biological processes such as metabolism in as much as they are ultimately indicative of "freedom" (3; see also Kass 1995).[2] Indeed, vitalism has often served as a mask or indicator of humanism, itself often with theological foundations. That is, claims of an oppositional or differential sort, in which "Life," "organism," "the animal" or "the living body" are opposed, often in foundation a list ontological terms, to "physical nature," "mechanical nature," "mechanistic materialism," "the world as machine" and so on, like Carolyn Merchant's *Death of Nature* (Merchant (1980); see Sutton and Tribble (2011) for an inspiring critique) often in the end have an anthropocentric motivation such as defending freedom, as in Jonas' case above, or those thinkers for whom materialism and scientific analysis are suitable

[1] "*Le normal et le pathologique*," (Canguilhem 1965b, p. 167). See also Canguilhem (1972, pp. 77, 155).

[2] I am not suggesting that Jonas was a panpsychist, but rather that what interests him is not Nature per se, but conscious, self-maintaining organisms as such—and then, by extension, a system which enables such organisms to exist (thanks to Darian Meacham for demanding this clarification). A philosopher familiar with Hegel might recognize here a form of the philosophy of nature in which organisms are relevant inasmuch as they are (weak, or provisional) forms of subjectivity, and ultimately of Spirit. It does not seem as if Jonas would have appreciated this similarity, but such concerns lie outside the remit of the present essay.

for "the material universe" but "yield disastrous results when applied to the inner, subjective world of human nature, human thought, and human emotions" (Hill 1968, p. 90). In contrast, Canguilhem was a *naturalist*, to use a term of art popular from the last decades: he approvingly quotes Spinoza asserting that we are *parts of Nature* and nothing more: we, as humans, or rational agents, or possessors of a pineal gland, do not form an *imperium in imperio* (Canguilhem 1965a, p. 95).

But my question here is, in what way does Canguilhem argue, biochauvinistically, for living bodies being special? One of the curious features of Goldstein's account we find again in Canguilhem's unique way of engaging with "organisms" and the question of their uniqueness: the way in which he wavers or moves back and forth between a cautious, *epistemological* position (reminiscent of the Kantian regulative ideal in the third *Critique*) in which organisms are real and special *because of the way we cognitively constitute them*, and a bold, *ontological* position in which organisms are real because of basic, intrinsic features which are just there. I shall not go into the details of Goldstein's account, which sounds more Heideggerian than anything else —for example, the claim in his "Concluding Remarks" that "the organism is a being enduring in time," curiously enough "in eternal time, for it does not commence with procreation, certainly not with birth, and does not end with death"—although to be fair these "existential" motifs crop up in Canguilhem too (Goldstein 1934/1995, p. 387).[3] But if we set that aside, Goldstein definitely contributed a new kind of approach which was, of course, holistic and organismic while nevertheless operating at a primarily heuristic, non-ontological level. As he says, "*The Organism* consists mainly of a detailed description of the new method, the so-called holistic, organismic approach. [...] We were confronted then with a difficult problem of epistemology. The primary aim of my book is to describe this methodological procedure in detail, by means of numerous observations" (Goldstein 1934/1995, p. 18).

However, this convenient distinction between the epistemological (projective, constitutive) vision of biological entities and the ontological vision (strong vitalist, "rational metaphysics" as Kant might have said), is somewhat muddied when Canguilhem introduces a further vitalist twist: that it might be an objective ("ontological") feature of living beings (i) that they are interpretive beings, à la Goldstein, and especially (ii) that they need to consider *other* entities as themselves organismic, purposive, vital (Canguilhem 1965a). There is also an existentialist *parfum* in Canguilhem's reflections (a further twist on the ontological dimension in [i]), when he describes this interpretive stance as essentially a kind of fundamental existential attitude.[4] One finds the properly biological or biomedical version of this "existentialism" in *The Normal and the Pathological*, with statements such as "the

---

[3]Interestingly, in one of his last papers, Goldstein pointed to the differences between his point of view and that of existential psychiatry: "I agree with the existentialist concept insofar as I also deny that biological phenomena, particularly human existence, can be understood by application of the method of natural science. But I differ as to the meaning of the term 'existence'. It means for me an epistemological concept based on phenomenological observations, which enables us to describe normal and pathological behavior and to give e definite orientation for therapy. It is a kind of philosophical anthropology" (Goldstein 1959, pp. 11–12).

life of a living being […] only recognizes the categories of health and illness on the level of experience, which is first of all an *épreuve* in the affective sense of the term —not on the level of science" (Canguilhem 1972, p. 131). We should notice here the appeal to a founding, subjective, dimension, although it is not clear if this should be treated as an ontologically specific region or not. That is, Canguilhem is neither listing "objective features" of living beings, like homeostasis, and claiming that they are "definitory," nor, conversely, is he opting for a fully subjectivist position, where "to live" is understand on the model of, or as interrelated with, "to know" as the property of a knowing subject. Is he closer to a Hegelian perspective, in which the organism is already a form of subjectivity? Again, this is not the place to decide such matters.

If we try to understand Canguilhem in relation to recent theoretical biology (including the "organizational" theories of A. Moreno et al., see Bechtel (2007), Mossio and Moreno (2010), Moreno and Mossio, 2015), using as a guiding question, "are organisms unique in the physical world? If so, why?", we arrive at a curious situation, in which he seems to be both more and less committed to the *uniqueness* of embodied, biomedical entities than other theoreticians. On the one hand, Canguilhem appears more cautious, and less crypto-dualistic than some prominent recent figures like Varela, who tend to fall into the category mistake of seeking to prove the uniqueness of the biological by providing some empirical criteria—a "laundry list," as it were, which frequently invokes Bernard's *milieu intérieur*, Cannon's notion of homeostasis, and more recently the work of Ganti, Luisi et al. on self-organization and autocatalytic processes (and organizational closure).[5] This is particularly odd when some of these figures invoke the authority of Kant in the Third *Critique* [as has become very common in this strand of theoretical biology, e.g. Weber and Varela (2002); Perret (2012); Simeonov et al. (2012)]. To put it bluntly, to provide an empirical set of criteria for why living beings are special and to claim that this fills in a Kantian framework, is not a good idea if this framework explicitly rejects the idea of giving empirical definitions of organism, inasmuch as Kant's organism concept is explicitly built around his notion of regulative ideal (Kant 1790/1987, § 73, 276; Wolfe 2010). For Kant, organism is a "reflective" construct rather than a "constitutive" feature of reality, and reflective judgments are "incapable of justifying any objective assertions" (Kant 1790/1987, § 67, 259; § 73, 277).

Kurt Goldstein and Canguilhem were, I think, on to something when they insisted that rather than say what is unique about the biological, we look to the *observer*: to be an organism is to have a *point of view* on organisms; one which produces intelligibility, which reveals organisms as meaning-producing beings (see,

---

[4]For more on the young Canguilhem as a humanist existentialist, a reader of Alain, prior to his turn to vitalism, see the precise analysis in Bianco (2013).

[5]For a rare acknowledgment of this problem, see Di Paolo (2009), where he criticizes Varela for "a hazy view of living systems as being defined by a list of properties (growth, reproduction, responsiveness" (p. 14). A nice extension of this point is in Machery (2012) (see especially his critical evaluation of those he calls "life definitionists," who "have constantly mixed folk intuitions with scientific considerations," p. 161).

Starobinski (1956, p. 5) who comments that "*comprendre nous met en présence d'une totalité signifiante*"[6]). Notice that this approach valorizes a *constructivist* dimension in the definition of life and the relevant individual and is not unlike the World Health Organization's notorious definition of health, which is broad enough to include all senses of well-being: "Health is a state of complete physical, mental and social well-being and not merely the absence of disease or infirmity."[7] That is, there may be biological "facts" or "invariants," but we are makers of our worlds. As to who this "we" might be—humans, higher mammals, all living creatures?—Canguilhem is never very clear how restrictive this concept is: like von Uexküll's *Umwelt*, could it apply to ticks and woodlice? He sometimes grants that "even for an amoeba, living means preference and exclusion," using the same phrase later in the book: "the life of a living entity, *even an amoeba*, only acknowledges the categories of health and sickness on the level of experience" (Canguilhem 1972, pp. 84, 131, emphasis mine). But most of the time he is interested in humans as subjective, embodied agents—the objects of medical science, caught between biological and social norms. And this is why I suggest that he can be called a humanist.

But on the other hand, this is not the final answer, or the argument-stopper: as I mentioned above, Canguilhem is also *more* biocentric or biochauvinistic than many of his contemporaries. This appears more clearly if we contrast Canguilhem with the fairly "disembodied" character of much of recent theoretical biology: in contrast, he *wants to be* a kind of vitalist. To be sure, Canguilhem is not the sort of thinker who seeks to discover "organismic laws" (like Elsasser 1961), lays out a laundry list of ontologically unique features, or most crudely, propounds a metaphysics of entelechies, like Hans Driesch, who converted his Chair in biology into one in philosophy in order to reinvent a jejune Aristotelianism based on his earlier experimental work in *Entwicklungsmechanik* (which Erik Peterson has described, fittingly, as 'bioexceptionalism' (Peterson 2012, 2013): an empire within an empire or "kingdom within a kingdom," as it were): a metaphysics of the sea urchin.

To be more precise, Driesch, who came out of the school of Wilhelm Roux's *Entwicklungsmechanik* (or study of the mechanisms of the developmental process), performed successful, and much-discussed experiments with sea urchin eggs, halving the two blastomeres (daughter cells) of the egg and successfully producing two whole embryos and larvae, complete in every respect. This total equality of the halved eggs he termed their "totipotency," and the cells derived from the egg he termed a harmonious equipotential system (Driesch 1914, p. 209). Faced with the evidence that there was no physical structure we can find in the sea urchin embryo

[6]Starobinski (1956, p. 5); the extent to which this includes non-human animals is open to discussion.

[7]Preamble to the Constitution of the World Health Organization as adopted by the International Health Conference, New York, 19–22 June 1946; signed on 22 July 1946 by the representatives of 61 States (Official Records of the World Health Organization, no. 2, p. 100) and entered into force on 7 April 1948. The definition has not been amended since 1948.

which is responsible for the "regulative" or "equipotential," force, he felt obliged to posit a vital force, the *entelechy*.[8] Tellingly, Driesch became so absorbed with this feature that he gave up experimental work to teach philosophy at the University of Leipzig, developing a form of vitalism, as he called it, focusing on the idea that *entelechies* exist in all living organisms. The choice of term was deliberate, for he believed one had to revive a vitalist thinking which had lain dormant since Aristotle (the Montpellier school does not appear in his historical surveys). Canguilhem comments on Driesch's "shift" from science to metaphysics as follows:

> The vitalist biologist who turns philosopher of biology thinks he brings a certain capital with him to philosophy, but in reality he brings to it only a land-income [*rentes*], which continually decreases in the market of scientific values – for the simple reason that research, in which he no longer participates, continues to move forward. Such is the case with Driesch's abandonment of scientific research for philosophical speculation and even teaching. What we have here is an unpremeditated abuse of confidence. The prestige of scientific work stems above all from its internal dynamism. The former scientist sees himself deprived of tills prestige in the eyes of active scientists. He believes he will preserve it among the philosophers. This must not be so. Philosophy, being an autonomous enterprise of reflection, does not honor any prestige at all, not even that of the scientist, or – even more rightly – that of the ex-scientist (Canguilhem 1965a, p. 94; I have used the translation in Canguilhem 2008a, pp. 68–69).

Canguilhem is not a metaphysician of entelechies, then; nor is he a quasi-religious defender of the sovereignty of organic life like Hans Jonas or his more simplistic disciple Leon Kass (Kass 1995); nor a defender of philosophical anthropology like Helmuth Plessner (here I refer back to my comment regarding the hidden or overt foundationalism in such forms of vitalism). In some respects, particularly in his 1966 essay "*Le concept et la vie*," which begins with a long reflection on Aristotle, he seems closer to Marjorie Grene and her attempt to return to Aristotelian teleology [Grene (1968, 1974); Grene herself wrote favorably about Canguilhem, see, Grene (2000)]. Unlike many of these thinkers, as well as phenomenologists of embodiment, Canguilhem has no appeal to a Romantic subjectivity, e.g. in the sense described (critically) by Jean-Marie Schaeffer: "In phenomenology, the understanding of embodiment (*corporéité*) is part of an approach that continues to accept the epistemic privilege of consciousness's self-investigation as axiomatic" or (affirmatively) by the enactivist theorist Evan Thompson: "Life realizes a kind of interiority, the interiority of selfhood and sense-making."[9] In explicit contrast to Varela and most of the above-mentioned thinkers (with the exception of Grene), Canguilhem does not have any problems with Darwinian evolution (Canguilhem 1972, p. 90; Méthot 2013), and indeed is not engaged in the project of "refounding," "regrounding" or otherwise reinventing a

[8] I note that Bergson (who was sometimes wrongly associated with Driesch under the banner of vitalism in the early twentieth century) attacked this claim of a life-force in all living organisms explicitly. Bergson asked: where is this force? at what level? He expressed doubts that nature could be interpreted strictly in terms of this internal "finality" (Wolsky and Wolsky 1992, p. 156f).

[9] Schaeffer (2007, p. 118), Thompson (2007, p. 238). Thompson often refers to "sense-making" as a distinctive feature of enaction, in autopoietic systems (e.g. p. 139).

new program for science. There are occasional, late exceptions which display a more reactive attitude towards the march of science, such as his remarks against some of psychology, cognitive science and cognitive neuroscience in the essay "*Le Cerveau et la Pensée*" (Canguilhem 1980/1992), which themselves extend criticisms already articulated in (Canguilhem 1958/2002c). But is he still a "biochauvinist," claiming that there is a special "biological space and time"?

All of this is really quite "dialectical," in the sense of being slippery, and almost circular—but in a productive sense. Namely, when a prominent figure like Andy Clark, who pushed cognitive science to take embodiment much more seriously in a variety of publications at least since *Being There* (Clark 1997), has to warn about the mysticism of "pressing the flesh" (Clark 2008), he is effectively stepping back from twenty years' worth of emphasis on what is unique about embodiment. When Di Paolo warns against the naïveté of "biochauvinism," ten pages later he speaks approvingly of another theorist (Michael Wheeler)'s concept of "vital materiality" (Di Paolo (2009, p. 20), referring to Wheeler (2010), the paper had been available for some years). Wheeler had used this term in opposition to what he calls *implementational* materiality. *Vital* materiality is meant to convey the sense of the necessarily biological features of certain types of organization.

Similarly, just when Canguilhem has finished warning the reader about the intellectual dangers inherent in positing that living beings are like an empire within an empire (*imperium in imperio*, Canguilhem 1965a, p. 95), he will then assert—as he does at length in "*Le concept et la vie*," that it is *Life itself*—written with a very capital L, that determines livings beings to act in these interpretive, purposive, normative, vital ways. Life "disconcerts logic" (Canguilhem 1977, p. 1). In a lecture in the problem of regulations in the organism and society, he says that:

> An organism is an entirely exceptional mode of being, because there is no real difference, properly speaking, between its existence and the rule or norm of its existence. From the time an organism exists, is alive, that organism is "possible," i.e., it fulfills the ideal of an organism; the norm or rule of its being [*existence*] is given by its existence itself. (Canguilhem 2002b, pp. 106–107)

An "entirely exceptional mode of being" sounds like ontological specificity.

He states what I loosely called the dialectical slipperiness of the relation between Life itself and the thinker's vitalism (a claim about ontology or about stances?) more sharply in *The Normal and the Pathological* itself: "It is life itself, in its differentiation between its propulsive behavior and its repulsive behavior, which introduces the categories of health and illness into human consciousness. These categories are biologically technical and subjective, not biologically scientific and objective" (Canguilhem 1972, p. 150). Notice here the subjectivism—the appeal to a foundational subjectivity—which I had earlier connected to a particularly anti-naturalistic trend in phenomenology, and the more recent theory known as enactivism, associated with Varela in particular, which often asserts that life is lived "outside of the physical": "Life is not physical in the standard materialist sense of purely external structure and function [...] [w]e accordingly need an expanded notion of the physical to account for the organism or living being" (Thompson

2007, p. 238). Indeed, Canguilhem himself, sounding less careful than usual, will sometimes say that "[i]n short, it is impossible for the objectivity of medical knowledge to cancel out (*annuler*) the subjectivity of the lived experience of the patient" (Canguilhem 1978/2002a, p. 409; this essay was added to the later edition of this book). Yet the subjectivity at issue is, to be fair, never disembodied, never some pure ego contemplating the reality of the flesh like a sailor in a ship.[10] Where Canguilhem differs sharply from the phenomenology of embodiment is that the latter is permanently tempted by a foundationalist distinction between *Leib* as interiority and *Körper* as exteriority (as Schaeffer notes in the passage cited above). From Merleau-Ponty to Varela and Thompson, such thinkers maintain that the lived body (which really is *the* body in their discourse) exists at least in part "outside of physical space" (Merleau-Ponty 1963, p. 209). Thus the living body—indeed, any organism—"is an individual in a sense which is not that of modern physics" (154).

Now, Canguilhem is in his own way, a thinker of embodiment, which I have noted in contrasting his view with both Driesch's (neo-)vitalism and Jonas's metaphysics of organism. But he has no need for these additional commitments to a "non-physical" dimension of Life. Indeed, I don't think Canguilhem, the medical doctor, would ever go as far as Deleuze and speak of a vitalism of the inorganic, a "powerful non-organic life,"[11] or, as contemporary theorists might, of "a vitality intrinsic to materiality as such," wherein the author recommends "detach[ing] materiality from the figures of passive, mechanistic, or divinely infused substance" (Bennett 2010a, p. xiii). Life is too central for him—not life-forces or entelechies, not cosmic or impersonal life, but the life of embodied agents. Similarly, the particularly *medical* emphasis in his vitalism (manifest in his focus on Bichat and related figures), which can be conveyed in the basic claim that all living beings die and get sick, with the implied, irreducibly *axiological* dimension, distinguishes it from forms of vitalism predicated on embryology and its mysteries: "the patient is a Subject" (with a capital Canguilhem 1978/2002a, p. 409; for more on Canguilhem on values and subjectivity, see Sholl, ms.). That is, a philosophical reflection on health and sickness, on the "normativity" of the organism and its experience (Goldstein-Canguilhem) is at some distance from a reflection on the egg, its potential and the metaphysics one can derive from it. Of course, not all scientific and theoretical reflections on the uniqueness of developmental systems need to appeal to a metaphysical uniqueness of life, even at their most holistic, organismic

[10]The image that the (immaterial) soul is in the (material) body like a sailor in a ship is something that Aristotle considers (*De Anima* II, i, 413a5) and that Descartes in the Sixth Meditation rejects, without mentioning Aristotle, and sounding for all the world like a phenomenologist: "Nature … teaches me, by these sensations of pain, hunger, thirst and so on, that I am not merely present in my body as a sailor is present in a ship, but that I am very closely joined and, as it were, intermingled with it, so that I and the body form a unit" (AT IX, 64 / CSM II, 56).

[11]See, Deleuze (1993, p. 164): "*La vitalité non-organique est le rapport du corps à des forces ou puissances imperceptibles qui s'en emparent ou dont il s'empare,*" and Deleuze and Guattari (1991, p. 172). In *Francis Bacon, Logique de la sensation*, the phrase "*la vitalité non organique d'un corps sans organe*" is partly credited to Wörringer and opposed to the phenomenological unity of the body (Deleuze 1981/2002, p. 31).

moments (Oyama 2010), and similarly, there is nothing inherently false about focusing on the unique features of biological systems, whether of the homeostatic sort (Bernard, Cannon, Luisi, Turner), the developmental (Oyama) or of the ecologically systemic sort (Odling-Smee).[12]

Conversely, and despite their shared affinity for Goldstein, it is more than unlikely that Canguilhem would verse into Catholic mysticism of the flesh, as Merleau-Ponty does in the *Phenomenology of Perception*: "Just as the sacrament not only symbolizes [...] an operation of Grace, but is also the real presence of God [...] in the same way the sensible has not only a motor and vital significance but is a way of being in the world [...] sensation is literally a form of communion."[13] I think Canguilhem's advocating of a core Spinozist tenet (we are all parts of Nature, there is no kingdom within a kingdom), his Nietzschean position with regard to life as the production of value(s), and his Darwinian recognition of the role of chance and evolution, to name three basic features of his thought, put him at odds with the above doctrine. This is so, even if, commenting in fact on Merleau-Ponty in a late lecture on Health, Canguilhem reflects with what I *think* to be a hint of distance, regret or irony on the limitations of a conceptualization of the living body as "inaccessible to others, accessible only to its titular holder" (2008b, p. 476); that is, he has referred to "commentator after commentator" who ascribes superiority to what is given as such, acknowledging the existence of a side of the living body that is "inaccessible to others, accessible only to its titular holder" (476).

This sense of privacy, of inaccessible interiority, is a crucial feature of many defenses of what organisms are and how they are different from machines: Leibniz for instance, for whom they differ from ordinary machines in possessing a "deeper source"[14]; or perhaps Kant when he stated rather confidently, and influentially, that "there will never be a Newton of a blade of grass" in the third *Critique* of 1790, having already claimed in the so-called "pre-critical" *Universal Natural History and Theory of the Heavens* of 1755 that "we will sooner understand the formation of all celestial bodies, the cause of their motions, in short, the origin of the entire present arrangement of the world-edifice, than we will come to know distinctly or

[12]For some philosophical discussion of these various recent models in biology, see Barberousse et al. (2009) and Normandin and Wolfe (2013).

[13]Merleau-Ponty (1962, p. 212). Novalis already identified the experience and conceptual paradoxes of the sense of touch with "the mystery of transubstantiation" (Novalis 1798/1987, p. 622). This fascination with the flesh as somehow apart from the physical world is present, prior to Merleau-Ponty, in the Husserl of *Ideas* II, and later, in Didier Anzieu and his notion of the "*Moi-Peau*," and Jean-Luc Nancy, with his "secularized Christian" fascination with embodiment *qua* incarnation. They seem to repeat verbatim the powerful mystical utterances concerning a body beyond this world, of figures such as the twelfth-century nun Hildegard of Bingen and the thirteenth-century Flemish poet and Beguine, Hadewijch (Dailey 2011). Granted, it is possible to derive other positions from Merleau-Ponty, notably in his earlier work *The Structure of Behavior*.

[14]Letter to Hoffmann of September 17, 1699, in Hoffmann (1749, I, pp. 49a-b), cf. *De ipsa natura* (1698, § 3, GP IV, p. 505), Leibniz (1969, p. 95).

completely the production of a single herb or of a caterpillar from mechanical grounds."[15] This is what Schaeffer meant in the passage I cited above, when he refers to the understanding of embodiment that holds as foundational the "epistemic privilege" of a self-aware consciousness (Schaeffer 2007, p. 118). Of course, not all claims that organisms are categorically different from machines amount to defining this difference in terms of a deeper interiority or selfhood. But increasingly, from the late eighteenth century onwards, and into twentieth-century phenomenology (and its embodied variants), the emphasis is on the latter, as is also manifest in Varela's insistence in his last essays on a "first-person science" (Varela and Shear 1999). We might say that the extent to which Canguilhem is committed or not, to the presence of a foundational subjectivity either "in the body" or as an irreducible feature "of the body," is the extent to which he is a phenomenologist.

Canguilhem was a self-proclaimed vitalist (although with a degree of irony), a "biochauvinist" in the sense that as a thinker of the normal and the pathological, of a "knowledge of life," as a disciple of Goldstein, he is one of the main figures of what was known as 'biophilosophy' in the mid-twentieth century—a project which differs from present philosophy of biology in a variety of ways (Gayon 2010), notably, that biophilosophy feels that philosophy, sometimes even metaphysics, can dictate its conditions to biology, since living beings have features (value? purposiveness? consciousness?) that remain inaccessible to quantitative science. In contrast, the philosophy of biology is very much a project engaged in conceptual clarification of "emerged" science, which it does not challenge. However, even qua biophilosopher, it bears noting that Canguilhem lacks the hostility to evolutionary thought found e.g. in Goldstein and Varela, just as he lacks the potentially reactionary appeal to return to a lost Aristotelian world (as in Jonas and Grene).

Some biophilosophers stand at a greater distance from mainstream science than others. Goldstein, sounding quite close to the ideas Canguilhem was to make famous in *The Normal and the Pathological*, holds that "an organism that actualizes its essential peculiarities or—which means the same thing—meets its adequate environment and the tasks arising from it, is 'normal'" (Goldstein 1934/1995, p. 325). Perhaps unconsciously paraphrasing Goldstein, Jonas in a late piece describes organisms as "things whose existence is their own achievement. That means that they only exist because of what they are doing," which he then explains as "their activity as such is their being" (Jonas 1992, p. 82). While this is not in line with mainstream biology (whether molecular, evolutionary, developmental, etc.), it is not explicitly anti-naturalist; and it is also a weak form of biochauvinism, in that it is less a *substance* (a set of empirical features), and more a *function* or *activity*

[15]Kant (1987), § 75, pp. 282–283; Kant (1755), Ak 1, p. 230. For a nice discussion which makes Canguilhem a phenomenologist see Gérard (2010); for an equally compelling reading which seeks to distance Canguilhem from phenomenology, see Sholl (2012) and especially Sholl (ms.). I am closer to Sholl's interpretation—and Canguilhem's rather pointed barbs at the expense of Husserl and in favour of Foucault (e.g. in Canguilhem 1967), should be taken into account here—but it must be recognized that there are elements in Canguilhem which lend themselves to Gérard's reading.

which is being invoked as uniquely organismic. In contrast, Raymond Ruyer's insistence on how the organism transcends the spatial realm, maintaining itself through time due to its "potential," which does not itself belong to the space-time world, is more of a revisionary metaphysics. For Ruyer, organisms possess a unity beyond spatial categories; they are fundamentally historical in character (Ruyer 1946, pp. 8, 14, 27, 58, 94). Ruyer appears to be afraid of a universe composed of inanimate matter, with shocks and displacements explainable exhaustively by the laws of mechanics—a universe in which the organism is no longer anything more than a machine: "If you are shocked by what amounts to a generalized 'theory of organism' [...] you had better see clearly that the choice is between this theory and that of a 'generalized molecule'" (Ruyer 1952, p. 166).

I have tried to distinguish between a series of views, not identical with one another, in which a valuative term variously called "the organism," "the (lived) body," "Life" and so on is presented as special in different ways, and usually opposed to the rest of physical nature. While Canguilhem shares the intuition that an organism is always "actualizing a potential," in a dynamic relation between a plurality of norms and an environment which is made "one's own" (an *Umwelt*), he does not oppose modern biology, and is certainly not seeking to "reintroduce the subject into biology," unlike Varela (Weber and Varela 2002, p. 117). He is arguing from properties of existing biological entities—sometimes cells, sometimes monsters or environments, but most often persons, whether considered as agents or as patients. As he says in the Introduction to the *Normal and the Pathological*, he is not so presumptuous as to claim that he could renew medicine by incorporating a metaphysics into it (Canguilhem 1972, p. 9). I have not tried here to articulate a "Canguilhemian philosophy of medicine" (some have: Trnka 2003); doubtless it would resemble in some important ways, reflection on the importance of a "patient-centred" medicine, and would pay close attention to the Goldsteinian and Canguilhemian focus on how the organism (or person, or patient) is a creator of norms (of stability, of health, of survival and so on), in a partly constructivist sense. Yet if we wish to take Canguilhem seriously, some of the metaphysics, the bio-chauvinism, the existential dimension in his thought take us beyond the practical concerns of an empirically focused philosophy of medicine.

Perhaps we should distinguish between three basic claims: *strong vitalism*, with a metaphysical foundation; *biochauvinism*, which is more of a "spontaneous scientific form" of vitalism, stripped of all or most of its metaphysical commitments but definitely tending towards a holistic, organismic perspective; and *Canguilhem's view*, which of course he never names, enjoying as he does the play of aporias and the mask of the scholar. We could speak of a non-metaphysical vitalism, or a "naturalized vitalism"[16]—but then we run into difficulties in accounting for the passages where he speaks of an irreducible, experiential dimension of life; we could say that to the biochauvinistic claims of theoretical biology, he adds an *existential*

[16]Thanks to Pierre-Olivier Méthot for this suggestion. For a related idea of a "functional vitalism" (as opposed to the metaphysical variety) see Wolfe (2011a).

dimension. Yet Canguilhem doesn't seem to succumb to the temptation of a bottomless interiority, inwardness or privacy and its concomitant transcendence. Somewhere in between the cold appeal of the inorganic, and the (hot?) mesmerism of transubstantiation—at some distance then from the fascination with a kind of transcendence of the flesh found in Merleau-Ponty, Varela or Thompson, where biochauvinism verges on the mystery of transubstantiation—Canguilhem's vitalism, *his* biochauvinism, his quirky appeals to the "truth of my body" (2008b, p. 475) if not his residual existentialism may hold some lessons for present-day thinking about embodiment, neither obsessively reductionist, nor whimsically holist.

Acknowledgments Versions of this paper have been presented at the Workshop on The Normal and the Pathological, University of Warwick, September 2011; Canguilhem's Philosophy of Life, KU Leuven, June 2012. I thank the organizers and audiences of those events, and Pierre-Olivier Méthot for their helpful comments.

References

Barberousse, A., Morange, M., & Pradeu, T. (Eds.). (2009). *Mapping the future of biology: Evolving concepts and theories*. Dordrecht: Springer.

Bechtel, W. (2007). Biological mechanisms: Organized to maintain autonomy. In F. Boogerd, F. J. Bruggeman, J.-H. S. Hofmeyr & H. V. Westerhoff (Eds.). *Systems biology: Philosophical foundations* (pp. 269–302). Amsterdam: Elsevier.

Bennett, J. (2010a). *Vibrant matter: A political ecology of things*. Durham: Duke University Press.

Bennett, J. (2010b). A vitalist stopover on the way to a new materialism. In D. Coole & S. Frost (Eds.), *New materialisms: Ontology, agency, and politics* (pp. 47–69). Durham: Duke University Press.

Bianco, G. (2013). At the origins of Georges Canguilhem's 'Vitalism.' Against the Anthropology of Irritation. In S. Normandin & C. T. Wolfe (Eds.), *Vitalism and the scientific image in post-enlightenment life science, 1800–2010* (pp. 243–267). Dordrecht: Springer.

Canguilhem, G. (1965a). Aspects du vitalisme [1946–1947]. In *La connaissance de la vie*, revised edition (pp. 83–100). Paris: Vrin. (First published 1952).

Canguilhem, G. (1965b). La connaissance de la vie, revised edition. Paris: Vrin. (First published 1952).

Canguilhem, G. (1967). Mort de l'homme ou épuisement du Cogito? *Critique, 242*, 599–618.

Canguilhem, G. (1972). Le Normal et le pathologique (3rd ed.). Paris: PUF. (First published 1943).

Canguilhem, G. (1977). La formation du concept de réflexe aux XVIIe et XVIIIe siècles (2nd ed.). Paris: Vrin. (First published 1955).

Canguilhem, G. (1992). Le Cerveau et la Pensée (1980). In E. Balibar, D. Lecourt, et al. (Eds.), *Canguilhem, philosophe, historien des sciences* (pp. 11–33). Paris: Albin Michel.

Canguilhem, G. (2002a). Puissance et limites de la rationalité en médecine (1978). *Études d'histoire et de philosophie des sciences concernant les vivants et la vie* (pp. 392–411). Paris: Vrin.

Canguilhem, G. (2002b). Le problème des régulations dans l'organisme et la société. In É. Canguilhem (Ed.), *sur la médecine* (pp. 101–125). Paris: Éditions du Seuil.

Canguilhem, G. (2002c). Qu'est-ce que la psychologie? (1958). In É. Canguilhem (Ed.), *d'Histoire et de Philosophie des Sciences* (pp. 365–381). Paris: Vrin.

Canguilhem, G. (2008a). *Knowledge of Life* (P. Marrati & T. Meyers, Eds., S. Geroulanos & D. Ginsburg, Trans.). New York: Fordham University Press.

Canguilhem, G. (2008b). Health: Crude concept and philosophical question (T. Meyers & S. Geroulanos, La santé, concept vulgaire et question philosophique (1988), Trans.). *Public Culture, 20*(3), 467–477.

Clark, A. (1997). *Being there*. Cambridge, MA: MIT Press.

Clark, A. (2008). Pressing the flesh: A tension in the study of the embodied embedded mind? *Philosophy and Phenomenological Research, 76*(1), 37–59.

Dailey, P. (2011). Children of promise: The bodies of Hadewijch of Brabant. *Journal of Medieval and Early Modern Studies, 41*(2), 317–343.

de Issekutz Wolsky, M., & Wolsky, A. A. (1992). Bergson's vitalism in the light of modern biology. In F. Burwick & P. Douglass (Eds.), *The crisis in modernism. Bergson and the vitalist controversy* (pp. 153–170). Cambridge: Cambridge University Press.

Deleuze, G. (1981). *Francis Bacon. Logique de la sensation*. Paris: Éditions de la différence, réédition, Seuil, 2002.

Deleuze, G. (1993). *Critique et clinique*. Paris: Minuit.

Deleuze, G., & Guattari, F. (1991). *Qu'est-ce que la philosophie?*. Paris: Minuit.

Di Paolo, E. (2009). Extended life. *Topoi, 28*, 9–21.

Driesch, H. (1914). *The History and theory of vitalism* (C. K. Ogden, Trans.). London: Macmillan.

Elsasser, W. (1961). Quanta and the concept of organismic law. *Journal of Theoretical Biology, 1*(1), 27–58.

Foucault, M. (1989). Introduction (1985). In Canguilhem, The Normal and the Pathological (C. Fawcett, Trans.). New York: Zone Books.

Gayon, J. (2010). Vitalisme et philosophie de la biologie. *Répha, 2*, 7–18. Reprinted in P. Nouvel (Ed.), *Repenser le vitalisme - Histoire et philosophie du vitalisme* (2011). Paris: PUF.

Gérard, M. (2010). Canguilhem, Erwin Straus et la phénoménologie: La question de l'organisme vivant. *Bulletin d'analyse phénoménologique, VI*(2), 118–145. http://popups.ulg.ac.be/bap.htm.

Geroulanos, S. (2009). Beyond the normal and the pathological: Recent literature on Georges Canguilhem. *Gesnerus, 66*(2), 288–306.

Giroux, E. (2010). *Après Canguilhem: définir la santé et la maladie*. Paris: PUF.

Goldstein, K. (1939/1995). *The Organism: A holistic approach to biology derived from pathological data in man* (A translation of *Der Aufbau des Organismus*, 1934). New York: American Book Company/Zone Books.

Goldstein, K. (1959). Notes on the development of my concepts. *Journal of Individual Psychology, 15*, 5–14.

Grene, M. (1968). *Approaches to a philosophy of biology*. New York: Basic Books.

Grene, M. (1974). *The understanding of nature: Essays in philosophy of biology*. Dordrecht: Reidel.

Grene, M. (2000). The philosophy of science of Georges Canguilhem: A transatlantic view. *Revue d'histoire des sciences, 53*(1), 47–63.

Hegel, G. W. F. (1970). *Encyclopedia of the philosophical sciences in outline* (1817), vol. 2 (A. V. Miller, *Philosophy of Nature,* Trans.). Oxford: Oxford University Press.

Hill, E. (1968). Materialism and monsters in the Rêve de D'Alembert. *Diderot Studies, 10*, 67–93.

Hoffmann, F. (1749). *Operum omnium physico-medicorum supplementum primum*. Geneva: Fratres De Tournes.

Jonas, H. (1966). The phenomenon of life. Towards a philosophical biology. New York: Harper & Row/Dell.

Jonas, H. (1992). *Philosophische Untersuchungen und metaphysische Vermutungen*. Frankfurt am Main: Insel.

Kant, I. (1755). Allgemeine Naturgeschichte und Theorie des Himmels. English edition: Kant, I. (1755). Universal Natural History and Theory of the Heavens. Cambridge: Cambridge University Press.

Kant, I. (1987). *Critique of Judgment* (1790) (W. Pluhar, Trans.). Indianapolis: Hackett.

Kass, L. R. (1995). Appreciating the phenomenon of life. *Hastings Center Report, 25*(7), 3–12.

Leibniz, G. W. (1969). *Opuscules philosophiques choisis* (P. Schrecker, Trans.). Paris: Vrin.

Machery, E. (2012). Why I stopped worrying about the definition of life… and why you should as well. *Synthese, 185*, 145–164.
Merchant, C. (1980). *The death of nature: Women, ecology, and the scientific revolution*. New York: Harper and Row.
Merleau-Ponty, M. (1962). *Phenomenology of Perception* (C. Smith, Trans.). London: Routledge Kegan Paul.
Merleau-Ponty, M. (1963). *The Structure of Behaviour* (A.L. Fisher, Trans.). Boston: Beacon Press.
Méthot, P.-O. (2013). On the genealogy of concepts and experimental practices: Rethinking Georges Canguilhem's historical epistemology. *Studies in History and Philosophy of Science, 44*, 112–123.
Moreno, A., & Mossio, M. (2015). *Biological autonomy. A philosophical and theoretical enquiry*. Dordrecht: Springer.
Mossio, M., & Moreno, A. (2010). Organisational closure in biological organisms. *History and Philosophy of the Life Sciences, 32*, 269–288.
Normandin, S., & Wolfe, C. T. (Eds.). (2013). *Vitalism and the scientific image in post-enlightenment life science, 1800–2010*. Dordrecht: Springer.
Novalis (1987). *Vorarbeiten* (1798), in *Werke, Tagebücher und Briefe*, ed. H.-J. Mähl and R. Samuel, 3 vols., vol. 2: *Das philosophisch-theoretische Werk*, Munich: Carl Hanser Verlag.
Oyama, S. (2010). Biologists behaving badly: Vitalism and the language of language. *History and Philosophy of the Life Sciences, 32*, 401–423.
Perret, N. (2012). A Symmetrical approach to causality in biology. *Philosophia Scientiæ, 16*(3), 177–195.
Peterson, E. L. (2012). 'Neither camp will have me': C. Lloyd Morgan, Joseph Needham, J. H. Woodger, and the early-20th century attempt to devitalize holism. In Presentation at conference on *Hasard, holisme et réductionnisme dans les sciences de la vie*, Paris, ENS, Centre Cavaillès (May 2012).
Peterson, E. L. (2013). The conquest of vitalism or the eclipse of organicism? The 1930s Cambridge organiser project and the social network of mid-twentieth century biology. *British Journal for the History of Science* (forthcoming).
Ruyer, R. (1946). *Éléments de psycho-biologie*. Paris: PUF.
Ruyer, R. (1952). *Néo-finalisme*. Paris: PUF.
Schaeffer, J.-M. (2007). *La fin de l'exception humaine*. Paris: Gallimard.
Sholl, J. (2012). The knowledge of life in Canguilhem's critical naturalism. *Pli, 23*, 107–127.
Sholl, J. ms. Problematizing a Phenomenology of Life: Goldstein, Merleau-Ponty and Canguilhem.
Simeonov, P. L., Brezina, E. H., et al. (2012). Stepping beyond the Newtonian paradigm in biology. In P. L. Simeonov, L. S. Smith, & A. C. Ehresmann (Eds.), *Integral biomathics* (pp. 319–418). Dordrecht: Springer.
Starobinski, J. (1956). *L'idée d'organisme*. Paris: Centre de Documentation Universitaire/Collège philosophique.
Sutton, J., Tribble, E. B. (2011). Materialists are not merchants of vanishing: Commentary on David Hawkes, 'Against Materialism in Literary Theory'. *Early Modern Culture* 9. http://emc.eserver.org/1-9/sutton_tribble.html.
Thompson, E. (2007). *Mind in life: Biology, phenomenology, and the sciences of mind*. Cambridge, Mass: Harvard University Press.
Trnka, P. (2003). Subjectivity and values in medicine: The case of Canguilhem. *The Journal of Medicine and Philosophy, 28*(4), 427–446.
Varela, F., & Shear, J. (Eds.). (1999). *The view from within. First person approaches to the study of consciousness*. Exeter: Imprint Academic.
von Uexküll, J. (2010). *A Foray into the worlds of animals and humans*, with *a theory of meaning* (1934) (J. D. O'Neil, Trans.). Minneapolis: University of Minnesota Press.

Weber, A., & Varela, F. J. (2002). Life after Kant: Natural purposes and the autopoietic foundations of biological individuality. *Phenomenology and the Cognitive Sciences, 1*, 97–125.
Wheeler, M. (2010). Mind, things and materiality. In L. Malafouris & C. Renfrew (Eds.), *The cognitive life of things: Recasting the boundaries of the mind* (pp. 29–37). Cambridge: McDonald Institute for Archaeological Research Publications.
Wolfe, C. T. (2010). Do organisms have an ontological status? *History and Philosophy of the Life Sciences, 32*(2–3), 195–232.
Wolfe, C. T. (2011a). From substantival to functional vitalism and beyond, or from Stahlian animas to Canguilhemian attitudes. *Eidos, 14*, 212–235.
Wolfe, C. T. (2011b). Vitalism. In M. Gargaud, et al. (Eds.), *Encyclopedia of astrobiology* (pp. 1749–1750). Berlin: Springer.

Chapter 13
Of (Auto-)Immune Life: Derrida, Esposito, Agamben

Michael Lewis

1 The Political Life

Why is there such a marked preference for speaking of bio-*ethics* rather than bio-*politics*, in traditional Anglophone analytic philosophy? It is as if life were something pure and unscathed, wholly natural and naturally whole, uncontaminated by politics, law, and power. It is the task of this essay to demonstrate that this is not the case and therefore it is not possible simply to address life on the level of the individual and the ethical. For life cannot be thought as whole and unscathed in its individual propriety. Life cannot be wholly immunised against what does not, properly speaking, belong to it. To think otherwise is to "naturalise" life, to think of life as a purely natural entity, which is to fall victim to ideology, since nature is never uncontaminated by culture, and life is never free of politics.

In speaking of the political nature of life we should immediately call to mind Aristotle's definition of man as "by *nature* a political animal" (*ho anthrōpos physei politikon zōion*) (*Politics* 1253a2–3, emphasis added) and Foucault's famous statement according to which a revolution has taken place in the history of this notion: "For millennia, man remained what he was for Aristotle: a living animal with the additional capacity for a political existence; modern man is an animal whose politics places his existence as a living being into question" (Foucault 1990 [1976], p. 143).

Some of the ideas contained in this essay were first presented at the University of Brighton (28th March 2011), the University of Warwick (January 18th 2011), and—albeit obliquely—at Manchester Metropolitan University (26th February 2009). I must thank Darian Meacham for his help with the final version.

M. Lewis (✉)
University of the West of England, Bristol, UK
e-mail: Mike.lewis@uwe.ac.uk

D. Meacham (ed.), *Medicine and Society, New Perspectives in Continental Philosophy*, Philosophy and Medicine 120, DOI 10.1007/978-94-017-9870-9_13

One could approach the political life of man from one of two points of view: that of the power which comes ever more intimately to govern life, and that of the life steadily being overwhelmed. Here, partly due to the nature of the present volume, I shall examine the latter. To this end, let us ask the following question: what must life *be* if it is capable of rendering itself vulnerable to the incursion of political power? Our exploration of this question will revolve around the notions of *immunity*—the "immune system"— and auto-immunity. The immune system is that which, by rights, might have been thought to protect the individual against such intrusions into the "body proper," our own flesh, while "*auto*-immunity" describes the way in which this immunity can always turn against itself, undermining the organism's immune defenses, for better or worse.

Autoimmunity describes the origin of a breach in the supposedly impermeable boundaries of the individual which opens that individual self to its "other," rendering the immune individual inherently *communal*, which is to say *political in its very organismic life*.

Our task here is to show how the immunity of the human animal must be understood not to oppose but to first make possible the most basic form of community. Our guides will be the two thinkers who have most profoundly explored this notion of immune and autoimmune life: Jacques Derrida and Roberto Esposito. To conclude, we shall address some questions to the "immunitary paradigm" by describing an alternative conception of life and its relation to the political proposed by Giorgio Agamben.

2 Immunity and Identity: The Philosophical Importance of Immunity

The philosophical question at stake in the notion of immunity is the question of identity: it concerns the most basic ontological unit, the most primitive thing in existence, the individual substance, and we shall see that it ends up placing the substantial character of this individuality—its self-sufficiency or completeness—in doubt.

Philosophy has for the greater part of its history defined identity in an oppositional way, and that is to say in terms of the opposition between self and what is not self, self and other. In order to function, this definition must presuppose the principles of non-contradiction and excluded middle, according to which—in this case —one cannot be both one's self and an other at the same time, and hence—given that there is no third possibility—the exclusion of the other fully defines what the self is. Thus the identity of each individual is determined by being opposed to the identity of every other individual. The self radically excludes all otherness: individuals are individual *substances* which do not depend on others for their existence, and they are radically separated from these others.

The notion of immunity has, broadly speaking, two senses: a biological sense and a legal or political sense. The relation of immunity to the individual substance is most clear in the case of biological immunity: the immune system is what protects the *identity* of the vital substance. The immune system constitutes the (porous and shifting) *boundary* between what belongs properly to oneself and what does not.

The immune system thus maintains a boundary between the vital systems of which it is a part and the outside, or, perhaps better, between the vital system and what threatens it, and this is what it means to have an "identity." As Esposito will point out, however, this boundary does not need to be understood, and in the end cannot be understood as it was in the early days of immunological science, and perhaps since the inauguration of philosophy, as a rigid, impermeable boundary. Biology—and not just biology—has in recent times given us a more intriguing way to understand this boundary, as one of a regulated *permeability*. On this account, a certain measure of alterity (otherness) is incorporated into the very identity (sameness) of the organism and installed as an essential part of the protective apparatus itself, as if one could not protect the identity of the self without incorporating a certain measure of otherness within it.

Immunity takes many forms. Here we shall be concerned with "adaptive immunity," in which contact with pathogens stimulates the development of antigens. Thanks to its "memory," the immune system can respond appropriately in the event of any future encounters with the same pathogens, or ones similar to it. More specifically, we shall address the intentional manipulation of the immune system through inoculation, in which a pathogen is deliberately and artificially introduced in order to stimulate immunity by means of an appeal to "immune memory." A classic example of inoculation may be found in the smallpox vaccination, where the human immune system is exposed to a different virus, that of cowpox, in such a way as to cause it to develop an immune response that will protect it not just against cowpox itself, but also against the more dangerous smallpox.

Hence the very notion of immunity will provide us—at the level of philosophy—with a new way of understanding *identity*, a self-identity that cannot be *opposed* to the other, but which is, at the most basic level, in community with others. In this way, by taking its lead from biology, philosophy alights upon the idea of a hospitality to the other which is essential to the very constitution of the self.[1]

This essay is an attempt to determine precisely how this immunity should be understood and how, in light of this notion, we should modify our philosophical concepts, particularly that of identity.

---

[1]The way in which a biological affair extends its relevance to ontology (and that is to say, philosophy) is captured by Esposito as follows, in relation to the most extreme disease of immune deficiency: "What is affected by AIDS [Acquired Immune Deficiency Syndrome] is not only a health protocol but an entire ontological scheme: the identity of the individual as the form and content of its subjectivity. [...] [T]he disease destroys the very idea of an identity-making border: the difference between self and other, internal and external, inside and outside" (2011 [2002], p. 162).

3 Auto-Immunity

We may approach a hospitable and non-hostile understanding of immunity by attending to the phenomenon of *auto*-immunity, immunity to one's self, which amounts to the self's attacking its own organs, tissues and processes, including the very immune system which was to have protected it and its identity. Autoimmunity would therefore be an immunity against one's *self*. I am specifically interested in the concept in the precise sense of the self's attacking the system which renders the maintenance of this self possible by separating it rigorously from its other—an immune response that weakens or destroys the organism's immunity.

We should here distinguish between the way "autoimmunity" is used in biology and the more basic ontological sense which philosophy gives to it. In the latter, the self undermines its own completeness, and this incompleteness means that the self is open to everything *other* from the very beginning. This openness and relationality is a permanent ontological state. This philosophical or ontological notion of auto-immunity finds expression in the biological sense of "autoimmunity" as the possibility that the organism might misrecognise certain parts of itself (cells, tissue, even entire organs) as foreign or threatening and hence to be rejected; but at the same time, the organism can also be deceived into misrecognising something foreign as its own, thus making possible the act of transplantation and all manner of artificial grafts. The difference between the philosophical sense of autoimmunity and the biological sense is that philosophical autoimmunity describes a permanent state that characterises all substances, while biological autoimmunity is a *possibility* which may or may not be actualised in a particular organism.

The reason why a substance and—more narrowly speaking—an organism might have this tendency towards autoimmunity can be clarified by considering the way in which immunisation functions in the form of inoculation: by deploying a non-lethal form or dose of a certain pathogen in order to build up an entity's defense *against* that very pathogen or ones similar to it—as in the case of the smallpox vaccine.

When it comes to poisons and pathogens, if the immune defenses are not instituted in this way, the borders of the individual will be subject to all manner of ingressions, and eventually the boundary will become obscured by continual trespass, before vanishing altogether: this is the moment of ontological disintegration and biological death.

4 Derrida on Autoimmunity

In our investigation of immunity and autoimmunity, we shall begin with Derrida. This is for at least two reasons: One is that he is the most prominent and important thinker to deploy this vocabulary, and he uses it to speak of the rethinking of the ontology of *substance* that deconstruction was engaged in from the very beginning.

This is significant for us since our concern here is precisely the way in which the notion and structure of immunity might force us to rethink identity or substantiality.

The second reason is that an investigation of Derrida will lead us onto the work of the contemporary Italian philosopher, Roberto Esposito, who takes up the problem of immunity where Derrida left off and then carries it in two important new directions and into two new contexts: the *historical* unfolding of immunity in relation to the problem of biopolitics, and the relation between immunity and *community*.

But first we need to become acquainted with the philosophical relevance of immunity as Derrida understands it. The *loci classici* for Derrida's comments on autoimmunity were all written in the last decade of his life: "Faith and Knowledge" (1996), "Autoimmunity: Real and Symbolic Suicides" (2001), and *Rogues* (2002).

In "Faith and Knowledge," from 1996, Derrida describes the way in which both religion and science (faith and knowledge) in their traditional forms rely on the notion of an absolute instance that would remain "immune" in the sense of "unscathed," untouched by otherness, and invulnerable to ingression: in other words, an instance of the purest sovereignty.

Derrida attempts to demonstrate the impossibility of such an immune instance by attending to the very logic of immunity itself, according to which it is always possible for immunity to turn back on itself and become *auto*immunity. In this way, the supposedly complete totality perforates and breaches its own totality. From the very start, deconstruction was concerned to show that anything which presents itself as a totality cannot do so without referring to some other thing from which it distinguishes itself; in other words, the substance has to enter into *relation* from the very beginning, and this is the very source of its own possibility. The necessity of such a recourse inevitably contaminates the pure autochthony and autarchy of any totality. The reference of the same—finite totality—to the other is a necessary relation. And this other in turn must refer to *another other* in order to constitute its own identity. And this process of referring will go on to infinity. Thus the identity of the same can never be entirely stabilised, determined once and for all. This means that the reference to the other lays one open to a loss of identity, an identity which one will never in truth have had. The novelty of "Faith and Knowledge" is its describing this self-undermining or self-deconstruction of an only putatively absolute instance in terms of *immunity* and its *autoimmune* recoil.

I shall cite three passages from this text in order to demonstrate that Derrida begins by speaking of the notion of immunity in the context of faith and knowledge, before going on to show how the same notion functions in the contexts of politics, law, Christianity, and biology. He will then suggest that, if one takes one's mark from the biological context, the notion of (auto)immunity can be generalised without limit to all identities.

Here are Derrida's words, which introduce the idea of the impossibility of absolute immunity in the case of religion:

> The same movement that renders indissociable religion and tele-technoscientific reason in its most critical aspect reacts inevitably *to itself*. It secretes its own antidote but also its own power of auto-immunity. We are here in a space where all self-protection of the unscathed, of the safe and sound, of the sacred (*heilig*, holy) must protect itself against its own

> protection, its own police, its own power of rejection, in short against its own, which is to say, against its own immunity. It is this terrifying but fatal logic of the *auto-immunity of the unscathed* that will always have associated science and religion. (Derrida 2002 [1996], pp. 79–80)[2]

These lines may be taken to describe the starting point of Roberto Esposito's project, and indeed the latter cites this passage in *Immunitas* (2011 [2002], pp. 52–53). In this connection, one should also note that Derrida here inserts a footnote on the *political* relevance of the notion of immunity, which associates immunity with *community* on exactly the same (etymological) grounds as Esposito: "The 'immune' (*immunis*) is freed or exempted from the charges, the service, the taxes, the obligations (*munus,* root of the common of community)" (Derrida 2002 [1996], p. 80n27).[3]

Derrida goes on to speak of the way in which the idea of immunity is then transplanted into the domains of law ("diplomatic immunity," for instance) and Christianity (the legal inviolability of the space of the temple), before moving on to the example which is most crucial to us here, a chronologically later use of the term "immunity" in the context of biological life. Here Derrida ventures an extremely helpful and clear definition of *auto*-immunity. In this passage, we should heed the way in which the reference to biological immunity *in particular* seems to authorise Derrida in asserting the *generality* of autoimmunity:

> It is *especially* in the domain of biology that the lexical resources of immunity have developed their authority. The immunitary reaction protects the "indemnity" of the body proper in producing antibodies against foreign antigens. As for the process of *auto*-immunisation, which interests us particularly here, it consists for a living organism, as is well known and in short, of *protecting itself against its self-protection* by destroying its own immune system. As the phenomenon of these antibodies is extended to a broader zone of pathology and as one resorts increasingly to the *positive* virtues of immuno-depressants destined to limit the mechanisms of rejection and to facilitate the tolerance of certain organ transplants, we feel ourselves authorised to speak of a sort of *general logic of auto-immunisation*. (Derrida 2002 [1996], p. 80, emphases added)[4]

---

[2]At least two important works in English have in recent years made the notion of autoimmunity their central focus: Martin Hägglund's *Radical Atheism* and Michael Naas's *Miracle and Machine*.

[3]Derrida gives a succinct account of this part of "Faith and Knowledge" in *Rogues*: "The formalisation of this autoimmune law was there carried out around the *community* as *auto-co-immunity* (the common of community having in common the same duty or charge [*munus*] as the immune), as well as the auto-co-immunity of humanity" (2005 [2003], p. 35).

[4]Here Derrida is perhaps abbreviating the full scope of "auto-immunity" in the biological sense: it refers not only to the immune system's attacking itself, but also to the immune system's attacking *other* parts of the organism and other processes that are taking place within it. That said, later in the same passage, Derrida might be seen as gesturing towards this when he speaks of the rejection of transplants, which at least seems to imply that an organism's immunity to itself can extend to parts other than the immune system itself. I am here indebted to Darian Meacham for his clarification of the biological sense of "auto-immunity".

It is crucial to note the way in which Derrida shifts from a negative to a positive version of autoimmunity: autoimmunity makes it possible for the integrity of the organism to be destroyed, it can precipitate the end of life, but it also opens up the possibility of prosthetic grafts, transplants, and implants, which can prolong life. The "intruder" to which one is hospitable may turn out to be an enemy or a friend. It is this duplicity in value that Derrida uses to authorise his *generalisation* of the logic of autoimmunity. The justification of this generalisation will become clearer as we go along.

In "Autoimmunity," six years later, in 2001, called upon to discuss the attacks of September the eleventh, Derrida recalls and redeploys this logic in the context of democracy and the anti-democratic threat to democracy which appears to come from outside but which is in fact an intrinsic consequence of democracy itself (in this context, American democracy).

Democracy will perhaps end up becoming the example of autoimmunity that Derrida privileges, even more than the biological, and indeed we might surmise that while it was the *double* (positive and negative) connotations of the biological sense of immunity that allowed him to generalise the notion, one of the most important results of this will have been that it allows him to understand the *political* form of autoimmunity to be found in democracy. Before himself quoting the passage I have cited on "the *auto-immunity of the unscathed*" (2002 [1996], pp. 79–80), Derrida comments on his earlier text as follows: "I there proposed to extend to *life in general* the figure of an autoimmunity whose meaning or origin first seemed to be limited to so-called natural life or to life pure and simple, to what is believed to be the purely 'zoological,' 'biological,' or 'genetic'" (2003 [2001], p. 187n7).

In his later quotation, to reflect the particular context into which this passage has been transplanted, Derrida underscores the word "terrifying" and goes on to suggest that, according to the logic of auto-immunity, the greatest threat of terror comes from within, in that destruction of the immune system which allows the relatively strict border between one's self and the outside to collapse, and along with it one's very identity, not because of an external enemy's attack, but as a result of internal corruption. "My vulnerability is thus, by definition and by structure, by situation, without limit. Whence the terror. Terror is always, or always becomes, at least in part, 'interior.' And terrorism always has something 'domestic,' if not national, about it. [...] [T]he enemy is *also always* lodged on the inside of the system it violates and terrorises" (2003 [2001], p. 188n7).

In *Rogues*, from the following year, 2002, the value of this generalised sense of autoimmunity for thinking about democracy becomes more clear. Here, Derrida shows in detail how the threat to democracy does not simply approach from outside, and neither is it merely a contingent defect of certain (totalitarian or imperialistic) democracies; rather, it is inherent to the very *idea* of democracy itself. Accordingly, he speaks of two (autoimmune) possibilities for a democratic process, two ways in which a democracy by its very nature is susceptible to becoming *non*-democratic:

(1) The first possibility is that the democratic process may elect a non-democratic party who have vowed, if elected, to abolish the very democratic process itself. Here the threat issues from the outside but is nevertheless a possibility that democracy lays itself open to as a result of its very essence.
(2) The second possibility is that democracy, in order to ward off this threat, suspends its own democratic character and cancels an election in which this eventuality is likely to occur (as was the case in Algeria in 1992). Thus democracy renders itself temporarily non-democratic in order to protect its identity *as* democratic. It infects itself with a measured dose of the poison which it is trying to immunise itself against.

One might think of these two autoimmune possibilities of democracy as the negative and positive values inherent to the very concept of democracy, since one would allow it to be abolished, while the other would temporarily hold it in abeyance in order ultimately to reinstate it. The two possibilities are not dissociable: that democracy *can* be suspended means that it can disfigure its own identity in order to preserve that identity, but always at the risk of losing it altogether (2005 [2003], pp. 30–3, cf. ibid. p. 35).

Derrida himself speaks explicitly of "immunisation" and then "auto-immunisation" in this context:

> [in Algeria, in 1992,] they decided in a sovereign fashion to suspend, at least provisionally, democracy *for its own good,* so as to take care of it, so as to immunise it against a much worse and very likely assault. […] [T]he hypothesis here is that of a taking of power, or rather, of a transferring of power (*kratos*) to a people (*dēmos*) who, in its electoral majority and following democratic procedures, would not have been able to avoid the destruction of democracy itself. Hence a certain suicide of democracy. Democracy has always been suicidal, and if there is a to-come for it, it is only on the condition of thinking life otherwise, life and the force of life. […] [/] There is something paradigmatic in this autoimmune suicide. (2005 [2003], p. 33)

5 Roberto Esposito: Legal and Biological Immunity

Roberto Esposito, along with Giorgio Agamben, is one of the most significant philosophers to have emerged from Italy in the last century. He takes Derrida's thought of immunity as his point of departure and immediately begins to develop it in a somewhat different direction, or at least to take it further than Derrida himself did, in a way that is inflected by the work on community undertaken by Derrida's friend, Jean-Luc Nancy.[5]

[5]This hesitation between a new direction and an explicitation reflects an ambivalence in Esposito's own position: "the category of immunisation that Derrida only hints at *or* takes in another direction is ushered back into the foreground, but in a new light" (Esposito 2011 [2002], p. 55, translation modified, emphasis added).

Esposito focuses on two aspects of the word "immunity," the legal and the biological, and, in a way that is reminiscent of Derrida's generalisation of immunity on the basis of its biological sense, Esposito will use a certain characteristic of the biological notion to rethink immunity, while taking it somewhat beyond Derrida in the direction of the relation between immunity and *community.*

Let us begin with the legal sense of immunity. The intrinsic relation between immunity and community is perhaps the most crucial insight of Esposito's work. This link is suggested by etymology, in that both words include the Latin root, "*munus,*" which Esposito defines as "an office—a task, obligation, duty (also in the sense of a gift to be repaid)" (Esposito 2011 [2002], p. 5).

The Latin language has at least two words for "gift": *munus*, which refers to a gift that is *given*—rather than a gift *received*, which is designated by the word "*donum*":[6] "the *munus* indicates only the gift that one gives, not what one receives" (Esposito 2010 [1998], p. 5, cf. ibid. p. 139). The *munus* is also a gift that, once given, obliges the recipient to reciprocate (2010 [1998], p. 5). This reciprocal obligation is what binds individuals together to form a *community* (*communitas*). By contrast, in the context of this *munus,* those who are "immune" are those exempt from this obligation to reciprocate, because they have not received the gift in the first place: they have no offices to perform. The immune are thus removed to a place outside of the community (2011 [2002], p. 5).

The real key to Esposito's account, however, is the biological interpretation of immunity, for he will use a certain interpretation of the biological immune system to rethink the relation between immunity and community in light of an *historical* situation characterised by an extreme immunisation affecting all areas of *social* life.

Esposito defines biological immunity as "the refractoriness of an organism to the danger of contracting a contagious disease" (2011 [2002], p. 7). And the way in which this is achieved is through "an attenuated form of infection [that] could protect against a more virulent form of the same type. From here came the deduction, proven by the effectiveness of the various vaccines, that the inoculation of non-lethal quantities of a virus stimulates the formation of antibodies that are able to neutralise pathogenic effects at an early stage" (2011 [2002], p. 7).

Already we can see that the immune system forms a boundary of a strange kind: in order to protect the integrity of the self, it gives entry to the forces of dissolution. In this way, the immune process is "structurally aporetic"[7] (2011 [2002], p. 8, cf. ibid. p. 159). Life can remain alive only by incorporating death. The opposition between life and death is thus no longer rigorous. Indeed, in philosophy, "life" has always tended to perturb the rigour of oppositions.

---

[6]Although, strictly speaking, *munus* may be understood as a *species* of the genus *donum* (Esposito 2010 [1998], p. 4).

[7]Esposito also says "homeopathic," since the cure for the poison is itself (something similar to) the poison or infecting agent (2011 [2002], p. 8).

6 The Two Interpretations of Biological Immunity

For Esposito, it is of crucial importance that biological immunity can be interpreted in two different ways: either as a militaristic defense against the foreign, or as an hospitable relation to the other.

To understand the importance of this, we need to know something of Esposito's broader project. Esposito's task is a political one, and it is a task which has been lent urgency by the historical moment in which we find ourselves. The solution to the problem can be given only if the problem is correctly interpreted, and throughout his great trilogy, *Communitas* (1998), *Immunitas* (2002), and *Bios* (2004), Esposito tries to show that the "key" which allows us to discern and explain the most significant phenomena of our situation is "immunity."

Once in possession of this key, we should be able to recognise that the way immunity is functioning today in the social world is based on a misunderstanding or disambiguation of the notion, which has led to its relationship with *community* being distorted. This misuse of immunity might be summarised under the heading of "security" or "defence," the way in which the securing of national and social life against a supposedly dire threat has become the primary concern of government. Esposito thus speaks of "the hypertrophy of the security apparatuses that are increasingly widespread throughout contemporary societies" (2011 [2002], p. 16).

Esposito interprets this as a destructive and self-destructive form of immunisation, in which the immunisation has accelerated to such a pace that it has begun to outrun the very threat which it was originally intended to ward off: "Instead of adapting the protection to the actual level of risk, [the "self-protective syndrome"] tends to adapt the perception of risk to the growing need for protection—making protecting itself one of the major risks" (ibid. p. 16). He concludes: "As in all areas of contemporary social systems, neurotically haunted by a continuously growing need for security, this means that the risk against which the protection is meant as a defense is actually created by the protection itself" (ibid. p. 141, translation modified). This is the point at which immunisation, understood as the construction of a rigid barrier between self and other, turns against itself and starts to endanger the very identity which it was supposed to be securing.

This exacerbation might be understood to result from a misunderstanding of the nature of the immune system according to the first of the *biological* interpretations that Esposito identifies: the immune system as a militaristic defense mechanism, absolutely refusing entry to all otherness (cf. ibid. p. 152). This is the misuse or disambiguation of "immunity" to which we referred earlier. This obsolete understanding may well be at the root of our political problems.

In any case, by means of this hyperbolic attempt at immunisation, the community ends up becoming autoimmune, attacking its own defences and leaving itself vulnerable to the forces that would bring about its disintegration. The excess of immunisation affects all levels of society from the international "globe," to the national community, to the individuals whose increasing privatisation and isolation from one another have been persistently analysed by Slavoj Žižek, amongst others, in terms of a "pathological narcissism" which results in an acute "fear of the other" (cf. Žižek 1994, pp. 7–8).

In light of this, the question that confronts us is how to restore community. Since community and immunity are inherently bound together, the answer to this question will need to tell us what community must be if it is not opposed to immunity. An immune system is indeed necessary to the integrity of the individual, and this integrity is in turn integral to the community itself, unless we think of community as a fusional substance without individuality. As we shall see, Esposito, following those "thinkers of community," Nancy and Georges Bataille in particular, but also Martin Heidegger, Immanuel Kant, and Jean-Jacques Rousseau (Esposito 2010 [1998], p. 15ff), thinks that this would eliminate the "com," "*cum,*" or "*sym-*" of community and hence eradicate community itself, properly understood. We need rather to rethink community in a *certain* conjunction with immunity which will allow us to avoid the two extremes of absolute individuation (immunity without community) and non-individuated fusion (community without immunity).

Thus we must not detach immunity from community, but rather "deepen[…] the internal contradiction" between them in order to stress the imbrication of immunity and community *in* its very aporetic character (Esposito 2011 [2002], p. 16). This will involve Esposito in an attempt to apply the *second* of the biological interpretations of immunity to the legal sphere, as if a more advanced and politically promising understanding of immunity had been developed in the science which hit upon the notion of immunity only later. As Esposito puts it:

> I have sought the answer to the question with which I began at the very heart of the protective mechanism […] on the *biological* plane, in the immune system that ensures the safeguarding of life in the body of each individual. Not because the biological immune system is a neutral or original object compared to the derivative or metaphorical nature of other forms of social immunisation. On the contrary […] its functioning has been the object of an excess of meaning that threatens to erase, or at least confuse, its distinctive traits. (2011 [2002], pp. 16–17, emphasis added)

The excess to which Esposito refers here is the militaristic interpretation of the immune system as a border defence, allergic to all otherness. This is to be contrasted with the chronologically later interpretation which understands the immune system as akin to hospitality: "more recent study of the structure and functioning of the immune system seems to suggest another interpretive possibility, one that traces out a different philosophy of immunity" (ibid. p. 17). This philosophy will explain how "this new interpretation situates immunity in a non-excluding relation with its common [or communal] opposite. The essential point of departure […] is a conception of individual identity that is distinctly different from the closed monolithic one" (ibid. p. 17).

Esposito links this advance in interpretation to the history of *technology* and suggests that this new understanding of immunity and identity "has been made possible, even inevitable, by advances in genetic and bionic technologies: rather than an immutable and definitive given, the body is understood as a functioning construct that is open to continuous exchange with its surrounding environment" (ibid. p. 17). And crucially, he states that, "the immune system may very well be the driving force behind this exchange" (ibid. p. 17). The immune system is thus not something opposed to the common, but is the very possibility of a genuine intertwining of self and other.

As proof of the validity of this new interpretation, Esposito offers the example of pregnancy and the fact that the mother's immune system under normal conditions does not reject the foetus it is carrying. Esposito avers that this refusal takes place not *in spite of* but *because of* the child's genetic heterogeneity, bestowed upon it by the father (ibid. p. 170). This is the phenomenon of "immune tolerance" (ibid. p. 166) and the related notion of "autotolerance," which stands in opposition to autoimmunity (ibid. p. 164): "if tolerance is a product of the immune system itself, it means that, far from [...] rejecting [what is] other-than-self, it includes the other within itself, not only as its driving force but also as one of its effects" (ibid. p. 167). What the example of pregnancy reveals is that an immune defence is not necessarily destructive; in this context, the mother's immune system is "engaged in a furious battle" with the child, but this struggle is precisely what keeps the child alive (ibid. p. 170). And indeed, the mother's own distinct identity is also sustained by the same conflict: "difference and conflict are not necessarily destructive. Indeed, just as the attack of the mother protects the child, the child's attacks can also save the mother from her self-injurious tendencies" (ibid. p. 171). This would explain why Esposito says that, "once its negative power has been removed, the immune is not the enemy of the common, but rather something more complex that implicates and *stimulates* the common" (ibid. p. 18, emphasis added; cf. pp. 169–71).

It is precisely this embracing of otherness as a condition for the formation of identity rather than its antagonistic opposite that renders the militaristic interpretation of the immune system implausible:

> At this point the whole immune dynamic takes on a shape that cannot be assimilated into the current interpretation: rather than acting as a barrier for selecting and excluding elements from the outside world, it acts as a sounding board for the presence of the world inside the self. [...] [The body's] boundaries do not lock it up inside a closed world; on the contrary, they create its margin, a delicate and problematic one to be sure, but still permeable in its relation to that which, while still located outside of it, from the beginning traverses and alters it. We could say that, contrary to all the military interpretations, the immune system is itself the instrument of this alteration. (ibid. p. 169, translation modified)

Esposito goes on to say that, "[a] perspective is thus opened up within the immunitary logic that overturns its prevailing interpretation. From this perspective, nothing remains of the incompatibility between self and other. The other is the form the self takes where inside intersects with outside, the proper with the common, immunity with community" (ibid. p. 171).

And it is at precisely this point that we should apply the biological interpretation of immunity to the political and legal form of immunity. Or perhaps, given that a literal community is *already* opened up at the biological level, such an application is not even needed, since the immune system itself will constitute the most elementary cell of a community between self and other, as if the biological were already *intrinsically* communal, and life always already political.

7 The Community

This, then, is how Esposito philosophically rethinks the immune system in terms of a porous logic of identity which he explicitly relates to our community with others; immunity *is* exposure and communication:

> [N]othing is more inherently dedicated to communication than the immune system. Its quality is not measured by its ability to provide protection from a foreign agent, but by the complexity of the response that it provokes: [...] this is perhaps the only—certainly the first—experience of the stranger in relation to but also in the very constitution of the proper. [...] [E]ach body is already exposed to the need for its own exposure. This is the condition common to all that is immune: the endless perception of its own finitude. (Esposito 2011 [2002], p. 174)

What we have in common is our mutual exposure, given to us by our immune systems, which expose us, in a measured way, to every form of otherness. This is Esposito's answer to the question, "can we imagine a philosophy of immunity that, without denying its inherent contradiction, even deepening it further, reverses the semantics in the direction of community?" (ibid. p. 165).

This leads us onto the way in which Esposito thinks this community of immune others, although here we can only touch upon its most prominent contours. As the subtitle of the introduction to Esposito's book devoted to the question of *communitas* indicates, this is a community of those who have "Nothing in Common."

This is an idea which Esposito inherits most immediately from Georges Bataille and Jean-Luc Nancy, and it is the one we have already broached in terms of the balance between absolute immunity and absolute community, individuation and dis-individuation. This new notion of immunity provides us with the theory of the "with" or the "com-" that we have been seeking. It will leave us with a community that is neither thought on the basis of a common property shared out between many individuals nor understood as an individual of a broader kind. Bataille and Nancy are heirs to Heidegger's deconstruction of the ontology of substance but they take that thought in a *communal* direction: their problem is how to think the relation between mortal singularities *without* substantialising or "reifying" that relation. If thought is condemned to think in terms of substances and their presence, according to an ousiological determination[8] that Esposito himself seems to take for granted here, we may speak of the "unthinkability of community" (2010 [1998], p. 1). Esposito describes this tendency of thought as its "mythological inclination" and expresses the problem as follows: "How are we to think the *pure relation* without supplying it with subjective substance? [...] [T]hat void tends to present itself in almost irresistible fashion as fullness" (ibid. p. 15). Perhaps this refers only to the

[8] I take this term from Miguel de Beistegui (2004, p. 36). It refers to the identification of being with presence or substance (*ousia*, in Greek) which Heidegger and others associate with the beginning of philosophy as metaphysics and which they locate in the work of Aristotle, if not Plato, or even Parmenides.

failure of *philosophical* thought, which can be averted by means of the recourse to the natural science of *biology*, for this relationship becomes thinkable precisely on the basis of the second interpretation of biological immunity that we have been exposing.

8 Esposito and Derrida: History and Community

Two features differentiate Esposito's thinking of immunity from Derrida's: first, the historical tale which attempts if not to explain then at least to show how the political events of modernity can be unified and narrated.[9] This allows Esposito to at least address the idea of history and the specificity of the present day in a way that one might suspect Derrida, who has expressed doubts about the very notion of "history," is unable to.[10] It is as if Derrida's thought remains fundamentally structural or

---

[9]If there *is* a philosophy of history in Esposito as distinct from a mere narration, it is perhaps to be found *in embryo* in his notion of technology. History would therefore be a history of technology, as if technology had brought us to the ambivalent moment in which we stand, between two interpretations of immunity. We have already seen Esposito suggesting that the second, "hospitable" interpretation "has been made possible, even inevitable, by advances in genetic and bionic technologies" (2011 [2002], p. 17).

The relation between politics and life would thus be given a particular historical form by the level of technology that has been attained and the kind of technology that has been developed: "the connection between politics and life is radically redefined by the unstoppable proliferation of technology" (2011 [2002], p. 146). We might interpret this as saying that the ways in which power can directly act upon bare life without mediation are greatly enhanced by the manner in which technological systems have now infiltrated the most intimate interiors of our bodies and our relation to those bodies.

Once again, Esposito credits Nancy with the link between community and technology, or more precisely, *technē* (2011 [2002], p. 150–53). *Technē* may indeed be identified with the exposure to the other governed by the immune system, since *technē* is precisely the moment at which the supposedly proper, natural body of the self opens onto the non-natural other (2011 [2002], p. 151).

[10]Speaking of Derrida's theory of fundamentalist religious movements as reactions to the globalisation that *religion* has embraced in recent times, Esposito says the following: "this is hardly sufficient to resolve the question of religious immunity. The entropic dialectic we have just described would itself appear to be the final outcome of a *much more ancient process,* one whose beginnings have been preserved in the original semantic stratification of the religious phenomenon" (2011 [2002], p. 53, emphasis added). These he discovers in a text by the linguist, Emile Benveniste, which Derrida cites, but the implications of which, according to Esposito, he does not fully explore.

To begin an adequate defence of Derrida on this point, one would have to examine his last two seminars on *The Beast and the Sovereign*, which do deal with a history, albeit a history of texts, which coincide to a large extent with those addressed by Esposito. One would also need to examine the way in which "Faith and Knowledge" in particular, and indeed all of the texts on immunity, are unquestionably driven by "contemporary" concerns—at least in their deployment of this vocabulary. And more fundamentally, as Derrida points out in his dazzling interview, "Politics and Friendship," one would need to examine his early work on historicism from a Husserlian point of view (Derrida 2002 [1989], pp. 156–57).

synchronous, a theory of the nature of identity and its self-undermining *at all times,* in a way that is not subject to an unequivocally determinable historical change. One might relate this to Derrida's and Esposito's respective theories of democracy since for Esposito it seems that an end to the autoimmune threat might well be reached when the intertwining of community and immunity is properly thought, while for Derrida, the autoimmune, anti-democratic possibility is inherent to the very *idea* of democracy, and is hence eternally a part of it.[11]

Secondly, Esposito's much more (explicitly) developed theory of the way immunity is entwined with community; in other words, the way in which the self-undermining of the totality of the individual in its propriety *opens* the individual to a communal relationship. It is perhaps for this reason that Jean-Luc Nancy is a more predominant reference in Esposito's work than Derrida.

9 Conclusion. Agamben: Of a Possible Survival Beyond Immunity

Let us relate what we have achieved so far to the question with which we began: the question of bio-politics and thus, at least indirectly, bio-ethics. Esposito, deploying his thinking of the "dialectical" relationship between immunity and community, delineates his own relation to biopolitics by differentiating his approach from Giorgio Agamben's:

> [W]hat does it mean to say that politics is enclosed within the boundaries of life? […] the answer to this question should not be sought in the folds of a sovereign power that includes life by excluding it [Agamben's position]. Rather, what I believe it should point to is an epochal conjuncture out of which the category of sovereignty makes room for, or at least intersects with, that of immunisation. This is the general procedure through which the intersection between politics and life is realised. (Esposito 2011 [2002], pp. 138–39)

[11]"Derrida, rather, gives it a much less optimistic, even tragic characterisation. More than immunity or immunisation, he always speaks of 'autoimmunity' […]. The contemporary political situation can indeed be interpreted in the light of a similar destructive and self-destructive process. On this point I am in complete agreement with him. […] [/] Nevertheless, certain relevant differences remain in relation to the formation of the category of immunity that in Derrida emerges as somewhat extemporaneous, in the sense that immunity is linked neither with the theme of community [Derrida in fact does indicate this connection, as we have seen—M.L.] (which Derrida rejects in favour of the weaker concept, from my point of view, of friendship), nor with that of biopolitics, which is utterly extraneous to his thought [in fact, the final seminars on *The Beast and the Sovereign* demonstrate this to be false, at least up to a point—M.L.]. This isolation of the category of immunity […] impedes Derrida from fully grasping the dialectical character of immunity […]. In fact, Derrida doesn't treat the long-standing modern character of the immunitary paradigm, which emerges as crushed in the contemporary period. On the other hand, it is precisely the indissoluble, albeit negative, relation with *communitas* that opens for me the possibility of a positive, communitary reconversion of the same immunitary *dispositif*' (Esposito 2006, pp. 53–55, translation modified).

Esposito helpfully locates his own position by means of a critique of his fellow theorists of biopolitics, Agamben and Antonio Negri. He finds that in Agamben, generally speaking, biopolitics is thought in a "negative, even tragic" fashion, and in Negri it is thought in a positive, "productive, expansive" way (Esposito 2006, p. 50). Neither position satisfies Esposito, and his own rethinking of the relation between life and politics, immunity and community, manages to account for the fact that biopolitics may take on a positive *or* a negative form, which, according to Esposito, the one-sided theories of Agamben and Negri do not:

> I have tried to move the terms of the debate by providing a different interpretive key that is capable of reading them [the positive and the negative connotations of "biopolitics"] together, while accounting for the antinomical relation between them. All done without renouncing the historical dimension, as Agamben does, and without immediately collapsing the philosophical prospective into a political one, as Negri does. As you know, this hermeneutic key, this different paradigm, is that of immunity. (Esposito 2006, p. 50)

Hence, "[t]o grasp the dual potential biopolitics holds for destruction or affirmation, we have to go back to its founding relationship with the immune system, which constitutes both its transcendental condition and its functional model" (Esposito 2011 [2002], p. 145, translation modified, cf. ibid. p. 150).

Nevertheless, a brief excursion through Agamben's work might lead us to a different conclusion. For is there not in Agamben's work a notion of life that does without the notion of immunity altogether, and which might produce an alternative vision of biopolitics that Esposito is unable to envisage?

What does Agamben say of the life which lays itself open to politics? Does his thought in fact move beyond the horizon of immunity? What interests Agamben most about life in its contemporary form, life and the particular way in which it has become the object of politics and political power, is its absolute vulnerability. Esposito—following Foucault—will have stressed the importance of the shift from a sovereign paradigm to a purely biopolitical one, a shift which involves the removal of all mediation between power and biological life (Esposito 2011 [2002], pp. 14–15; pp. 112–13). Formerly this relation was mediated by a legal system of rights and laws which ensured that the citizen was subject to political power in their *public* form, but their private life, which included the reproductive capacities of *biological* life, remained within a separate sphere (cf. Agamben 1998 [1995], pp. 1–11). Biopolitics in its contemporary guise is defined by the collapse of this distinction. Even the most basic of the human being's biological functions is now immediately subject to political domination.

The most extreme, "paradigmatic" figure of this biopolitical situation is *homo sacer*, a figure defined in Roman law according to the ambiguity of the Latin adjective "*sacer*" which means both "sacred" and "condemned," a man guilty of a certain crime as a result of which they may be killed with impunity, but not ritually killed, not sacrificed (Agamben 1998 [1995], pp. 71ff). In other words, they are living and nothing more: "mere life," barely alive, without being possessed of the least dignity, rights, or legal protection. Theirs is a life of pure exposure to the power of another, an other who enjoys an absolute power of decision over the survival of that life.

According to Agamben, the nature of life is potential. The same goes for *homo sacer* but in this case, life has been reduced to a minimal and utterly passive potential: "its capacity to be killed" (ibid. p. 8). It is subject to an external sovereign power to such an extent that both its survival and its perishing are beyond its control. It thus remains below the level of an animal in the sense that its very instinct for survival has been destroyed and yet it cannot commit suicide while it remains suspended in life by the hesitation of those who can exterminate it at will. The place in which the possible reduction of life to the level of *homo sacer* was most starkly brought to light was the concentration camp, metonymised by the name "Auschwitz" (ibid. pp. 114ff).

The crucial feature of *homo sacer* for our purposes is that, despite having just one possibility remaining, its own death at the hands of another—it nevertheless survives. It still lives. What are we to say of this in the context of immunity? Here we have a figure of life whose every form of defence has been broken down, it lacks even a will to survive in its individual integrity. It is as if in *homo sacer* we find a victim of Acquired Immune Deficiency Syndrome nevertheless surviving, absolutely at the mercy of powers beyond his or her control: in this case, technological life-support and synthetic drugs, rather than the executing sovereign Other.

Is such a figure thinkable on either Esposito's or Derrida's account? Without an immune system, the identity of the living individual is supposed to disintegrate, and death to ensue. But Agamben locates an extremely surprising—in fact, empirically testified—kind of life which nonetheless endures even at this level: one thinks also of the marvellous example which he cites from Jakob von Uexküll, of the tick that lives for eighteen years without any stimulation at all (Agamben 2004 [2002], p. 47). It is as if life were a potential, a power for living that could somehow survive *without* immune defences, as a pure exposure and awaiting. As if, even when subjected to the absolute and unmediated power of an other, subsisting only in the hush before its sentence is pronounced, in the stay of execution before the coming of an unpredictable though certain event—death—life endured.

Here we might discern the influence of one of Agamben's teachers, Martin Heidegger. For the latter, the anticipation of an unpredictable end is a relation to death which characterises every human "life" even *before* that "life" has received any biological determinations, and perhaps even before that individual living substance can be understood as having any real or metaphorical "immune system." This would imply that life was first of all an exposure and a potential, a vulnerability to an invincible power, ultimately death itself, but at the same time nevertheless empowered by this possibility that will always remain outstanding, to the very end, even in the face of a complete collapse of the immune system. The one possibility that is always yet to come, a power we therefore retain for precisely as long as we are alive, is that of dying, and this is an absolutely solitary possibility, unique to each one of us, which leaves us *without* relation: "death reveals itself as that *possibility which is one's ownmost, which is non-relational, and which is not to be outstripped.* As such, death is something *distinctively* impending" (Heidegger 1962 [1927], p. 294).

The issue between Heidegger and Agamben will ultimately revolve around the question of whether this is essentially a power we have mastery over, or at least a possibility which is the source of our *active* power, or whether this power can, in extreme biopolitical situations of the kind Agamben describes, be given over to another, as a result of which we would be essentially related *to* this other, even here, but—contrary to Esposito's idea of community—in a relationship that would be asymmetrical.

But in either case, this suggests that life can be understood in a way that is ultimately more basic than all considerations of its immunity and community—if there is a relation to the other, it does not have the symmetry of communal being-with, and it is unrelated to immunity—in terms of a non-biological power exposed to the possibility which always stands at the border of life and which maintains the individual integrity of the substance even in the absence of any immune defences: and that is its own dying.

To be sure, this might all seem to confirm the negative, if not tragic characterisation of Agamben's thought which Esposito proposes, and to indicate the necessity of thinking life as an intimate mutual belonging of immunity and community. But if it offers *both* a theory of life prior to immunity *and* a way of thinking relation prior to the immunitary-communitary combination, then we should take it extremely seriously.

References

Agamben, G. (1991 [1982]). *Language and death: The place of negativity* (K. E. Pinkus & M. Hardt, Trans.). Minneapolis: University of Minnesota Press.

Agamben, G. (1998 [1995]). *Homo sacer: Bare life and sovereign power* (D. Heller-Roazen, Trans.). Stanford: Stanford University Press.

Agamben, G. (1999 [1998]). *Remnants of Auschwitz: The witness and the archive* (D. Heller-Roazen, Trans.). New York: Zone Books.

Agamben, G. (1999). *Potentialities: Collected essays in philosophy* (D. Heller-Roazen (Ed., Trans.)). Stanford: Stanford University Press.

Agamben, G. (2000 [1996]). *Means without end: Notes on politics* (V. Binetti & C. Casarino, Trans.). Minneapolis: University of Minnesota Press.

Agamben, G. (2004 [2002]). *The open: Man and animal* (K. Attell, Trans.). Stanford: Stanford University Press.

Aristotle. (1989). *Politics* (H. Rackham, Trans.). Cambridge: Harvard University Press.

de Beistegui, M. (2004). *Truth and genesis: Philosophy as differential ontology*. Indianapolis: Indiana University Press.

Derrida, J. (1989 [2002]). Politics and friendship (Interview with Michael Sprinkler). In E. Rottenberg (Ed. & Trans.), *Negotiations: Interventions and interviews, 1971–2001*. Stanford: Stanford University Press.

Derrida, J. (1994 [1993]). *Spectres of Marx: The state of the debt, the work of mourning and the new international* (P. Kamuf, Trans.). London: Routledge.

Derrida, J. (2002 [1996]). Faith and knowledge: The two sources of "religion" at the limits of reason alone. In S. Weber & G. Anidjar (Ed. & Trans.), *Acts of religion*. London: Routledge.
Derrida, J (2003 [2001]). Autoimmunity: Real and symbolic suicides—a dialogue with Jacques Derrida (P. A. Brault & M. Naas, Trans.). In G. Borradori (Ed.), *Philosophy in a time of terror*. Chicago: University of Chicago Press.
Derrida, J. (2005 [2003]). *Rogues: Two essays on reason*. (P-A. Brault & M. Naas, Trans.). Stanford: Stanford University Press.
Derrida, J. (2008). *The animal that therefore I am* (M-L. Mallet & D. Wills, Ed. & Trans). New York: Fordham University Press.
Derrida, J. (2009 [2008]). *The beast and the sovereign*, Volume I [2001–2002] (G. Bennington, Trans). M. Lisse, M-L. Mallet & G. Michaud (Eds.). Chicago: University of Chicago Press.
Derrida, J. (2011 [2010]). *The beast and the sovereign*, Volume II [2002–2003] (G. Bennington, Trans.). Chicago: University of Chicago Press.
Düttmann, A. G. (1996 [1993]). *At odds with AIDS: Thinking and talking about a virus* (P. Gilgen & C. Scott-Curtis, Trans.). Stanford: Stanford University Press.
Esposito, R. (2006). Interview with Timothy Campbell. (A. Paparcone, Trans.) *Diacritics*, *36*(2), 49–56.
Esposito, R. (2008 [2004]). *Bios: Biopolitics and philosophy* (T. Campbell, Trans.). Minneapolis: University of Minnesota Press.
Esposito, R. (2010 [1998]). *Communitas: The origin and destiny of community* (T. Campbell, Trans.). Stanford: Stanford University Press.
Esposito, R. (2011 [2002]). *Immunitas: The protection and negation of life* (Z. Hanafi, Trans.). Cambridge: Polity.
Esposito, R. (2012 [2007]). *Third person* (Z. Hanafi, Trans.). Cambridge: Polity.
Esposito, R. (2012 [2010]). *Living thought: The origins and actuality of Italian philosophy* (Z. Hanafi, Trans.). Stanford: Stanford University Press.
Esposito, R. (2013 [2008]). *Terms of the political: Community, immunity, biopolitics* (R.N. Welch, Trans.). New York: Fordham University Press.
Foucault, M. (1990 [1976]). *The history of sexuality, 1: The will to knowledge* (R. Hurley, Trans.). London: Penguin.
Hägglund, M. (2008). *Radical atheism: Derrida and the time of life*. Stanford: Stanford University Press.
Heidegger, M. (1962 [1927]). *Being and time* (J. Macquarrie & E. Robinson, Trans.). Oxford: Blackwell.
Lacoue-Labarthe, P., & Nancy, J-L. (1997). *Retreating the political*. (S. Sparks Ed.). London: Routledge.
Naas, M. (2012). *Miracle and machine: Jacques Derrida and the two sources of religion, science, and the media*. New York: Fordham University Press.
Žižek, S. (1994/2005). *The metastases of enjoyment: Six essays on women and causality*. London: Verso.

Chapter 14
The Psychopathology of Space: A Phenomenological Critique of Solitary Confinement

Lisa Guenther

1 The Rise of the Supermax Prison

Since the mid-1980s, supermax prisons have multiplied across the United States, with 57 facilities in current operation, and at least 80,000 prisoners held in some form of "restricted housing" or solitary confinement.[1] The rapid growth of the supermax prison industry both reflects and helps to accomplish a shift in US penal policy from the goal of rehabilitation to the task of perpetual control. Advocates portray supermax prisoners as "the worst of the worst": serial killers, rapists and terrorists who pose a threat to the safety of guards, inmates, and society at large. But the decision to isolate a prisoner is not based on the crime for which they were convicted, and it is not made in the presence of a judge or lawyers; it is an administrative decision internal to the prison and subject to periodic review. Most prisoners end up in control units as a result of breaking prison rules or because they have been identified as the member of a gang. The process of gang member identification and "debriefing" (or the formal renunciation of gang membership) is so fraught that prisoners at Pelican Bay, Corcoran, Red Onion, and other supermax prisons in California and across the country have engaged in periodic hunger strikes

[1]It is difficult to determine with any exactness how many prisoners are currently held in supermax confinement in the US, or even how many supermax prisons exist at the federal and state levels. See Tapley (2010) for a detailed analysis of the available data. The first supermax prison in the world was established in 1983 in Marion, Illinois, when the entire prison was locked down in response to the murder of two guards. The first purpose-built supermax was Florence ADX, which opened in Colorado in 1985. Supermax prisons have now been built in at least ten other countries: Canada, Mexico, Brazil, Columbia, the UK, Ireland, Denmark, Malaysia, Saudi Arabia and Australia. See Gomez (2006) for a historical and political account of the emergence of supermax prisons.

L. Guenther (✉)
Vanderbilt University, Nashville, USA
e-mail: Lisa.guenther@vanderbilt.edu

D. Meacham (ed.), *Medicine and Society, New Perspectives in Continental Philosophy*, Philosophy and Medicine 120, DOI 10.1007/978-94-017-9870-9_14

since spring 2011 to protest their conditions.[2] Supermax prisons are also notorious as destinations for politically active prisoners or perceived leaders within the general prison population.[3] Once a prisoner has landed in a supermax unit, it can be extremely difficult to get out; even minor infringements or perceived infringements of prison rules can set back one's date of release into the general prison population, sometimes indefinitely. And yet, most prisoners, even "the worst of the worst," will eventually be released from prison. Those who are considered too dangerous to be reintegrated with other prisoners during their sentences are released directly onto the street, often without counselling, medication, job prospects, or even photo ID—just $100 cash and a bus ticket (Yáñez-Correa and Jennifer 2012).

"Supermax prison" is an unofficial term for what are officially called Security Housing Units or Special Housing Units (SHU), Control Units (CU), High Security Units (HSU), Communication Management Units (CMU), Administrative Segregation (Ad-Seg), Administrative Maximum (Ad-Max or ADX), restricted housing, and so forth. Such units may be found anywhere from maximum security prisons to county jails; they are usually set apart from the rest of the prison in "pods" branching out from a central command station. The common feature of so-called supermax units is the degree of isolation from other prisoners and from the world. Prisoners spend between 22 and 23½ h a day in their cell, the size of which typically ranges from 6 × 8 feet to 8 × 12 feet. The cell is usually painted white or pale grey to reduce visual stimulus. Furnishings consist of a bed, a table and seat, a toilet, and a sink—all bolted in place. There is often a non-breakable mirror above the sink. There are either no windows at all or just a small, narrow window that lets in light but affords little or no view of the outside. Artificial lights may be dimmed at night, but they are rarely, if ever, turned off. Surveillance cameras also run continuously, and in many control units, prisoners communicate by intercom with correctional officers, psychiatrists, and even medical doctors. There is a slot in the door, called a cuffport or "pie flap," through which food trays are exchanged and the prisoners' hands are cuffed or uncuffed for trips outside the cell. These slots can be bolted from the outside, in part to prevent prisoners from "bombing" the guards with cocktails of their own feces or urine.[4]

When prisoners engage in forms of resistance such as refusing to "cuff up" or to return their meal tray, they can be forcibly extracted from their cells by an emergency response team in riot gear. They may be pepper-sprayed or tasered and put in four-point restraints (with both hands and arms fastened to the ground) or in a

---

[2]See Reiter (2010) for a detailed discussion of these issues.

[3]The former warden of Marion Penitentiary, Ralph Arons, admitted that "[t]he purpose of the Marion Control Unit is to control revolutionary attitudes in the prison system and in the society at large" (cited Shaylor 1998, p. 398). See James (2003, 2005) for writing by US political prisoners such as George Jackson, Assata Shakur, Mumia Abu-Jamal, Leonard Peltier, Susan Rosenberg, Marilyn Buck, Laura Whitehorn and Alan Berkman, all of whom have been held in maximum or supermax level prisons.

[4]See Shalev (2009), Rhodes (2004), and Haney (2003) for a more detailed account of the history and conditions of supermax prisons.

restraint chair. Officers are entitled to perform strip searches of inmates—including cavity searches—if they suspect the inmate of possessing contraband items. Often, these searches are conducted as a matter of routine when prisoners return from the showers, the exercise yard, or even from non-contact visits. The exercise yard is often not much bigger than the cell. It is typically made of concrete or tightly-woven security mesh walls that offer little or no view of the outside and only a small glimpse of sky. These yards are often called "dog runs" because of their resemblance to an outdoor kennel. Depending on the prisoner's level of good behavior, they may be given access to books, radio, television and/or non-contact visits with loved ones. Often, the only "television" available in a supermax prison is a closed-circuit broadcast of training videos and religious programming.

What would it be like to have one's bodily contact with others reduced to the fastening and unfastening of restraints through a slot in the door, punctuated with the most intimate probing of the surface and depths of one's body?[5] Not to be able to speak to anyone except through intercom, or by yelling through a slot in the door? To be kept in solitude, and yet exposed to constant surveillance and to the echoing noise of other prisoners?[6] What would it be like to be blocked from the lived experience of open, unrestricted space? Not to see the sky or the horizon for days, weeks, even years on end? Not to know if it's day or night apart from the schedule of one's feedings and allotted exercise times?[7]

Many prisoners speak of their experience in supermax prison as a form of living death.[8] On one hand, their bodies still live and breathe, eat and defecate, wake and sleep (often with difficulty). On the other hand, a meaningful sense of living

[5]A supermax prisoner interviewed by Lorna Rhodes says: "I've got some people out there I know from the streets and I know they're going to give me a hug. But I won't be able to because it's embedded in my mind that when people touch me it has a negative effect, you know, that every time somebody touches me it's a cop" (Rhodes 2004, p. 34).

[6]Anthropologist Lorna Rhodes says of her own experience visiting a control unit: "Echoing in their hard-edged interior, their shouts are a blur of rage-saturated sound" (Rhodes 2004, p. 22). One of the prisoners interviewed by Rhodes says: "They put you in an environment where you can't talk to anybody else, you can't have any contact… unless you yell or scream… The only thing you hear is the keys jingling" (31).

[7]A supermax prisoner interviewed by Rhodes says: "Your lights are on all day… it really kind of dulls all your senses… It makes you numb. You get easily mad. You feel that everything they do is just to make you mad…" (Rhodes 2004, p. 30).

[8]Gomez writes: "The CU — and its more recent progeny, Special Housing Units (SHU) — collapsed the legal and physical space between life and politics — and between punishment and death" (Gomez 2006, p. 60). "Designed as a breathing coffin, the CU was/is a space of permanent living death" (61). See also Caleb Smith's work on the early US penitentiary, which he described as "a 'living tomb' of servitude and degradation as well as the space of the citizen-subject's dramatic reanimation. Its legal codes divested the convict of rights; its ritualized disciplinary practices stripped away his identity; it exposed him to arbitrary and discretionary violence at the hands of his keepers; it buried him alive in his solitary cell. But it also promised him a glorious return to citizenship and humanity. It mortified the body, but it also claimed to renovate the soul. Its ideal subject was one who, in the words of one great Philadelphia reformer [Benjamin Rush], 'was dead and is alive'" (Smith 2009, p. 6).

embodiment has for the most part drained out of their lives; they've become unhinged from the world, confined to a space in which all they can do is turn around or pace back and forth, blocked from an open-ended perception of the world as a space of mutual belonging and interaction with others. Stephen Tillich, a Washington state inmate, says of his experience in the Control Unit: "It's like being in a tomb" (Rhodes 2004, p. 113). Angela Tucker, confined in the SHU at Valley State Prison for Women (VSPW) says: "It's like living in a black hole" (Shaylor 1998, p. 386).[9] Jeremy Pinson, a prisoner at Florence ADX, says, "you feel as if the world has ended but you somehow survived" (Greene 2012). While many prisoners feel like they are treated like animals rather than human beings, others do not even feel like they are treated as well as animals; they feel more like "baggage" or "inventory" in a warehouse.[10] Even the prison staff often relate to prisoners as things rather than living beings. One officer describes his work receiving inmates into a Washington state prison this way: "We are just like the guys who work loading docks – we're trying to *move* stuff" (Rhodes 2004, p. 101).

In clinical terms, the effects of supermax confinement are known collectively as "isolation sickness" (Scott 1969), RES (Reduced Environmental Stimulation), or the brutally frank SHU (Security Housing Unit) syndrome (Haney 2003, p. 137; Grassian 1983, p. 2003). Typical symptoms include affective disorders such as anxiety, paranoia, uncontrollable rage, and depression; cognitive disorders such as confusion, inability to focus, oversensitivity to stimuli, obsessive rumination, hallucinations, and other perceptual distortions; physical disorders such as headaches, lethargy, insomnia, digestive problems, heart palpitations, fainting spells, and bodily aches and pains; and in extreme cases, psychotic breakdown, self-mutilation, and suicide (Grassian 1983, 2006; Haney 2003). In Craig Haney's study of 100 prisoners in the SHU at Pelican Bay supermax prison, over 80 % showed signs of the following nine symptoms: anxiety, headaches, lethargy, insomnia, ruminations, irrational anger, oversensitivity to stimuli, confused thought process, and social withdrawal (Haney 2003, pp. 133–134). Thirteen further symptoms were found in over half of the prisoners.

Many of the symptoms associated with SHU syndrome overlap with post-traumatic stress disorder (PTSD) and with the typical effects of sensory deprivation and social isolation in the "free world" (Haney 2003, p. 130, 132). But there is also a range of "social pathologies" produced by the specific situation of punitive isolation

[9]Shaylor comments: "[T]he "blackness" of the SHU is reflected in both its racialized nature and the darkness of the cells themselves; the degree of force within the SHU is experienced by the women through physical brutality and sexual violence; the space of the SHU is oppressively small; mental stability is warped; the experience of passage of time is transformed; and communication flowing both into and out of the SHU is severely restricted" (Shaylor 1998, p. 415).

[10]Denise Jones, an inmate at Valley State Prison for Women, argues: "They treat us like animals. No, you wouldn't treat an animal the way they do us here. I am sure they don't treat their dogs the way they treat us" (Shaylor 1998, pp. 395–396). Mark Medley, a maximum security inmate at Maryland State Prison argues that prisoners are moved into different cells as part of a managerial plan rather than for the sake of rehabilitation or even security: "It's just that they have to liquidate their inventory as a matter of storage space" (Baxter et al. 2005, p. 215).

in a supermax unit. Haney notes the phenomenon of "prisonization" whereby prisoners who manage to adapt to the situation of extreme control find it difficult to adjust to life outside the control unit; the structure of their life, their relation to space and time, their social relations with others, and even their own identity, is so thoroughly organized by the prison regime that they find it difficult or impossible to initiate or sustain their activity without it (Haney, 2003, p. 139). Haney writes:

> [T]he absence of regular, normal interpersonal contact and any semblance of a meaningful social context creates a feeling of unreality that pervades one's existence in such places. Because so much of our individual identity is socially constructed and maintained, the virtually complete loss of genuine forms of social contact and the absence of any routine and recurring opportunities to ground one's thoughts and feelings in a recognizable human context leads to an undermining of the sense of self and a disconnection of experience from meaning. (Haney 2003, p. 139)

Haney leaves the relation between "a feeling of unreality" and "the absence of regular, normal interpersonal contact and any semblance of a meaningful social context" unexplained, as if we already knew what this meant, given that human beings are "social animals." But the meaning of sociality, and the relation between meaning and sociality, is precisely what needs to be explained if we are to understand the harm of extreme isolation and to develop strategies for both abolishing its use and supporting the recovery of isolated prisoners.

We need a phenomenological language to understand the meaning of the empirical data gathered by Haney and others, and to engage with prisoners' own descriptions of their experience, or unravelling of experience, in prolonged solitary confinement. In what follows, I will outline the theoretical framework for a phenomenological analysis of solitary confinement and explore one strand of this analysis in greater detail: the relation between space, sociality, and psychopathology in the testimony of prisoners and in Merleau-Ponty's account of "pure depth." It may seem odd to focus on depth as a bioethical or biopolitical problem, but as I hope to show, the experience of a world in depth, with dimensions that I experience as "there" even when they are not directly accessible to me, is a key feature of the "meaningful social context" that Haney invokes but does not explain. By reflecting on the experience of depth and its foreclosure in extreme isolation, we can begin to develop a bioethical and biopolitical language for articulating both the violence of solitary confinement and the social, political and ethical texture of everyday perceptual life.

2 Outline for a Phenomenology of Solitary Confinement

The challenge of phenomenology is to reveal, through a careful description of lived experience, the transcendental structures that make this experience possible and meaningful. One of the first things I notice when I reflect on my lived experience is that it is *mine*: I experience the world in the first person, as a consciousness whose thoughts, perceptions, memories, and so forth, belong first and foremost to me. No one but me has direct access to my own conscious processes: I think, therefore

(I know that) I am. For Husserl, this Cartesian insight provides irrefutable evidence for the existence of consciousness as an absolute condition for the possibility of any experience whatsoever, and also of any meaningful experience. And yet, there is more to first-person experience than the "I think." If we reflect again on first-person experience, then we also notice that consciousness is consciousness *of something*: a robin's nest, a philosophy textbook, a number, a memory.... Even when I reflect on my own consciousness processes, as in phenomenological reflection, my consciousness is oriented towards something other than the pure act of reflecting. The relational, orientational character of consciousness is just as essential to the structure of experience as the existence of first-person consciousness; experience is unthinkable without something to be experienced. This is not to say that the object of experience must *exist* in order to be thought, imagined, or remembered. Rather, Husserl maintains the priority of transcendental consciousness over the world to which it is essentially correlated; the intentional act, or noesis, constitutes the intentional object, or noema, without being constituted by it. To put this somewhat differently, the world depends on consciousness, but consciousness does not depend on the world. Husserl goes so far as to say that the world could be destroyed, and transcendental consciousness would still remain as an absolute residuum:

> [I]t is quite conceivable that it is not only in single instances that experience through conflict dissolves into illusion, and that every illusion does not as it were de facto proclaim a deeper truth [...] it is conceivable that our experiencing function swarms with oppositions that cannot be evened out either for us or in themselves [...] that a world, in short, exists no longer [...]. [L]et us think of the possibility of the non-Being which belongs essentially to every Thing-like transcendence: it is then evident *that the Being of consciousness*, of every stream of experience generally, *though it would indeed be inevitably modified by a nullifying of the thing-world, would not be affected thereby in its own proper existence*. (Husserl 1983, p. 137)

Such a nullification of the thing-world would destroy "certain ordered empirical connexions, and accordingly also systems of theorizing reason which take their bearings from these" (137). But it would not destroy consciousness itself, with its "fleeting concentration-centres" and "rough unitary formation" (137). Husserl concludes that "*no real thing*, none that consciously presents and manifests itself through appearances, *is necessary for the Being of consciousness* (in the widest sense of the stream of consciousness)" (137). Rather, the being of the world depends on the absolute being of consciousness.

This may seem absurd: How can consciousness exist if the world does not? Who would "be there" as a subject of experience, if concrete subjects did not already exist in the world? Husserl's claim becomes less counter-sensical if we recall that he is interested, at least in his earlier, foundational work, in reflecting on the relation between meaning and experience, and in tracing the concreteness of lived experience back to its transcendental conditions. Just as the empirical tree can burn down or be turned into lumber without affecting the meaning of the tree for consciousness, so too could the whole world be destroyed, without affecting the meaning of the world for consciousness. The stakes of Husserl's transcendental idealism are high for our own reflections on the phenomenology of solitary confinement. If we follow the phenomenological method this far, then we could never hope to find the *meaning* of experience through empirical investigation. Consciousness is not just "a little tag-end of the world" (Husserl 1991, p. 24), to be studied with the same empirical methods that we bring to the study of natural sciences such as biology, chemistry, and physics, or even to the empirical methods of the social sciences. Rather, consciousness is the transcendental condition for the possibility of any meaningful experience whatsoever, and we must reflect on the structure of consciousness in a way that is appropriate to its transcendental status. This does not exclude the empirical sciences or diminish their importance; it merely grounds them in the more fundamental transcendental science of phenomenology. And since consciousness is essentially correlated to a world, the intricate structures and levels of worldhood are of vital interest to phenomenology, especially in its investigations of the lifeworld in which the full social person dwells.[11]

There is much more to be said about the phenomenological method, but I want to begin focusing on the possibilities and limits of this method for an analysis of solitary confinement. What are we to make of Husserl's claim that the Being of consciousness would not be affected by the destruction of the "real" world, given the first-person testimony of prisoners in solitary confinement? Consider Jack Henry Abbott's reflections on the 14–15 years that he spent in solitary confinement:

> [S]omething happens down there in the hole, something like an event, but this event can only occur over a span of years. It cannot take place in time and space the way we ordinarily know them. (Abbott 1991, p. 45)
>
> My body communicates with the cell. We exchange temperatures and air currents, smells and leavings on the floor and walls. I try to keep it clean, to wash away my evidence, for the first year or so, then let it go at that. (46)
>
> If you are in that cell for weeks that add up to months [Abbott is referring to a strip-cell consisting of nothing but an open toilet in the center, sprayed around with urine and feces], you do not ignore all this and live "with it"; you *enter* it and become a part of it. (29)[12]

[11]The lifeworld is the social, cultural, and historical context which forms the (often unacknowledged) background in relation to which we form our individual beliefs. Like the natural attitude, the lifeworld requires clarification and critique; but we cannot transcend the lifeworld, nor should we assume that true knowledge consists in breaking with socially-inherited meanings to obtain a purely objective, ahistorical grasp of reality. Rather, the lifeworld is what grounds a meaningful experience of oneself, others, things, and events in a shared context where there are multiple perspectives, sometimes consonant and sometimes conflicting. Husserl describes the lifeworld as follows: "We, as living in wakeful world-consciousness, are constantly active on the basis of our passive having of the world; it is from there, by objects pregiven in consciousness, that we are affected; it is to this or that object that we pay attention, according to our interests; with them we deal actively in different ways; through our acts they are "thematic" objects" (Husserl 1970, p 108).

[12]Abbott called himself a "state-raised convict" (Abbott 1991, pp. 3–22). The son of a Chinese prostitute and an Irish sailor, he had already spending time in juvenile detention at age 9, was sent to an industrial school at age 12, and was sentenced for up to 5 years at age 18 for cashing a check for insufficient funds. While in prison, he killed a fellow inmate in prison and received an indeterminate sentence of 3–20 years.

> Solitary confinement can alter the ontological makeup of a stone. (45)

Consider also Stuart Grassian's 1982 interviews with prisoners in the SHU at Walpole State Penitentiary:

> Melting, everything in the cell starts moving; everything gets darker, you feel you are losing your vision. (Grassian 1983, p. 1452)
>
> They come by [for breakfast] with four trays; the first has big pancakes – I think I'm going to get them. Then someone comes up and gives me tiny ones – they get real small, like silver dollars. I seem to see movements – real fast motions in front of me. Then seems like they're doing things behind your back – can't quite see them. Did someone just hit me? I dwell on it for hours. (1452)
>
> I can't concentrate, can't read. . . Your mind's narcotized. . . sometimes can't grasp words in my mind that I know. Get stuck, have to think of another word. Memory is going. You feel you are losing something you might not get back. (1453)

What do prisoners in solitary confinement risk losing, to the point of not getting it back? How does prolonged sensory and social isolation undermine prisoners' capacity to think clearly, to perceive stable objects, to remember, and even to distinguish between what they did and what was done to them? What is the relation between the sensory and the social here, between the capacity to perceive things as stable, persistent and real, and the chance to experience other embodied subjects in a shared world? And how have some prisoners managed to retain some sense of meaningful experience—to the point where they are still able to speak about it at all—even in the absence of what Haney calls "regular, normal interpersonal contact" and "a meaningful social context"?

The psychiatric language of RES or SHU syndrome can only go so far in explicating what Abbott calls an "ontological event" that seems to blur the distinction between consciousness and world, and to unravel the essential structure of transcendental consciousness. But can phenomenology do any better? To the extent that we accept Husserl's claim that consciousness would "*not be affected thereby in its own proper existence*" but only "modified" by the destruction of the thing-world, we risk marginalizing the experience of prisoners in extreme isolation and underestimating the violence to which they are exposed *in their very being*—to the point where some prisoners take their own life rather than persisting in the living death of isolation (Husserl 1983, p. 137). And yet, Husserl's acknowledgement that under such conditions, consciousness is no longer able to distinguish between truth and illusion, and that our "experiencing function swarms with oppositions that cannot be evened out either for us or in themselves" (137) resonates with the confusion, both cognitive and ontological, described by prisoners in solitary confinement.

There are many ways to undertake the challenge of a phenomenological response to the testimony of prisoners in solitary confinement.[13] In what follows,

[13] I have explored several of these in Guenther (2013). It's also important to note the limitation of phenomenology in accounting for social structures such as racism and poverty, which distribute the risk of incarceration and punitive isolation in radically unequal ways. While I agree with Husserl that a transcendental account of consciousness is necessary to account for the very

I will take up one possibility: a reading of the French phenomenologist, Maurice Merleau-Ponty's account of the relation between intercorporeal depth and psychopathology in *Phenomenology of Perception.*

3 Bodies in Depth

> Experience discloses beneath objective space, in which the body eventually finds its place, a primitive spatiality of which experience is merely the outer covering and which merges with the body's very being. To be a body is to be tied to a certain world, as we have seen; our body is not primarily *in* space: it is of it. (Merleau-Ponty 1962, p. 171)

For Merleau-Ponty, the body is both *in* space and *of* it. What does this mean, and why is the spatiality of the body more primary than its insertion into space? The body is a spatial object; it can bump into things, it has objective being. But it is also the site of lived experience; I feel things not just *in* my body but *as* a body. To modify Heidegger's account of Being-in-the-world, the body is not "in" the world the way that water is in a glass; rather, it is the perspective from which my experience of space, and even of my own body as a spatial being, unfolds. I perceive the world not as a god hovering above the world, nor as a robot passively recording raw data, but as a being who is wholly intervolved with a world in relation to which I am both constituted and constituting: an organism subject to the laws of physics, but also an active participant in the unfolding of the world's meaning and its history. In phenomenological discourse, constitution does not mean fabrication or causation; the world is not merely an idea of consciousness, nor is consciousness merely the outcome of naturalistic processes. Rather, the *meaning* of the world is constituted by consciousness, within a particular context of givenness which includes the givenness of a particular kind of body with physiological structures and capacities which remain open to development and enhancement over time. On one hand, I have a visual apparatus whose function and operation can be adequately described from a third person perspective in terms of physiological structures and processes. On the other hand, the lived experience of vision both presupposes this physiological level and exceeds it, demanding a different methodology to describe how vision unfolds *for* someone, beginning with the most immediate level of experience for any consciousness, namely first person experience. I do not indiscriminately take everything in at the same level or to the same degree; rather, I am drawn to certain things rather than others, picking out some things as objects in the foreground and placing others in the background. These levels shift according to what concerns me most at this or that moment, and I am not always the one who determines my own concerns; the relation between body and world unfolds as a conversation, in a dynamic tension between passive givenness and active constitution. Merleau-Ponty puts it this way:

(Footnote 13 continued)
possibility of meaningful experience, I strongly believe that this transcendental analysis must be supplemented by a critical practice of social scientific research.

> Besides the physical and geometrical distance which stands between myself and all things, a 'lived' distance binds me to things which count and exist for me, and links them to each other. This distance measures the 'scope' of my life at every moment. (286)

In this sense, the experience of depth is not merely perceptual in a cognitive sense, but also affective or emotional. I am *moved* by things, and not everything moves me in the same way. Affective depth marks the emergence and unfolding of meaningful space, space that matters to what Heidegger would call my Being-in-the-world. To care about things—to be structured *as* care—is to be open to the way some aspects of the world leap out at me and seize me, while others recede into the background or even escape my notice. Depth, then, is not just a matter of three-dimensional space; it involves the invisible dimensions of meaning and feeling, which both unfold from an experience of the spatial world and also evade any attempt to represent them on a grid or graph. I mean "depth" to refer to the dimension opened up by the interplay of what is presented in lived experience and what it not presented, and perhaps not even representable, but is nevertheless appresented in some intrinsic connection to what is directly perceived. For example, I perceive the front of a statue and apperceive the back, which remains hidden from me; I perceive a dog running after a rabbit and apperceive its consciousness (and the consciousness of the rabbit); I perceive a shadow in the corner and apperceive a threat (or perhaps a welcome relief from the sun). Each of these is, in its own way, an example of depth because each involves the opening of a virtual dimension in the midst of the actual, which fleshes out an experience of the world *as* a world, namely, as both the context for everyday perception and as what overflows any given perception, as an open-ended horizon of possibility.

The basic phenomenological coordinates of the body-in-depth are the "here" and the "there." My body is the primordial "here" from which I encounter every "there"; it is the root of my intentional consciousness and of my existence as a living being. The "here" of my bodily perspective is both utterly inescapable and utterly mobile; it is both a root and a vehicle for my open-ended exploration of the world. Movement is a vital component of this experience:

> [M]y body is geared onto a world when my perception presents me with a spectacle as varied and clearly articulated as possible, and when my motor intentions, as they unfold, receive the responses they expect from the world. (250)

This "gearing of the subject onto his world [...] is the origin of space" (251). As I move through the world, interacting with objects and other subjects, a constantly-changing but consistently-patterned series of profiles or glimpses of the world unfolds from the perspective of my embodied consciousness. Each of these profiles is partial, revealing some aspects of the world while concealing others; I can never see the front and the back of an object simultaneously, but as I move around, my body "gears into" the heterogeneous texture of the world, and I gain a sense of the object as a whole that exceeds what I can experience in any given moment, but that nevertheless has a coherence or wholeness of its own. Precisely because perception is partial and perspectival, it is also inexhaustible; I can never complete my perception of even a simple object like a cup or a table, since it is only accessible to me through a blend of presence and absence.

But the main thing that my body gears into is not a thing at all; it is the body of another person, another starting-point for an experience of the world. The body of the other is the "there" to which my own body—my "here"—is essentially correlated. Likewise, my "here" is experienced as "there" for another person's "here." Merleau-Ponty calls this structure *intercorporeality*. It suggests that our bodies are never exclusively our own; my "here" calls out for your "there," and vice versa. My own experience of the world is intertwined with the bodies of others, both present and absent, who occupy the places from which I, too, could experience the world, but never *as* that other person. So even when I am alone, as in a solitary confinement unit, my experience of the world is still structured through the here-there relation of intercorporeality. The question is: What happens to this intercorporeal structure when someone is deprived of *concrete* everyday experiences of a space shared with other embodied subjects? How does an extreme manipulation of what we could call the empirical world—the concrete living environment—affect the transcendental structures of experience, and vice versa?

Merleau-Ponty calls the body of another person "the completion of the system" through which I make sense of the world (352). It is the anchor that stabilizes my experience of space, and allows me to experience a meaningful difference between objective reality and subjective fancy or hallucination. Every time I hear a sound and see another person look towards the origin of that sound, I receive an implicit confirmation that what I heard was something real, that it was not just my imagination playing tricks on me. Every time someone walks around the table rather than through it, I receive an unspoken, usually unremarkable, confirmation that the table exists, and that my own way of relating to tables is shared by others. When I don't receive these implicit confirmations, I can usually ask someone—but for the most part, we don't need to ask because our experience is already interwoven with the experience of many other living, thinking, perceiving beings who relate to the same world from their own unique perspective. This multiplicity of perspectives is like an invisible net that supports the coherence of my own experience, even (or especially) when others challenge my interpretation of the world. For Merleau-Ponty, the structure of intercorporeality is so fundamental that it shapes the meaning of objects, even when I am alone:

> In the cultural object, I feel the close presence of others beneath a veil of anonymity. *Someone* uses the pipe for smoking, the spoon for eating, the bell for summoning, and it is through the perception of a human act *and another person* that the perception of a cultural world could be verified. (348, emphasis added)

But without a concrete, everyday experience of another person, the traces of intercorporeality in the object becomes like a haunting, and it is not clear who is the ghost—myself or the other.

When we isolate a prisoner in solitary confinement, we deprive them of the intercorporeal network of support that sustains the meaning of their experience. They may still perceive the table and chair that is bolted in place in their cell, and they may still have the memory of what tables and chairs mean for other people. But their capacity to distinguish between these objects as *there-for-me* and *there-for-others* (or *objectively* there), is structurally undermined through prolonged solitary confinement. The "there" that would otherwise anchor the prisoner's experience of the world from "here" has been pulled up, casting them adrift without a clear orientation point for intersubjective verification, or for the support of others to help clarify the distinction between perception and hallucination, truth and illusion. What can we say about this unraveling of meaningful experience from a phenomenological perspective?

4 Pure Depth and Psychopathology

In his discussion of spatial and social depth, Merleau-Ponty raises the possibility of an experience of "pure depth": depth without a determinate object, "a spatiality without things" (283). He calls this experience of pure depth "night":

> Night is not an object before me; it enwraps me and infiltrates through all my senses, stifling my recollections and almost destroying my personal identity. I am no longer withdrawn into my perceptual look-out from which I watch the outlines of objects moving by at a distance. Night has no outlines; it is itself in contact with me; it enwraps me and its unity is the mystical unity of the *mana*. Even shouts or a distant light people it only vaguely, and then it comes to life in its entirety; it is pure depth without foreground or background, without surfaces and without any distance separating it from me. (283)

Night is the name for an experience of space unhinged from determinate objects and from the limits or outlines that distinguish self from non-self. Recall the experience of prisoners in prolonged solitary confinement: the strange feeling of death in life, in which one's body begins to "communicate" with the cell, the outlines around things seem to melt, and the cell walls themselves begin to waver. Could the experience of endless day, as in the 24-h illumination of the supermax cell, be tantamount to an experience of night? Is supermax confinement an experience of pure depth, or is it an experience of space deprived of depth? And how exactly could we determine the difference?

For Merleau-Ponty, the experience of night seems fecund and generative; it exposes us to the pre-personal matrix from which our bodies individuate and to which they remain attached by a mystical umbilical cord. But even here, the experience of night is highly ambivalent; it stifles my reflections and threatens to destroy my personal identity just as much as it connects me to the *mana* of pure depth:

> Sometimes between myself and the events […] the lived distance is both too small and too great: the majority of the events cease to count for me, while the nearest ones obsess me. They enshroud me like night and rob me of my individuality and freedom. I can literally no longer breathe; I am possessed. (286)

The experience of pure depth can be suffocating as well as liberating; affective depth, the site of mattering, can invert into a radical loss of meaning where nothing counts anymore. Supermax daylight, no less than the experience of night, threatens to destroy the prisoner's sense of personal identity—not because it is free from limits, but because it is confined to such strict limits that the open-ended field of experience that defines the world, and defines both self and other as co-inhabitants of a shared world, begins to disintegrate.

What anchors and stabilizes the experience of pure depth is the correlation of an individuated, embodied perspective—a "here"—with a world of stable, determinate objects—a "there." Merleau-Ponty calls this "clear space"—"that impartial space in which all objects are equally important and enjoy the same right to existence" (287). Clear space is not opposed to night; it remains connected to pure depth, "thoroughly permeated by another spatiality thrown into relief by morbid deviations from the normal" (287). Nor is it drained of affective significance, as Shiloh Whitney observes:

> Our perceptual distance from the things that populate our world is not guaranteed. It depends on our ability to care, to become acquainted with affective entities that polarize space in their own right. This in turn lets us achieve "lived distance": a margin of respectful affective distance from things and others…. (Whitney 2010, p. 14)

Clear space is the sane, rational space of a world shared in common with others, a world in which things matter, but where their precise meaning is subject to constant mediation and negotiation. It is a sense of space maintained by both an engagement with the world and a capacity to sleep or withdraw from the world. Merleau-Ponty writes: "During sleep […] I hold the world present to me only in order to keep it at a distance, and I revert to the subjective sources of my existence" (Merleau-Ponty 1962, p. 284). Sleep is the escape that both reconnects me to the experience of primary spatiality—to the night—and also allows me to retain and even recover my sense of personal identity, my distinction from the night, the root of my own subjective existence. The temporal rhythm of alternating night and day, sleep and waking, release and return, sustains the fabric of embodied subjectivity in a world that is experienced in depth, somewhere between the extremes of pure depth and objective space. But an exposure to pure depth without the stabilizing rhythm of night and day can undermine the subject's capacity for a meaningful experience of the world.

Merleau-Ponty cites schizophrenia as an example of those "morbid deviations from the normal" produced by an overexposure to the pure depth night. He presents schizophrenia less as a mental illness than a phenomenological disorder of Being-in-the-world rooted in a pathological experience of space: "The schizophrenic no longer inhabits the common property world, but a private world, and no longer gets as far as geographical space […]. [T]he world can no longer be taken for granted" (287). For one reason or another—Merleau-Ponty does not speculate on the etiology of the disease—schizophrenia unhinges the patient from a common world, afflicting him with an experience of the world not shared with other people. We could say that schizophrenia removes the patient from "clear space":

> What protects the sane man against delirium or hallucination, is not his critical powers, but the structure of his space: objects remain before him, keeping their distances and, as Malebranche said speaking of Adam, touching him only with respect. What brings about both hallucinations and myths is a shrinkage in the space directly experienced, a rooting of

> things in our body [rather than in a shared world], the overwhelming proximity of the object, the oneness of man and the world, which is, not indeed abolished, but repressed by everyday perception or by objective thought, and which philosophical consciousness rediscovers. (291)

The schizophrenic is exposed to a prolonged experience of night: an experience that unravels the meaning of "experience" understood phenomenologically as the subjective basis for knowledge of the objective (i.e. intersubjective or intercorporeal) world. Clear space, with its consistent correlations between self and other, body and world, keeps the night at bay; it carves "places" out of the pure depth of spatiality, and it institutes stable but flexible limits on the proximity and distance of things. In so doing, it preserves a hollow within the world for the reception of a body, and a hollow within the body for the reception of a world. Of course, clear space can also be reified into objective or grid space when the rationalist subject attempts to deny or overcome the lived experience of depth, in which case rationality also becomes a source of pathology. But there is a place (quite literally) for an experience of clear space somewhere between night and the grid of objective space.

Merleau-Ponty's analysis of schizophrenia in *Phenomenology of Perception* sheds light on the phenomenological dimensions of SHU syndrome as a pathological experience of space, and so of embodied subjectivity. If schizophrenia is a pathology of space in which in which the world shrinks to the limits of my own private experience, and so destabilizes my sense of reality to the point where "the world can no longer be taken for granted," then prolonged solitary confinement amounts to a production of something like schizophrenia in the prisoner (287). But if this is the case, then supermax confinement is not a solution to the problem of finding a place to keep "the worst of the worst" from harming others. It is—among other things—a technology for producing what one could call mental illness, if "mental" were not too narrow a term to express the complex intertwining of body, mind and world that I have just described. Prolonged solitary confinement in a control prison threatens to exhaust the otherwise inexhaustible horizons of perceptual experience by blocking the prisoner's concrete experience of depth in its spatial, affective and social dimensions. It leaves the prisoner feeling like her life has been drained of meaning, like she is dead within life, no longer *of* space but merely *in* it.

The prisoner who is shut up in her solitary cell and monitored from a distance by video camera 24 h a day is rendered anonymous in the sense of being reduced to a nameless, faceless existence in which one is constantly reminded that one does not matter to anyone. But she is also denied access to anonymity of in the sense of being able to slip out of place or to "sleep," withdrawing from the fixity of her 8×10 cell, and withdrawing from the meanings attached to that cell: "the worst of the worst," "beyond rehabilitation," "a hopeless case," and so on. To put this another way: The prisoner in solitary confinement is denied the *incompleteness* of perceptual Being-in-the-world, the double incompleteness of the body-thing system and the self-other system, both of which sustain the sense of a world with inexhaustible horizons. She is confined to her own side of the otherwise open circuit between her own perceiving body and the heterogeneous field of the world, understood as "the field of fields" (351), the one world shared in common. Cut off from an open-ended experience of space and a non-coercive experience of others, the supermax prisoner risks losing the sense of herself as a subject of meaning and as a self-organizing and auto-affective Being-in-the-world. She is forced into a position that Merleau-Ponty argues does not exist except as a fiction devised by the intellectualist philosophers of cognition: namely, the theoretical position of the Cartesian cogito, an absolute individual whose existence is self-verifying and non-relational.[14] In other words, the supermax prisoner is forced into an ideal(ist) position in which non-incarcerated subjects never actually find themselves, but which the prisoner is expected to adopt through a coercive rearrangement of space: the position of a solitary, non-relational individual made to bear the full weight of her own existence, made "accountable" for everything she does, says and is, and for the "choices" she makes in a situation that is structured from top to bottom by domination and control.[15] When the prisoner fails to accept or sustain this impossible position, or to be stuffed into a faulty theoretical construct, s/he is punished for non-compliance. The punishment, of course, is more time in solitary confinement. The issue here is that the supposed justification for solitary confinement—that a subject be left alone to reflect on the contents of her transparent thoughts—is based on a problematic Cartesian conception of consciousness which overlooks, to a large extent, the embodied and intersubjective nature of subjectivity. The evidence for this is that subjects do not tend to reflect upon themselves while in solitary confinement, but literally come apart. Solitary confinement damages or destroys the relational structure of the subject in ways that undermine the possibility of meaningful reflection, and that are sometimes irreparable.

5 Pathology and Resistance

By way of conclusion, I want to consider a scene witnessed by anthropologist Lorna Rhodes on her first visit to a Washington State penitentiary. Rhodes observes an inmate, Jamal Nelson, in the solitary exercise yard. He is swinging his arms from side to side in widening circles until his knuckles start hitting the concrete walls. He continues to swing, splattering the concrete with blood, relentlessly marking the limits of the space allotted to him, as if oblivious to the pain and even to the walls themselves (Rhodes 2004, p. 3). What would drive someone to do this? We could invoke mental illness or SHU syndrome, and we could list the typical symptoms of such an illness or syndrome. These clinical diagnoses are important, especially in

[14] Of course, even the cogito needs to discover another absolute point beyond itself—the God of the Third Meditation—in order to secure a stable and reliable knowledge of the world. I discuss this point in relation to the ethical and epistemological issues raised by solitary confinement in Chapter 9 of *Solitary Confinement: Social Death and its Afterlives* (Guenther 2013).

[15] See Rhodes (2004) on the neoliberal logic of choice in supermax prisons and the double bind produced for prisoners who have almost no control over their situation, and yet must bear full accountability for their actions.

the context of class action suits on behalf of prisoners' rights; but without a phenomenological supplement, they fail to capture the complex relations of self, other and world that are at stake in Nelson's experience. Recall the ontological "event" that Jack Henry Abbott describes in his own first-person account of solitary confinement, whereby his body began to "communicate" with the cell, as if he had no choice but to "*enter* it and become a part of it" (Abbott 1991, p. 29). The person who bashes his own body against the walls of a cell is both refusing and confirming the logic of punitive individualism that structures supermax embodiment. The self-battering body makes a statement of sorts: these walls may confine me absolutely, but I absolutely refuse to be confined! There is a difference between my body and space—a "there" to which my "here" is correlated—and I will find it, even if I have to hurl myself against it, or even destroy myself in the process.[16] This kind of resistance may be self-defeating, or even self-destructive; but it remains an eloquent expression of the depth of emotional and ontological harm that prolonged solitary confinement can inflict on a person.

Some prisoners do manage to resist the violence of solitary confinement, sustaining a sense of place even within the evacuated, exhausted space of supermax confinement. Robert King, a member of the Angola Three who spent 29 years in solitary confinement in a dimly-lit 9 × 6 cell, writes:

> Some days I would pace up and down and from left to right for hours, counting to myself. I learned to know every inch of the cell. Maybe I looked crazy walking back and forth like some trapped animal, but I had no choice – I needed to feel in control of my space. (King 2010)

Like the act of bashing one's body into walls, the habit of pacing both resists and reinscribes the limits of place that block an experience of intercorporeal depth. But unlike bashing, pacing develops a more sustainable coping mechanism, a way of feeling "in control of [one's] space" even if one does not have the power to change places. Pacing is a bodily attempt to "take the measure" of the cell or cage, and in some way to take control over something that cannot be controlled.[17] The subject who paces is both refusing to sit still within his allotted space, and refusing to destroy his bodily integrity by bashing against the walls. It is a way of insisting that one is still a living, moving being, even though the world has been diminished to the point where one is no longer able to live and move freely and non-pathologically. Pacing

---

[16]Self-mutilation is a common response to prolonged solitary confinement. One of the prisoners interviewed by Grassian in 1983 says: "I cut my wrists – cut myself many times when in isolation. Now, it seems crazy. But every time I did it, I wasn't thinking – lost control – cut myself without knowing what I was doing" (Grassian 1983, p. 1453). Grassian comments on this impulse: "Many became grossly disorganized and psychotic, smearing themselves with feces, mumbling and screaming incoherently all day and night, some even descending to the horror of eating parts of their own bodies" (Grassian 2006, p. 351).

[17]See David Morris's discussion of pacing in *The Sense of Space*: "The lion does not first take the measure of its cage in objective units, and then, finding it small, pace its confines; its elliptical, perpetual stride already is the 'measure' of its environment, the 'measure' of an environment in which there is no striking distance, no safe remove; correlatively, the caged lion's stride is the 'measure' of an animal warped by confinement" (Morris 2004, p. 20).

does not express an acceptance of limits, but rather a nervous retracing of them, a habit formed around the impossibility of habituating oneself to what is an intolerable situation. In this sense, it is a way of coping—but even this coping mechanism is still a pathology that can become its own compulsive trap. Habits of adaption to the narrow and solitary space of a supermax unit can become habits of maladaption to life outside of prison, or even in the general prison population. Many prisoners find that their time in confined space and solitude expands the amount of personal space they need after they get released. It is as if the inmate's sense of personhood had expanded to fit the narrow constraints permitted to it, and even though the cell walls were a barrier to freedom and connection, he had adjusted to them, and maybe even identified with them in order to form a zone of comfort or safety (see Rhodes 2004, p. 34). As Robert King says, "I talk about my 29 years in solitary as if it was the past, but the truth is it never leaves you. In some ways I am still there" (King 2010).

Deprived of a regular, concrete experience of other embodied subjects in mutual interaction, and blocked from a regular, concrete experience of spatial distance or variable depth, the prisoner in solitary confinement risks coming unhinged from the world and thrown into a pathological experience of space that resonates with Merleau-Ponty's account of schizophrenia. The supermax unit is precisely that: a unit, a block of objective grid space that a living, moving, embodied Being-in-the-world is forced to occupy as if she were a piece on a chessboard, an absolute individual separable from the society of others and from the "larger place" of the world. This unit is measurable in feet or in "paces"—six by nine, eight by twelve—and yet the embodied *experience* of this space could never be expressed in terms of length and width, but only as the blocked experience of foreclosed depth that their occupants that are forced to undergo in solitude. The irony is that—tragically, absurdly—the supermax prisoner is one of the only living beings whose experience of space aligns with the account of objective grid space given by Cartesian rationalists. Nonincarcerated subjects are free to invest in the fiction of the solitary cogito with its clear and distinct ideas, all the while relying on their embodied experience of affective and intercorporeal depth to sustain a meaningful sense of Being-in-the-world. Only incarcerated subjects are forced to actually *exist* in such fictions, or to be broken by them. What the testimony of prisoners and the work of Merleau-Ponty helps us to see is that SHU syndrome is more than a mental illness afflicting individual subjects; it is a social, phenomenological and ontological pathology for which the language of psychiatry is both necessary and insufficient.

References

Abbott, J. H. (1991). Introduction. In N. Mailer (Ed.), *In the belly of the beast: Letters from prison*. New York: Vintage Books.

Baxter, C., Brown, W., Chatman-Bey, T., Johnson, H. B, Jr, Medley, M., Thompson, D., et al. (2005). Live from the panopticon: Architecture and power revisited. In Joy James (Ed.), *The new abolitionists: (Neo) slave narratives and contemporary prison writings* (pp. 205–216). Albany, NY: SUNY Press.

Gomez, A. E. (2006). Resisting living death at Marion penitentiary, 1972. *Radical History Review, 96*(Fall), 58–86.
Grassian, S. (1983). Psychopathological effects of solitary confinement. *American Journal of Psychiatry, 140*(11), 1450–1454.
Grassian, S. (2006). Psychiatric effects of solitary confinement. *Journal of Law and Policy, 22*, 325–383.
Greene, S. (2012). The gray box: An investigative look at solitary confinement. *Dart Society Reports*, January 24. Accessed July 9, 2012. http://www.dartsocietyreports.org/cms/2012/01/the-gray-box-anoriginal-investigation/
Guenther, L. (2013). *Solitary confinement: Social death and its afterlives*. Minneapolis: University of Minnesota Press.
Haney, C. (2003). Mental health issues in long-term solitary and 'supermax' confinement. *Crime & Delinquency, 49*(1), 124–156.
Husserl, E. (1970). *The crisis of the european sciences and transcendental phenomenology: An introduction to phenomenological philosophy* (D. Carr, Trans.). Evanston, IL: Northwestern University Press.
Husserl, E. (1983). *Ideas pertaining to a pure phenomenology and to a phenomenological philosophy: First book: General introduction to a pure phenomenology* (F. Kersten, Trans.). Dortrecht: Kluwer Academic Publishers.
Husserl, E. (1991). *Cartesian meditations: An introduction to phenomenology* (D. Cairns, Trans.). Dortrecht: Kluwer Academic Publishers.
James, J. (Ed.). (2003). *Imprisoned Intellectuals: America's political prisoners write on life, liberation, and rebellion*. New York: Rowman & Littlefield.
James, J. (Ed.). (2005). *The new abolitionists: (Neo) slave narratives and contemporary prison writings*. Albany, NY: SUNY Press.
King, R. (2010, August 28). Experience: I spent 29 years in solitary confinement. *The Guardian* [Online]. Available: http://www.guardian.co.uk/lifeandstyle/2010/aug/28/29-years-solitary-confinement-robert-king.
Merleau-Ponty, M. (1962). *Phenomenology of perception [PhP]* (C. Smith, Trans.). London: Routledge & Kegan Paul.
Morris, D. (2004). *The sense of space*. Albany, NY: SUNY Press.
Reiter, K. A. (2010). *Parole, snitch, or die: California's supermax prisons and prisoners, 1997–2007*. ISSC Fellows Working Papers. UC Berkeley: Institute for the Study of Social Change [Online]. Available: http://escholarship.org/uc/item/04w6556f.
Rhodes, L. A. (2004). *Total confinement: Madness and reason in the maximum security prison*. Berkeley, LA, London: University of California Press.
Scott, G. (1969). The prisoner of society: Psychiatric syndromes in captive society. *Correctional Psychologist, 3*(7), 3–5.
Shalev, S. (2009). *Supermax: Controlling risk through solitary confinement*. Portland, OR: Willan Publishing.
Shaylor, C. (1998). It's like living in a black hole: Women of color and solitary confinement in the prison industrial complex. *New England Journal on Criminal and Civil Confinement, 24*, 385–416.
Smith, C. (2009). *The prison and the American imagination*. New Haven and London: Yale University Press.
Tapley, L. (2010). The worst of the worst: Supermax torture in America. *Boston Review*, Nov/Dec. Accessed December 28, 2010. http://www.bostonreview.net/BR35.6/tapley.php.
Whitney, S. (2010). *A new conception of intentionality: Pure depth as affective orientation*. Paper presented at the Merleau-Ponty Circle Annual Meeting.
Yáñez-Correa, A., & Jennifer, L. (2012). On the perils of reentry following solitary confinement and possible solutions. *Grits for Breakfast*. September 25 [Online]. Available: http://gritsforbreakfast.blogspot.com/2012/09/on-perils-of-reentry-following-solitary.html.

Part V
Eugenics and Enhancements

Chapter 15
The Right to Be Impaired and the Legacy of Eugenics: A Critical Reading of the UN Convention on "Disability" Rights

Christien van den Anker

1 Introduction

The links between medicine and society can be viewed from many perspectives yet their relationship should always be seen as contested and political. Here I use human rights as my starting point. A sociological account of human rights should address the contested human rights discourse and its possibilities for emancipation as well as domination. Silences are not simply absences, but constitutive features of discourse and practice which inform issues of inclusion, exclusion, and participation (Bhambra and Shilliam 2008). The rights of "disabled" persons have long been a silence in human rights discourse, despite the atrocities against them and many other groups during World War II that informed the development of the UN human rights framework. However, the experimental gassing of 275,000 Germans labeled as "disabled" under the Nazi T4 program (Baker 2002) predating the war was not widely known, although the Allied governments had at least known of the death camps since 1944 (Swiebocki 2002). Therefore, despite the human rights agenda of the UN being conceptually linked to eugenics by using its worst outcomes as a point of reference, the rights of people targeted by disability oppression were not yet explicitly included as a matter of international concern.

The international codification of the rights of "disabled" persons developed after their appearance within national systems as part of anti-discrimination laws (Kanter 2003). The same is true for European-wide policy on disability rights (Mabett 2005, p. 97). Only in 2007, after a long campaign, did the UN International Convention on the Rights of Persons with Disabilities come into force.

Sociology and social policy also engaged with "disability" relatively late compared to perspectives on gender and race equality (Beckett 2005). This is evidenced by sociological handbooks being completely silent on the issue from the 1970s until

C. van den Anker (✉)
University of the West of England, Bristol, UK
e-mail: Christien.vandenanker@uwe.ac.uk

D. Meacham (ed.), *Medicine and Society, New Perspectives in Continental Philosophy*, Philosophy and Medicine 120, DOI 10.1007/978-94-017-9870-9_15

the 1990s (Worsley 1970; Joseph 1990). Currently, sociological literature recognizes various models of "disability." Sociologists distinguish between the medical model which holds that disabilities are abnormalities in need of curing and the social model of disability which holds that barriers to full functioning are social and don't need to be addressed by altering human bodies and minds through invasive procedures or medication. Although the social model of disability developed outside mainstream sociology, sociology has analyzed the disability rights movement (Beckett 2006) and the ways in which society impacts on the construction of identities. Similarly, the concepts of inclusion/exclusion are frequently used in sociological studies of social policy. The literature now includes many applications of a wide variety of sociological theories of disability (Bickenbacha et al. 1999). For example, from a functionalist paradigm, disabled individuals have inherently pathological conditions that can be objectively diagnosed, treated, and in some cases ameliorated. A structuralist paradigm explains disability as a product of oppositional structures within a socio-political system that produces disability through inequities and social injustice. In contrast, a postmodern paradigm negates the likelihood of objective reality, assumes that ambiguity is at play in the world, and destabilizes notions about oppositional power relations by revealing the tensions and paradoxes of the social world (Gabel and Peters 2004).

This chapter analyses the impact of eugenics on current models of "disability" and the rights of people targeted by disability oppression and contributes a proposal for transformation in line with critical social theory's aim of avoiding perpetuation of forms of domination and oppression. I use the overlapping methods of autoethnography of illness/impairment and sociological phenomenology of tracing lived experience combined with discourse analysis of the Convention (Stark and Brown Trinidad 2007). As Tierney (1998) asserted, "autoethnography confronts dominant forms of representation and power in an attempt to reclaim, through self-reflective response, representational spaces that have marginalized those of us at the borders" (66). Autoethnography can also be seen to encourage empathy and connection beyond the self of the author and contributes to sociological understandings (Sparkes 2002). Self-reflexive writing and related qualitative methodologies have been contested for not being representative, objective or generalizable. Yet, these objections rely on models of science that have themselves been criticized by constructivism and postmodernism and mainstream sociology still struggles to treat these methodologies fairly (Miller et al. 1998; Holt 2003). Autoethnography has also matured enough to address ethical issues raised by its methods (Harrison 1993) and its use in sociology has been recommended (Stanley 1993).

My argument runs as follows. Section 2 sets out the discovery of the social model of disability and legacies of eugenics following my diagnosis with young onset Parkinson's disease. Section 3 shows what the original eugenics movement entailed and portrays the wider context of "selective breeding" and "enhancement of the species" beyond the Nazi period. It also responds to critics who argue that eugenics can have benign interpretations. Section 4 assesses the Convention for its underlying models of disability and links to eugenics thinking. Section 5 sketches the implications of a fully inclusive model of society. I conclude with a summary of the argument and a call for inclusion as the principle to universalize the rights of people affected by disability oppression.

2 Becoming 'Disabled': Experiencing the Legacies of Eugenics

In disability discourse, there is a distinction made between the medical and the social model of disability. I discovered the validity of the social as well as the medical model of disability and the remnants of eugenics thinking through the experience of being diagnosed with young onset Parkinson's disease (PD) at the age of forty-three in August 2009. I quickly learned two important lessons. Firstly, it is not the physical effect of having Parkinson's disease that creates the biggest challenges for me at the moment, but the attitudes of others and the policies governing the availability of resources and rights. Secondly, many unexpected and worrying attitudes and feelings in myself and others around the right to exist as a "disabled" person became visible to me. I will illustrate these lessons in turn. Of course, they are individual and may not be felt in the same way by others.

PD initially caused tremor, stiffness in muscles, back and neck ache, slowness, incontinence, constipation, rigidity especially at night, confusion, difficulty prioritizing, exhaustion and low mood. Now I also have trouble swallowing, my vocal volume is low at times and I stumble or lose balance more frequently. I can still do most things but not as quickly, intensively or for as long as before. I've been told that symptoms will become symmetrical over time and the trajectory is that of a degenerative disease: symptoms vary individually and deteriorate despite being responsive to conventional medical intervention through drugs and brain surgery. My symptoms were initially reduced by systematic and frequent emotional expression in counseling, physical exercise and assuming leadership over my medical team. Now they also respond to a combination of three drugs.

The actual symptoms affect my life in a variety of ways. Experiencing tremor, stiffness or slowness induces feelings of anger and loss. Receiving information that the disease is "progressive" creates fear of the future. Yet, generally these have so far also been incentives to find practitioners, like for example an acupuncturist and a chiropractor who figured out together that my acute and severe back pain was caused by asymmetrical tension in the muscles. Treatment complemented by exercises reduced the muscle tension and eliminated episodes of pain. A good chair at work, memory foam mattresses and pillow and persistent attendance of Pilates classes are contributing to the prevention of pain. Similarly, I found ways forward that have made constipation, incontinence, sleeplessness and confusion nearly disappear. A practical solution like an electronic planner and a personal assistant have helped with organizational skills and prioritizing. Neither the physical experience of PD nor accessing resources is therefore the biggest challenge right now:

society is. The attitudes of other people and institutions present a time-consuming and emotionally hard journey.

Reactions of people to illness vary widely. Carel (2007) describes some of the excessively rude ones, for example that people out of fear, anxiety and pity actually ask how long she has got to live. They are relieved that this is someone else's story. I experienced a range of reactions in people from urgently wanting to help, expressing excessive sadness for me, telling of others who are ill, telling of how glad they are to have healthy bodies or telling of their own health issues; trying to tell me what to do to cure myself or make my symptoms go away. Some people can only see me as ill; they don't accept me talking about other aspects of my life; moreover, they require me to only show loss and upset at my illness and refuse to allow stories of overcoming some of the symptoms or learning something as a result of having this different identity. Yet, I'm not my condition. I want to be able to share all aspects of my life and thinking—not only PD. Fortunately, many people also show real care. On my first conference trip after diagnosis friends offered a warm welcome and made helpful suggestions around assisting me to address the physical challenges without seeing me as my illness only. It showed me how consciously caring means both engaging with the changed circumstances and respecting the whole person. Their care brought more tears than the frustration about being ill. And most recently I have experimented with increased physical challenges with allies who are willing to support me while they recognize that they are in an oppressor role towards me if they are able-bodied. Allies are friends, family or practitioners who are committed to supporting me and have the wider perspective of inclusion to resist the pressures of "disabling" society. They are pleased to discover with me how strength, flexibility and stamina can improve despite a degenerative neurological condition. They also respond helpfully when I fall off my bike or need assistance getting out of a river while canoeing due to my body stiffening up.

I'm not affected so much (yet) by PD but more by disability oppression. One time I was told by a close friend not to "harp on about inclusion." When I presented a first draft of this paper at a conference with medics and philosophers I was told that "some lives aren't worth living." These attitudes form part of the context in which my new identity is formed, both around beliefs about myself, and around perceptions of what is possible in a life with PD. The social expectations are that symptoms are consistent: needing assistance one day but not the next is hard. Even when no comments are made, I feel self-conscious when I lie down to rest my back most of an evening and then I participate in a game of rounders (a British game rather similar to baseball). These contrasts and shifts are accompanied by changes in my mood and sensing a variety of expectations in different people. The invisibility of many symptoms sometimes leads to having to justify making use of special facilities, whereas the visibility of symptoms sometimes makes it impossible to be an innocuous part of the group. It is interesting to experience how the amount of visibility that I perceive as helpful can vary: in some groups it is a good approach to state upfront why I move differently whereas elsewhere it is preferable to just blend in. However, I notice that I can blend in less than I think and people notice things about my physique and mental capacity at times. Still, there is always pressure to not be too disabled as well as not being disabled enough.

As far as support and resources are concerned, in practice many of the systems of support have developed into principles to fit in with rather than as flexible based on the support needed. For example, the reasonable adjustment of having a personal support worker has cost so much time on bureaucratic fights that it is tempting to give up.

Since it has become clearly visible to me how the symptoms are not the biggest interference with my life but the reactions of people to it, I have explored where these feelings stem from. My symptoms bother others more than me, as they are an "anomaly." Carel (2007) concludes that once you are ill, you become fair game. Others begin to perceive you as weak and unimportant, an object of pity and fascination. Yet for me even empathy and uninvited assistance are oppressive. I perceive people either resistant to help in the way I ask for, or overeager to help, which again excludes me as an agent of decision-making.

The hardest lesson, however, is to find attitudes in myself and others that expose our (internalized) criticism of disabled people which I have traced back to eugenics ideology. In order to spot my own feelings, I observe the feelings of my allies first. What are friends, family and other allies scared of? They dramatise the diagnosis as a big upset, create distance from me, and become afraid of making mistakes, i.e. upsetting my feelings. Yet, it is more important to make contact than to get it "right"—as I often explain to them, in my experience the anger with allies for "mistakes" is often an expression of the anger at being ill. Allies get afraid of being associated with the "weak and needy" and then they make me assimilate or compromise on my needs. Especially hard to be around are my slowness and my messy eating or general clumsiness which touch on social taboos related to being independent, rational adults. This goes back to the deeply ingrained fear of selection for destruction. This may be related to inherent fear of non-survival due to dependency which is exacerbated by political targeting of groups positioned as "weak" or "inferior." Indications are being "different" physically or socially, being slow or being "hard to understand" in speech. Even acting as an ally to the "weak" could endanger life in this situation. Fear of being "guilty by association" still creates distance between people from a very young age in the context of bullying in schools (Kliewer and Drake 1998).

What am I scared of? I have become aware of deeply distressing legacies of eugenics in my own attitude towards "disability," including my own illness. I doubt my right to exist, I am afraid of becoming dependent on others, and I realized that if my mother had known of my disability she would have aborted me. These fears were most clearly felt at a visit to former Nazi concentration camps Auschwitz and Birkenau in Poland where killing of the "weak" actually happened. The pressure to fit in and be perfected is also present in the experiences with medical staff. Pressure to take drugs that reduce symptoms, lack of attention for my improved well-being due to exercise and alternative medicine and disrespect of my thinking are ongoing struggles. They also ask incredulously if I "still work" which increases my fear of exclusion. The idea of disability was of course for a long time seen as a problem of the disabled person and not one imposed by society through reductionism and isolationism (Liachowitz 1988).

These feelings of potential exclusion from society and ultimately from life itself put a pressure not only on those who can't keep up but on everyone else still trying. The effects are visible in people constantly speeding up, competing with others, striving for more money, more physical "perfection" and pressures on parents trying to "perfect" their children, both physically and in terms of education and mental health standards. These are all elements of practice discussed in the enhancement debate. In counseling work in Israel I gained an insight that the pressures of perfection are very strongly felt there. Nahman also describes the culture of perfection affecting Jewish couples in Israel who receive fertility treatment with the ova of Rumanian women (Nahman 2013). When explored in workshops, it becomes clear that these pressures are related to legacies of eugenics and on the impact of the Nazi experiments in the name of eugenics. I believe that this discovery of a legacy of eugenics in my own experience informs us that eugenics ideology is still impacting on thinking about disability.

3 Legacies of Eugenics—Lived Experience During the Nazi-Period and Now

Eugenics is a term used frequently in the ethical debate on new genetic technology, yet often without detailed accounts of its consequences (Buchanan et al. 2000, p. 8). This section therefore shows the implications of eugenics in the 1930s and during WWII when disabled people were used for forced labour, sexual exploitation, tortured, killed and used for medical experiments.

Historically, the eugenics movement is nearly exclusively associated with national-socialism in Germany. Yet, this movement was older and much more widespread than that. It was the mainstream ideology at the time and included many in the socialist and social democratic left who supported state intervention in reproduction (Paul 1984, 567). The eugenics ideology did not end with the Allied victory over Germany, Italy, Spain, Vichy France and Japan. Eugenics remained the dominant approach to medical interventions on disabled people and migration policies. Even now people are affected by restrictive rights and limited access to reproductive care based on ethnic, religious or national characteristics; and the technological developments in genetics and reproduction have sparked off an intense debate on the ethics of preventing births, interrupting pregnancies and invasive surgery for "improvement" of bodies (Rembis 2009). Showing the horrific implications illustrates that if there are legacies of eugenics ideology in current thinking about "disability" then this is a major moral problem.

The word "eugenics" as first used by Francis Galton (1822–1911) literally meant "well-born" and was conceptualized as "good in stock, hereditarily endowed with noble qualities." Galton's American disciple Charles B. Davenport (1866–1944) referred to eugenics as "the improvement of the human race by selective breeding." In the first thirty years of the twentieth century eugenics movements developed in over thirty-five countries but they proved strongest in Britain, Germany, Scandinavia and the US (Adams et al. 2005, p. 234). The ideas enjoyed a good scientific reputation and offered hope to eliminate physical, mental and emotional disease through control of reproduction. Eugenicists urged states to adopt policies encouraging the reproduction of the "fit" and discouraging the reproduction of the "unfit" (Barrett and Kurzman 2004, p. 497). The legacy of the eugenics movement lies in three main areas: (1) sterilization laws based on prevention of disease as well as anti-social behavior cost arguments, (2) research into genetic factors of physical and mental disease as well as addiction, criminal or antisocial behavior and (3) quota on migration based on ethnicity and nationality, for example on Philippine immigrants (Tyner 1999). In the US the eugenics advocate Laughlin wrote a model sterilization law as a basis for thirty state sterilization laws. "The model law allowed for the compulsory sterilization of inmates and patients in public institutions, prisons, mental hospitals and reformatories who were deemed to be genetically unfit. […] By 1935, more than 20,000 people had been sterilized under these laws and by the 1960s, the number had grown to more than 60,000" (Adams et al. 2005, p. 238).

During the Nazi regime in Germany eugenics ideology involved mass killing, forced abortion, sterilization and rape of particular groups of people who were seen as racially or socially inferior. However, the first people targeted for destruction were German disabled children, for whom parents could apply to have them "euthanized," and disabled or mentally impaired adults killed under *Aktion* T4. The selection criteria for extermination were stipulated by the Nazi psychiatrists as hereditary illness, incurability, and incapacity to work productively (Hohendorf et al. 2002). This still focused on the "genetic purity" of the Aryan race, but now in terms of ability to function in society. Despite abortion being illegal, it was sanctioned by the "Hereditary Health Courts" in cases of "racial treason" (conception of a child from one "Aryan" and one Jewish or "colored" parent) and to prevent hereditary diseases (David et al. 1988, 91). Arguments for applying eugenics to socially inferior groups, who display criminal or addictive behavior were also developed in Sweden in the debate on forced sterilization (Spektorowski and Mizrachi 2004).

The daily, lived experience of eugenics during the Nazi era is illustrated by Miklos Nyiszli who was an assistant to Dr Joseph Mengele in Auschwitz and Birkenau. Mengele was in charge of selection: dividing arriving transports of Jews between the gas chamber and forced labor. Immediate death was reserved for "undesirables" according to Nazi ideology. This meant Jews were generally targeted but being strong and valuable as a worker could temporarily (on average three months to a year) save your life. The old, young, physically and mentally disabled did not make it through selection. There is a clear link between the Nazi racial theory with a capitalist work ethic: those who did not work were not allowed to live. Forced labor was both supporting the war effort and used to lure people to death camps without excessive force. (Nyiszli 2001, p. 147) By portraying the movement of people as a supply of labour, the Nazi regime could play into displaced people's hopes that the information they had on death camps wasn't true.

Another temporary reprieve was selection for medical experiments on twins, people affected by stunted growth and *noma sacieci* (a form of gangrene on the face and mouth) (Nyiszli 2001, p. 21). The goal of this research was to increase the birthrate of "super humans" who were destined to become the "master race" by every mother giving birth to twins. These experiments were scientifically very superficial. Mengele therefore moved on to post-mortem examinations, yet in order to compare the twins, he killed them to ensure simultaneous death (43). Eva Mozes Kor describes the experiences she and her twin sister had of the medical experiments by Mengele where he aimed to "learn how to create blond-haired, blue-eyed babies in multiple numbers to increase the German population" (Kor and Rojany Buccieri 2009, p 40). Mengele injected twins with life-threatening diseases and tested cures on them. He also attempted to change eye color and to change boys into girls and vice versa (45–46). Eva describes how she gets injected with a serious disease and against all odds survives. Others were not so lucky and their healthy twin was murdered with a shot of chloroform into the heart for comparative autopsies to take place (Kor and Rojany Buccieri 2009, p. 68). The ongoing fascination with twins is in itself an oppressive attitude, as it overlooks the separateness of persons when consistently confusing one person with another and it hurts dignity to be seen as a novelty instead of two persons who happen to be born at roughly the same time or who look more alike than ordinary siblings. Logically we can expect there to be legacies of eugenics around medical and genetic research into multiple births, too. For example, the separateness of persons is definitely violated by uncaring attitudes towards embryos who are seen as superfluous, back up or replacements for lost ones in in vitro fertilization. Yet, this is not to say that embryos or fetuses have inalienable rights either.[1]

Later accounts show post-war and ongoing instances of eugenics ideology. Immigration is an important area where eugenics thinking is still employed. This is a direct legacy of German eugenics advocates giving scientific backing to racial testimonials in 1935, which were meant to prove one's "Aryan" ancestry (Adams et al. 2005, p. 245) and the 1924 adoption in the US of the Johnson-Reed Immigration Restriction Act restricting immigration from Poland, Hungary, the Balkans and Russia, which Laughlin had testified to be "genetically inferior stock" (238). These quotas later restricted the influx of Jewish refugees who fled anti-Jewish oppression after 1933. Currently, immigration restrictions are being tightened and access to basic human rights for migrants is being reduced. Undocumented migrants in Sweden are entitled to access to public health services only in cases of medical emergency and only if they pay the full price (Khosravi 2010a, p. 105). Reproductive rights are among those most affected.

[1]Jürgen Habermas makes an important point about the distinction between an embryo or fetus not being "something for us to dispose over" while also not having "inalienable human rights" (Habermas 2003, p. 31).

> Exclusion from the healthcare system especially affects undocumented female migrants, who comprise 60 per cent of those using the informal healthcare system; the main health problems they suffered were gynaecological. […] Denying undocumented migrants' health care is an attempt to govern the reproduction of an undesirable population (Khosravi 2010b, p. 119)

However, even beyond lack of access to care, in Sweden undocumented women are actively discouraged from becoming pregnant. "Many of my female informants told me how they were 'advised' by different actors, from Migration Board officers to lawyers and even NGO activists, to not have a child. Even asylum seekers were encouraged not to have children during the asylum process" (Khosravi 2010b, p. 119).

These practices of discouraging pregnancy for female migrants tie in with the eugenics view of "selective breeding" and form the complementary part of anti-immigration policies towards "inferior races." This continues the long tradition of state-sponsored eugenic practice in Sweden. Alleged "social democratic" eugenics in Sweden were supposedly made free of racial bias—at least in theory—but in practice this was I think much less the case. Moreover, forced sterilization of women with learning difficulties and family planning programs targeting lower social classes were implemented in Sweden (Broberg and Roll-Hanssen 2005) Other practices that still show the effect of eugenics thinking are the continued use of tests on unborn babies to determine their genetic "health" (Hampton 2005; Parens and Asch 2000) and the practice of selective implantation, abortion and even infanticide on babies with genetic "defects" (Khalili-Borna 2007; Dixon 2008). Moreover, the underlying principle of a strong gene pool and healthy individuals also affects many people through pressure to conform, be strong and alter individual "anomalies" both through physical and mental intervention.

Another example is the forced sterilization of disabled people in the US (Pfeiffer 1994). People with learning difficulties were sterilized up to 1965 in North Carolina (Castles 2002) and the forced sterilization law in California was repealed in 1979 but was applied to women of Mexican, Puerto Rican and Native American descent up to that time in a drive against poverty (Stern 2005). The European Roma Rights Centre (ERRC) recently reminded the UN that the Czech Republic continues to deny compensation to Romani women who are victims of coercive sterilization, and has failed to take adequate steps to prevent coercive sterilizations from occurring in the future. The ERRC submitted a report on coercive sterilization to the Committee on the Elimination of Discrimination Against Women at the Committee's 47th session in Geneva. Although the policy is no longer in place, Romani women continued to be sterilized without their consent in the Czech Republic and Slovakia, with cases as recent as 2007.[2]

[2]See the website of the European Roma Rights Centre http://www.errc.org [last accessed 8 August 2013].

Eugenics thinking is dangerous not only because under extreme circumstances it led to genocide but because still now it has popularity as an underlying principle of medicine and immigration policy. Eugenics thinking denies moral boundaries around what is done to prevent the conception or birth of "disabled" people and allows for termination of the existence of "disabled" people. It treats people as means based on an economic perspective on what it means to be contributing to society, instead of as ends in themselves (Buchanan et al. 2000). Worryingly, this type of thinking is still present in contemporary approaches to "disability" as well as immigration rules and the reproduction of people targeted by racism. However, some philosophers argue that there are benign conceptions of eugenics. Sparrow summarizes the position held by the "new eugenicists" as follows:

> [...] there is little reason to fear the scientific application of genetic technologies to human beings, as long as the choice of whether and how to use them is left up to individuals. They argue that a "new" or "liberal" eugenics, which would be pluralistic, based on good science, concerned with the welfare of individuals, and would respect the rights of individuals, should be distinguished from the "old" eugenics, which was perfectionist, unscientific, concerned with the health of the "race" and coercive. According to the advocates of the new eugenics, the horrors associated with the old eugenics should not prevent us from embracing the opportunities offered by recent advances in the biological sciences.' (Sparrow 2011, p. 32)

From the past, however, we already know that individual choice can become constrained. Moreover, desires and expectations are socially constructed, so the "free" choice of "enhancement" operations must be publicly debated and a policy developed that protects human rights.

The bioethicist Alex McKeown explains how the idea of "well born" can be interpreted within the frame of the "new eugenics":

> The word "eugenics" may have an appalling legacy, but this is a contingent historical fact rather than something which necessarily follows from the desire of our children to be "well born." Being "well born" can have a multiplicity of meanings, not all of which correspond to something as discriminatory as a picture of a "master race."(McKeown, personal communication)

However, it is not the interpretation of eugenics as "well born" that causes the problems sketched here; it is the combination of "eu" (good) with "genics" (genes) that raises the issue of what boundaries to enforce concerning medical interventions, including in the area of reproduction, to "improve" people individually or as a "nation" or "race." The whole principle that population control is a legitimate concern for governance is controversial yet remains rather under-discussed except in the area of some social approaches to global public health (Mann 1997). Yet, as McKeown rightly points out, it is also due to the perfectionist thinking of eugenics approaches that these boundaries become problematic. Let's now look at the presence of these different underlying principles and models in the Disability Rights Convention.

4 Models of Disability Underpinning the Disability Rights Convention: Eugenics or Inclusion?

Disability in one form or another is experienced by ten percent of the world's population, according to the UN (Kanter 2003). However, despite human rights being equally applicable to all according to the Universal Declaration and all subsequent UN Conventions, disabled people still face discrimination. A human rights focus is important as they may be instrumental in empowering the individual and creating societal change (Brennan 2005, pp. 93–94). An important victory for the disability rights movement is the establishment of the UN Convention on the Rights of Persons with a Disability (hereafter: the Convention). The Convention was opened for signature on 30 March 2007, and entered into force on 3 May 2008. Here I assess the Convention for its underlying model of disability rights and show that it relies on both the medical model and the social model of disability. Moreover, I show it has inherent legacies of eugenics despite also calling for inclusive education and participation in society.

At first sight, the Convention seems to rely on a progressive understanding of disability as it contradicts the previous exclusion of disabled people in isolated living and work places. Initially disabled people's rights in national jurisdictions were focused on protection. These paternalistic efforts assumed lack of decision-making capacity of disabled persons. (Quinn 1999, p. 5) These types of policy regimes were based on a medical model of disability which was criticised for keeping disabled people outside of mainstream society (Brennan 2005, p. 94). In contrast, the social model of disability aims for removing societal barriers and maintains that it is the physical and cultural environment that creates "disability."

While the "social" model is now widely accepted, some scholars object to the separation between impairment and disability which they propose should be overcome by embodying disability within a social framework (Beckett 2006, p. 735). A similar call for a relational model is made by Shakespeare. He further points out that the social model of disability has only invited legal reform and identity politics aimed at the removal of societal barriers in law and attitudes (Shakespeare 2006). Others have argued that a transformative approach, viewing the exclusion of non-standard workers from the labour market as a structural societal barrier to the participation of "disabled" people, fits in with the social model, too (Gleeson 1997). Further criticism of the social model of disability argues that: "To be born with a genetic mutation which restricts autonomy because it causes serious mental or physical retardation, chronic pain, or dramatically limits lifespan cannot be said to be disadvantageous purely because of the way in which society is ordered" (McKeown 2012; personal communication).

In response to that line of criticism, I point to the impossibility and moral inappropriateness of trying to determine objectively which lives are worth living. There are enough examples of so-called able-bodied people with superfluous resources who are deeply unhappy and enough examples of so-called disabled people who are fully interested in life. Besides, the medical model of disability is often wrong about the expected "progress" or "life expectancy" of conditions. Whereas it is likely (and illustrated by anecdotal evidence) that most people living with long-term conditions experience frustration from time to time about barriers to activity in their life, this is a universal experience between "disabled" and "able-bodied" and not a reason for medical intervention. Moreover, if society provided more outlets for frustration, there might be less frantic searching for invasive surgery. After all, aspirations are also socially constructed.

The social model of disability simply argues that a large source of frustration and inequality of people managing long-term conditions is society itself; it does not deny that it may be a valid choice to use medication or other medical interventions to improve symptoms or try to slow down an illness. Moreover, barriers are a complex mix between the physical conditions of the person(s) experiencing them and characteristics of the environment. The environment in this case means both the physical world and the world of expectations and beliefs. For example, when people ask me "Do you still work?" They expect that living with a long-term illness prevents me from working. They do not realize that the barriers are not only the physical environment and the expectations resting on those who work full-time. Their own expectations behind such questions (that having a "degenerative disease" causes life changes) are part of the oppressive thinking around "disability" in most contemporary societies. I interpret these questions more as fear of not being able to work themselves rather than relevant to me. This fits in with another fear that becomes clearly visible to me when people emotionally react to my long-term condition: their fear of being ill themselves. Because the link between not working and long-term conditions is so immediate in people's eyes, their anxiety about independence is projected into the question they ask.

Having established the important distinction between the medical and the social model of disability, I now return to the assessment of the UN Convention on the Rights of Disabled Persons (the Convention). The Convention reflects the social model of disability when it states in its Preamble: "(e) Recognizing that disability is an evolving concept and that disability results from the interaction between persons with impairments and attitudinal and environmental barriers that hinders their full and effective participation in society on an equal basis with others." Article 1 declares the Convention's objective is "to promote, protect and ensure the full and equal enjoyment of all human rights and fundamental freedoms by all persons with disabilities, and to promote respect for their inherent dignity." It conceives of disability as being inclusive of, but not limited to "long-term physical, mental, intellectual or sensory impairments." Moreover, it firmly grounds the Convention in the social model of disability by stating that it arises from "interaction with various barriers may hinder their full and effective participation in society on an equal basis with others" rather than as an inherent limitation. Because these conceptual norms are set forth in the purpose article of the Convention, it follows that UN Member States cannot enter permissible reservations to the normative contents of this article (Stein and Lord 2007, pp. 24–5).

Despite its grounding in the social model of disability, there are remnants of the medical model of disability in the Convention, too. This can be seen in two major ways: by the reliance of the Convention on the conception of human rights grounded in liberal political discourse which has been shown to exclude at least some disabled people from participation based on their reliance on a concept of human nature that is rational and autonomous (Nussbaum 2006). The Preamble even states that autonomy and independence are important for people with disabilities, yet it does not specify a right to care or guardianship in cases of dependence, except for legal representation (Art. 12). In the general principles (Art. 4), choice, independence and participation are mentioned but not care or support. Despite the allowance for "specific measures" in the article on non-discrimination (Art. 5), equality of opportunity is not defined, so it is likely to be interpreted in its liberal conception, whereas others would include equalising measures beyond competition for jobs. Moreover, although the Convention specifically legislates against segregated living (Art. 19) and schooling (Art. 24), and confirms the right to family life (Art. 23), it omits to specify who counts as a person due human rights protection and therefore it doesn't outlaw selective abortion, prenatal genetic testing or prioritising able-bodied fertilised eggs for implantation. Despite the only almost explicit reference to eugenics in the right not to be part of medical or scientific experiments without consent (Art. 15), the article on the "Right to Life" (Art. 10) does not protect the right to life of unborn disabled children. Of course, the right to life for unborn children is controversial, yet my point is that whatever your position on it, the Convention is silent on the issue. This is peculiar as the prevention of the conception of disabled children, the allowance of termination of the pregnancy and the infant death due to neglect of disabled children are all large threats to their right to life which should have been addressed in the first international Convention on the rights of disabled persons.

Finally, Article 4, on General Obligations, states that the implementation of the Convention is programmatic with regard to social and cultural rights, i.e. that States can take measures to the "maximum of available resources," which leaves a gap in resources for implementation of the right to social protection, specific measures to ensure equality of opportunity and the call for universal design.

Moreover, there are precedents that when poorer states can't afford the funds for implementation of international agreements, the richer states provide assistance—this ought also to be a reason for the richer states to do so in the case of building up capacity and facilities in the area of disabled persons' rights. These kinds of international obligations are part of a cosmopolitan model of human rights that could contribute to principles of global public health which go beyond the methodologically nationalist model that is presently dominant (van den Anker 2005).

At present the individualism behind the medical model still informs the social model of "disability." The social model equally has a predominantly individualist methodology, looking at barriers for individuals to participate in society instead of at the societal principles that act as barriers to human functioning more generally. For example, the social model is often used to argue for individual labor participation instead of for fundamental changes to the organization of work. To give one national example, UK equality legislation requires individual "reasonable adjustments" to be made by employers to facilitate labor participation of people managing long-term conditions, yet there is hardly any investment in the equivalent of collective "reasonable adjustments" towards health and well-being, such as providing enough rest at work or inviting staff to harvest from the employer-produced harvest (on work-based allotments, for example) are easy ways of implementing this vision.

Therefore, the Convention is an example of the more general dilemmas of universal human rights law where member states do not easily take the lead on the kind of initiative that would address the impact of the capitalist work ethic pervading most contemporary societies. This ethics sets an increasingly fast pace of life that hampers full social participation for most human beings, including those of us puzzling out our needs due to long-term conditions.

Therefore, there are reasons for concern about the principles underlying the Convention. The Convention codifies current dominant attitudes towards disability rights as mainly concerned with enabling to participate equally in society. This perspective raises the question of what space there is for equal participation without assimilation to the "normal" standard in capitalist societies. These concerns tie in with the legacies of eugenics viewing disabled people as "unfit." In the final part of this chapter I now turn to a proposal for a different basis for the rights of people challenged by long-term conditions. I argue that a principle of inclusion has implications for the medical and social model of disability rights. It would also resolve the methodological individualism present in current approaches whereas it would create more space for thinking well about all people as a complete and complex person rather than viewing us mainly as our condition with our "disability" as a problem to solve.

5 Implications of Inclusion for Disability Rights

Zola called for the universalizing of disability policy as the entire population is "at risk" of chronic illness and disability (Zola 1989: 401). His argument is not based on equality for disabled people but on the recognition of an ageing population in richer societies. This is a good starting point to assess what inclusion means for people on a continuum of impairment (Nussbaum 2006). The social model of disability is too often used as shorthand which allows policies such as the UN Convention to focus solely on social inclusion from a reductionist capitalist perspective, i.e. as labor participation. Policy makers can then interpret the equal right to access to employment with the duty to contribute to society in economic terms. That attitude easily leads to the exclusion of non-working people targeted by disability oppression. Yet, inclusion means adapting not only the physical access to society but also its perceptions, modes of relating as well as it structural systemic transformation. Social inclusion is deeply affected not only by the right to life, to reproduce, to participate in culture and doing meaningful work; it also requires the reflection back that your state of being is valuable and your insights are worth communicating. (Frank 2000) This means that alternative modes of communicating, designing spaces and collaborating are required.

Inclusion is interpreted in different ways in the literature. For example, inclusion can have an emphasis on participation in cooperative frameworks where the most dominant framework is the market system (Buchanan et al. 2000, p. 258). Beckett (2009) argues for building an inclusive society by educating non-disabled children to develop positive attitudes towards disabled people. The goal of the disability movement has been to broaden the understanding of "inclusive education" to more than simply "integrating" disabled children into mainstream schools and instead ensuring that schools and classrooms become truly inclusive environments (Beckett 2009, p. 318). The Centre for Studies on Inclusive Education for example conceptualizes it as "founded upon a moral position which values and respects every individual and which welcomes diversity as a rich learning resource."[3] Mason (2000) holds that "[...] 'inclusion' is not a definable state, but a set of principles, which can be applied to anything. It is not essentially about "disability," but about building a sustainable future for all of us." Micheline Mason's view on impairment and building an inclusive society has taught me the most about the underlying values needed to make progress on this goal. Moreover, I was allowed to practice in workshops led by her. Those experiences come closest to my intuition about inclusion and have helped me to build my argument for human societies and rethinking not only the medical model of disability but also the social model.

In order to create inclusive societies, the exclusionary legacies of eugenics affecting people targeted by disability oppression need to be understood. Rieser and Mason (1990) model how values and policies are interrelated. Children acquire prejudices against disabled people from adults, the media, and the way society is organized. As adults they reinforce and legitimize the misinformation in policies and practices over which they have some control (Rieser and Mason 1990, p. 7). In Beckett's words there is an ongoing cycle of socialization, leading to the reinforcement of the disabling society in turn leading to further socialization (Beckett 2009, p. 320). These insights help to start to unlearn the oppression of people with long-term conditions, even if held by us challenged by impairments ourselves. Like any oppressed group, the internalized oppression makes us self-critical, critical of others under similar circumstances and occasionally grumpy with allies (Bishop 2002).

The inclusion movement started campaigning against segregated education which is an understudied legacy of eugenics (Baker 2002, p. 671). Through their engagement with schools, inclusion activists developed the view that the pace of capitalism is inhumane and excludes increasing numbers of people. We should see our needs (to rest, to go slow, to be seen as unique) not as individual "anomaly" or a "special need" but as an enrichment of everyone's experiences. It makes sense for a group to collectively ensure everyone's needs are met. In line with the principle of universal design, where accessibility is not a special entrance or toilet but all design is accessible, all needs would be seen as part of a set to collectively satisfy. Making disability rights accessible and developing a society based on inclusion, requires that the emotions holding eugenics-based attitudes in place need to be examined in

[3]See, www.csie.org.uk/inclusion [last accessed 8 August 2013].

self-reflection and expressed in order to heal from war, genocide, slavery and forced labor. My own experience making a start with this emotional work shows that it can result in a bigger perspective for life with an impairment as well as for social change beyond disability oppression. For example, I have a more active life since my diagnosis than before and I'm putting in place time for relaxation, exercise, connecting to people and contributing to social change that illustrate life is not over when diagnosed with a "degenerative disease" like Parkinson's. It took me three years to integrate the perspective that the future is unknown and there are many things I can do to have my focus on being more alive than ever before.

6 Conclusion

This chapter traced the ongoing effects of eugenics on the 2006 UN Convention on the Rights of Persons with Disabilities. I used the overlapping methods of auto-ethnography of impairment and sociological phenomenology of tracing lived experience combined with discourse analysis of the convention to show how eugenics is still present in current thinking that informs the Convention. Despite its emphasis on participation of "disabled" people in society, implicit acceptance of a capitalist work ethic in the Convention coincides with the eugenics vision that those who do not work, shall not eat, which conflicts with a principle of inclusion. The article ended with a sketch of implications for disability rights of adopting a stronger principle of inclusion compared to recent sociological conceptions and indicated the transformations required for its realization. If we don't address how we are influenced by eugenics then we unknowingly cross ethical boundaries. We are only able to imagine, campaign for and create real inclusion through healing from past hurts. An inclusive society will most likely include care and assistance as well as equal worth and dignity; respect for and accessibility of rights depends on the transformation of economic and social structures based on a culture of inclusion.

References

Adams, M. B., Garland, E., & Weiss, S. F. (2005). Human heredity and politics: A comparative institutional study of the Eugenics Record Office at Cold Spring Harbor (United States), the Kaiser Wilhelm Institute for Anthropology, Human Heredity and Eugenics (Germany), and the Maxim Gorky Medical Genetics Institute (USSR). *Osiris, 20*, 232–262.

Anker, C. van den (2005). Human rights and cosmopolitanism In R. Smith & C. van den Anker (Eds.) *Essentials of human rights* (pp. 67–69). London: Hodder Arnold.

Baker, B. (2002). The hunt for disability: The new eugenics and the normalization of school children. *Teachers College Record, 104*(4), 663–703.

Barrett, E., & Kurzman, C. (2004). Globalizing social movement theory: The case of eugenics. *Theory and Society, 33*(5), 487–527.

Beckett, A. E. (2005). Reconsidering citizenship in the light of the concerns of the UK disability movement. *Citizenship Studies, 9*(4), 405–421.

Beckett, A. E. (2006). Understanding social movements: Theorising the disability movement in conditions of late modernity. *The Sociological Review, 54*(4), 734–752.

Beckett, A. E. (2009). Challenging disabling attitudes, building an inclusive society: Considering the role of education in encouraging non-disabled children to develop positive attitudes towards disabled people. *British Journal of Sociology of Education, 30*(3), 317–329.

Bhambra, G. K., & Shilliam, R. (Eds.). (2008). *Silencing human rights. Critical engagements with a contested project*. New York and Basingstoke: Palgrave Macmillan.

Bickenbacha, J. E., Chatterji, S., Badley, E. M., & Ústun, T. B. (1999). Models of disablement, universalism and the international classification of impairments, disabilities and handicaps. *Social Science and Medicine, 48*, 1173–1187.

Bishop, A. (2002 [1997]) *Becoming an ally. Breaking the cycle of oppression*. Halifax, Nova Scotia, Canada: Fernwood Publishing.

Brennan, F. (2005). Disability and Human Rights. In R. Smith & C. van den Anker (Eds.), *The essentials of human rights* (pp. 93–97). London: Hodder Arnold.

Broberg, G., & Roll-Hanssen, N. (Eds.). (2005). *Eugenics and the welfare state. Sterilization policy in Denmark, Sweden, Norway and Finland*. East Lansing, Michigan: Michigan State University Press.

Buchanan, A., Brock, D. W., Daniels, N., & Wikler, D. (2000). *From chance to choice. Genetics and justice*. Cambridge, New York, Melbourne and Madrid: Cambridge University Press.

Carel, H. (2007). Havi Carel: My 10-year death sentence. In *The Independent*, 19 march. Accessed July 20, 2011 from http://www.independent.co.uk/news/people/profiles/havi-carel-my-10year-death-sentence-440805.html.

Castles, K. (2002). Quiet eugenics; sterilization in North Carolina's institutions for the mentally retarded, 1945–1965. *The Journal of Southern History, 68*(4), 849–878.

David, H. P., Fleischhacker, J., & Hohn, C. (1988). Abortion and Eugenics in Nazi Germany. *Population and Development Review, 14*(1), 81–112.

Dixon, D. P. (2008). Informed consent or institutionalised eugenics? How the medical profession encourages abortion of foetuses with down syndrome. *Issues in Law and Medicine, 24*(1), 3–59.

Frank, A. W. (2000). Illness and autobiographical work: Dialogue as narrative destabilization. *Qualitative Sociology, 23*(1), 135–156.

Gabel, S., & Peters, S. (2004). Presage of a paradigm shift? Beyond the social model of disability towards resistance theories of disability. *Disability and Society, 19*(6), 585–600.

Gleeson, B. J. (1997). Disability studies: A historical materialist view. *Disability and Society, 12*(2), 179–202.

Habermas, J. (2003). *The future of human nature*. Cambridge: Polity Press.

Hampton, S. J. (2005). Family eugenics. *Disability and Society, 20*(5), 553–561.

Harrison, B. (1993). A note on ethical issues in the use of autobiography in sociological research. *Sociology, 27*(1), 101–109.

Hohendorf, G., Rotzoll, M., Richter, P., Eckart, W., & Mundt, C. (2002). Victims of Nazi euthanasia, the so-called T4 action. First results of a project at the German Federal Archives to disclose records of killed patients. *Nervenarzt, 73*(11), 1065–1074.

Holt, N. L. (2003). Representation, legitimation, and autoethnography: An autoethnographic writing story. *International Journal of Qualitative Methods, 2*(1), 18–28.

Joseph, M. (1990). *Sociology for everyone*. Cambridge: Polity.

Kanter, A. S. (2003). The globalisation of disability rights law. *Syracuse Journal of International Law and Commerce [online]., 30*(2), 241.

Khalili-Borna, C.A. (2007). Technological advancement and international human rights: Is science improving human life or perpetuating human right violations? *Michigan Journal of International Law, 29*, 95.

Khosravi, S. (2010a). An ethnography of migrant 'illegality' in Sweden: Included yet excepted? *Journal of International Political Theory, 6*(1), 95–116.

Khosravi, S. (2010b). *The 'illegal' traveler: An auto-ethnography of borders*. Basingstoke: Palgrave.

Kliewer, C., & Drake, S. (1998). Disability, eugenics and the current ideology of segregation; a modern tale. *Disability and Society, 13*(1), 95–111.

Kor, E. M., & Rojany Buccieri, L. (2009). *Surviving the Angel of Death. The story of a Mengele Twin in Auschwitz Terre Haute*. IL: Tanglewood.

Liachowitz, C. H. (1988). *Disability as a social construct: Legislative roots*. Philadelphia: University of Pennsylvania Press.

Mabett, D. (2005). The development of rights-based social policy in the European Union: The example of disability rights. *Journal of Common Market Studies, 43*(1), 97–120.

Mann, J. M. (1997). Medicine and public health, ethics and human rights. *Hastings Center Report, 27*, 6–13.

Mason, M. (2000). *Incurably human*. London: Inclusive Solutions.

McKeown, A. (2012). Response given in the Watershed, 12 Dec 2012.

Miller, S. M., Wilson Nelson, M., & Moore, M. T. (1998). Caught in the paradigm gap: Qualitative researchers' lived experience and the politics of epistemology. *American Educational Research Journal, 35*(3), 377–416.

Nahman, M. (2013). *Extractions. An ethnography of reproductive tourism*. Basingstoke and New York: Pagrave MacMillan.

Nussbaum, M. (2006). *Frontiers of justice. Disability, nationality, species membership*. Boston: MA Harvard University Press.

Nyiszli, M. (2001). *I was Dr Mengele's assistant*. Oswiecim: Auschwitz Museum.

Parens, E., & Asch, A. (2000). *Prenatal testing and disability rights*. Washington, DC: Georgetown University Press.

Paul, D. (1984). Eugenics and the left. *Journal of the History of Ideas, 45*(4), 567–590.

Pfeiffer, D. (1994). Eugenics and disability discrimination. *Disability and Society, 9*(4), 481–499.

Quinn, G. (1999). The human rights of people with disabilities under EU Law. In P. Alston (Ed.), *The EU and human rights*. Oxford: Oxford University Press.

Rembis, M. A. (2009). (Re)Defining disability in the 'genetic age': Behavioural genetics, 'new' eugenics, and the future of impairment. *Disability and Society, 24*(5), 585–597.

Rieser, R., & Mason, M. (1990). *Disability equality in the classroom: A human rights issue*. London: ILEA.

Shakespeare, T. (2006). *Disability rights and wrongs*. London: Routledge.

Sparkes, A. C. (2002). Autoethnography: Self-indulgence or something more? In A. Bochner & C. Ellis (Eds.), *Ethnographically speaking: Autoethnography, literature, and aesthetics*. New York: AltaMira.

Sparrow, R. (2011). A not-so-new eugenics: Harris and Savulescu on human enhancement. *Hastings Center Report, 41*(1), 32–42.

Spektorowski, A., & Mizrachi, E. (2004). Eugenics and the Welfare State in Sweden: The politics of social margins and the idea of a productive society. *Journal of Contemporary History, 39*(3), 333–352.

Stanley, L. (1993). On auto/biography in sociology. *Sociology, 27*(1), 41–52.

Stark, H., & Brown Trinidad, S. (2007). Choose your method: A comparison of phenomenology, discourse analysis, and grounded theory. *Qualitative Health Research, 17*, 1372–1380.

Stein, M. A., & Lord, J. E. (2007). Jacobus tenBroek, participatory justice and the UN convention on the rights of persons with disabilities. *Texas Journal on Civil Liberties and Civil Rights, 13*(2), 167–185.

Stern, A. M. (2005). Sterilised in the name of public health. Race, |immigration, and reproductive control in modern California. *American Journal of Public Health, 95*(7), 1128–1138.

Swiebocki, H. (2002). *London has been informed. Reports by Auschwitz Escapees*. Oswiecim: Auschwitz Museum.

Tierney, W. G. (1998). Life history's history: Subjects foretold. *Qualitative Inquiry, 4*, 49–70.

Tyner, J. A. (1999). The geopolitics of eugenics and the exclusion of Philippine immigrants from the United States. *Geographical Review, 89*(1), 54–73.

Worsley, P. (Ed.). (1970). *Introducing sociology*. Harmondsworth: Penguin books.

Zola, I. K. (1989). Toward the necessary universalizing of a disability policy. *The Millbank Quarterly, 67*(22), 401–428.

Chapter 16
Being Machine: Two Competing Models for Neuroprosthesis

Corry Shores

1 Introduction

Some posthumanists see the potential in forthcoming enhancement technologies to alter human beings so much that we would no longer recognize them as members of our species (Birnbacher 2008, pp. 97–98). One sort of enhancement technology are prosthetic devices that would replace or increase normal human functioning, for example computer chips implanted in the brain or robotic arms controlled with our minds. On account of neuroplasticity, our brains would gradually reconfigure themselves so that we may use the prosthesis as though it were biologically a part of us. And, if our bodily organs can be replaced by mechanical counterparts, then piece-by-piece, as our body ages and its malfunctioning parts are replaced, one might gradually become less a human and more a machine, and one with extraordinary non-human abilities. There are even developments in brain simulation that could allow a computer to handle the functioning of large parts of one's brain, opening the possibility that one's whole brain might be "uploaded" to continue performing its functions on a computer connected to a robotic body. If the process of body-part replacement were slow and gradual enough that our minds and bodies always have ample opportunity to adjust to the new prosthetic devices, is it not conceivable that we could make a complete and continuous transition from human to machine using these technologies?

The author would like to thank Roland Breeur of the Husserl Archives, University of Leuven for his comments on earlier versions of this paper.

C. Shores (✉)
Ankara University, Ankara, Turkey
e-mail: corryshores@gmail.com

D. Meacham (ed.), *Medicine and Society, New Perspectives in Continental Philosophy*, Philosophy and Medicine 120, DOI 10.1007/978-94-017-9870-9_16

Andy Clark's and David Chalmers's "extended mind hypothesis" provides a theoretical account for our bodily and cognitive extension into external technologies, and Clark as well as therapeutic prosthetic researchers draw from Merleau-Ponty's philosophy of the body to explain how such devices become a part of our body schemas. But is Merleau-Ponty's "organic" view of the body really the best theoretical framework to explain how our bodies are becoming more and more robotic? I will argue instead that Deleuze's and Guattari's "machinic" model is a more promising theoretical basis for the notion of posthuman enhancement and also for successful therapeutic prosthesis usage.

2 Extending Minds and Bodies

Andy Clark and David Chalmers advance their theory of cognitive extension in their paper "The Extended Mind." Here they argue that cognition is a process that is not necessarily limited to the confines of the skull. Cognition, they explain, results from the workings of a cognitive system, like the system of interacting parts of the brain. Yet, our cognitive systems are not necessarily limited just to the brain, because for example we make use of gestures or postures when cognizing, or we use our fingers when calculating quantities (Clark and Chalmers 2002, p. 645). As well, we often use external implements like pencil and paper, calculators, and computers in conjunction with our brain's workings.

To clarify, Clark and Chalmers have us consider three different cases of cognition: 1. *brain alone*: a person sits behind a computer screen displaying geometrical shapes, and she must mentally rotate them to see which sockets they fit into; 2. *brain and external device*: someone in the same situation may instead press a button to display the shapes' rotations; and 3. *brain and internal device*: a future person can instead use a neural implant to rotate the image as fast as the computer in the previous case (643–644). The authors think that both the uses of the imagination and the neural implant are clearly instances of cognition. But in the second case, the button rotation performs the same computational action that the neural implant performs, only in this case the mechanism is external to the agent. In fact, the way that the brain and button interact in order to rotate the image is much like how the relevant parts of the brain interact when we instead use our imaginations. Now, if the brain's cooperating parts are considered a cognitive system, is there any reason to think that brains cannot interact with external devices in order to create broadened cognitive systems? Clark and Chalmers reply with their parity principle: "If, as we confront some task, a part of the world functions as a process which, were it to go on in the head, we would have no hesitation in accepting as part of the cognitive process, then that part of the world is (for that time) part of the cognitive process" (644, following the rendering in Clark 2008, p. 77).

Their MOMA thought experiment will illustrate the criteria for cognitive extension. Inga learns there is an art exhibit at the Museum of Modern Art, and she remembers MOMA is on 53rd Street. Otto has Alzheimer's, but he always carries his trusty notebook to record such useful information. He consults his notes and sees the correct address. Both people have the belief that MOMA is on 53rd Street; the only difference is that the cognitive system storing and recalling Otto's beliefs involves an external implement. Otto's case, then, fulfills Clark's and Chalmers's three criteria for extended cognitive systems:

> [T]he human organism is linked with an external entity in a two-way interaction, creating a *coupled system* that can be seen as a cognitive system in its own right. [1] All the components in the system play an active causal role, and [2] they jointly govern behavior in the same sort of way that cognition usually does. [3] If we remove the external component the system's behavioral competence will drop, just as it would if we removed part of its brain. Our thesis is that this sort of coupled process counts equally well as a cognitive process, whether or not it is wholly in the head. (Clark and Chalmers 2002, p. 644; enumerated distinctions, Menary 2010, p. 3)

Clark's response to one of Adams' and Aizawa's critical objections will help us clarify the nature of the parts' couplings. These critics open with the joke, "Question: Why did the pencil think that 2 + 2 = 4? Clark's answer: Because it was coupled to the mathematician" (Adams and Aizawa 2010, p. 67). Clark reminds them that not all the parts of the system need to be conscious; rather, they at least need to be *causally coupled* so to jointly contribute to the cognitive activity of the larger system they compose.

This coupling at work in extended cognitive systems is continuously and mutually modulatory. "Continuous reciprocal causation occurs when some system S is both continuously affecting and simultaneously being affected by activity in some other system O" (Clark 2008, p. 24). To illustrate the causal dynamics, Clark has us imagine a radio whose sound-output modulates the very same signal telling it what to play, which would bring about "a truly complex and temporally dense interplay between the two system components" (Clark 1997, p. 163). To envision this example another way we might consider how speakers placed near a turntable produce vibrations that affect those very same sounds it is playing. When causal influences are mutual, simultaneous, and continuous, it is impossible to disentangle one causal pole from the other so to place them into a linear chain of causal events. Rather, the interactive parts form a new systemic whole whose workings are best understood not in terms of linear mechanistic interactions but rather as a complex dynamical system. For example, the way fish swim illustrates how their causal couplings with water dynamics produces a larger "machine."

> The extraordinary efficiency of the fish as a swimming device is partly due [...] to an evolved capacity to couple its swimming behaviors to the pools of external kinetic energy found as swirls, eddies and vortices in its watery environment [...]. These vortices include both naturally occurring ones (e.g., where water hits a rock) and self-induced ones (created by well-timed tail flaps). The fish swims by building these externally occurring processes into the very heart of its locomotion routines. The fish and surrounding vortices together constitute a unified and remarkably efficient *swimming machine*. (Clark and Chalmers 2002, p. 646, emphasis mine)

For human beings, these causal couplings link brain, body, and world into new systemic wholes. Clark illustrates the reciprocal causality involved in human couplings with the examples of dancers and musicians.[1]

> Think of a dancer, whose bodily orientation is continuously affecting and being affected by her neural states, and whose movements are also influencing those of her partner, to whom she is continuously responding! Or imagine playing improvised jazz in a small combo. Each musician's playing is influencing and being influenced by everyone else. (Clark 2008, p. 24)

If we merely examined the musicians each independently of the others in the jazz band, we would be unable to explain how their reciprocal affections produced the music as a whole.

Yet even though the component parts of such systems are disentangleable, they nonetheless remain unique. For Clark, the interfaces mediating the interactions between parts on the one hand mark the limits of each component while on the other hand mesh them together to constitute a larger system. He explains this by building from the terminology John Haugeland employs when analyzing sensory interfaces. Like Clark, Haugeland thinks that the embodied human mind is thoroughly embedded in the world.

Haugeland first has us consider what makes a television much more systematic than a block of marble. The difference lies "in the nature of the *discontinuities* within the whole, and the character of the interactions across them" (Haugeland 1998, p. 212, emphasis mine). There are three essential characteristics of system components, and he illustrates with the example of transistors in a television set. 1. *A system component has restricted channels of affection*: the transistor has an input and an output contact-wire on each end, and the only way the other parts can affect it, and it them, is by means of these contacts. 2. *Its interactions with other parts are well-defined, reliable, and relatively simple*: only electrons flow through the transistor and not chemicals, for example. And 3. *On its own scale it is a self-contained system with its own parts, but on a higher scale its functioning is interdependent with all the other components of a system*: a resistor plus a capacitor do not make a system, but "a suitable larger arrangement of resistors, capacitors, and transistors might add up to a pre-amp—which could in turn be a component in a higher-level system" (212–213).

For the task of "dividing systems into distinct subsystems along nonarbitrary lines," Haugeland distinguishes the following mutually defined terms (211). A *system* is a relatively independent and self contained composite whose parts, its *components*, affect one another through *interfaces*, which are the points of "interactive 'contact' between components such that the relevant interactions are well-defined, reliable and relatively simple" (213). The preamp in his example then is by

[1]Deleuze also uses the examples of the music group and dancers in a similar way to illustrate Spinozistic differential composition. Different bodies can form composite bodies whose power is in part a matter of how much the components can differentially relate while sustaining their mutually affective contact. We do not address these ideas here, but they further support our description of and argumentation for machinic composition. See for example Shores (2012).

itself a system made of its component electronic parts, but insofar as it is a part of a whole stereo system, it is seen as a component that is incomplete on its own.

So when we are examining how the preamp interacts with the other stereo components, we are no longer concerned with the interfaces between resisters and so forth but rather between amp and preamp. When analyzing the system on a higher scale, the internal electronic component interfaces are set aside from primary concern, and so the preamp is no longer regarded so much as a composite system itself but more as one among other relatively solid units in a larger composite system. Yet this principle of unity on a higher order, which causes intervening interfaces on lower one to fade from consideration, is not why Haugeland thinks that our cognitive systems are seamlessly integrated with their environing world. Haugeland notes that perception in artificial intelligence is seen as transduction, meaning that at the interface where the sensor receives information, it reduces all the near infinity of bits of possible information to make a much simpler single detection like "there is a sleeping brown dog." The narrow channel of information that an artificial perceptual interface can handle is thus "low bandwidth." However, the perceptual systems of living organisms are not limited by such a "bottlenecking" of the information; they can take in untold quantities of informational bits at once, and for this reason their perceptual capacities are instead "high-bandwidth" (220–221). But, this high bandwidth capacity of biological perception is not like the transistor's interface that only allows very simple interactions, so Haugeland concludes that our perceptual systems are not interfaced with the world.

Yet according to Clark, Haugeland is mistaken to say that the flow across interfaces can only be simple. So even though Clark agrees that sensation involves direct agent-environment couplings, he is not ready to conclude that there are no interfaces. Clark has us instead combine the concept of interface as being a point of affective contact between components with the concept of super high-bandwidth information flow. This very intimate, mutual affectivity allows for parts to cooperate together as a larger system (Clark 2008, pp. 32–33).

Our perceptual interfaces, then, enable the immense flow of sense information to modify our body's workings in real time so that we may form coupled systems with the environing things in our world. In fact, Clark explains that his notion of continuous reciprocal causation is much like phenomenologist Merleau-Ponty's "whole organism-body-world synergies" (Clark 1997, p. 171). As an illustration of this, Clark refers to Merleau-Ponty's example of the perceptual dynamics involved if one were to hold an animal using some sort of capturing device. Merleau-Ponty provides this example to show how our reactions to a stimulus help give a stimulus its form in the first place. Merleau-Ponty notes how a cat's ear flattens when it is bent but twitches when it is tickled (Merleau-Ponty 1963, p. 11). The response is not directly and immediately mechanical, but rather the cat must wait a short period to properly sense the form of the stimulus' motion so that it makes the proper response. He has us think about how phones worked in his time, where apparently you dialed a name rather than a number. If we first dial an *O*, the automatic switchboard knows that within its listing there is only a limited set of possible second letters, so it only becomes receptive for those characters, and so on with each additional letter until there can only be one possible connection. Then the switchboard "responds" appropriately to its "stimulus" by connecting to the proper receiver, after this brief interval of processing (14). The cat's ear, likewise, discerns the form of the stimulus' touch-motion, moment by moment, with each step changing its mode of receptivity, including changes in the shape and position of the ear, until it has sensed enough that it may enact the proper response. But all the while, part of that response were the motions which altered its receptivity to the stimulus. Merleau-Ponty elaborates this with the captured animal illustration, and Clark suggests as an example a hamster in tongs. In order to keep the animal in the device, our hand responds appropriately to the motions it feels the animal making, but those very same motions condition the way the stimulus is perceived.

> When my hand follows each effort of a struggling animal while holding an instrument for capturing it, [...] each of my movements responds to an external stimulation; but [...] these stimulations could not be received without the movements by which I expose my receptors to their influence. "... The properties of the object and the intentions of the subject... are not only intermingled; they also constitute a new whole." (13, quoting Weizsäcker's *Reflexgesetze*)

So let's use Clark's suggested example. Imagine we catch a hamster with tongs, and it lengthens itself so its body narrows to slip out of the grips. Our hands sense the decrease in the animal's width, and we tighten our hold so to keep it captured. But, consider if we had never changed the strength of our hold. The hamster would have slipped out, rendering us insensitive to the lengthening that allowed it to escape. Thus, the tightening of our grip was simultaneously both the cause for us being able to sense the hamster narrowing while at the same time being our response to its narrowing. Merleau-Ponty clarifies somewhat with his next example. Consider when something catches our eye and we look to it. This interesting object can be said to cause our eyes' behavior of moving toward it; however, we would not have noticed it in the first place had we not already moved our eyes into its vicinity and had been in a mode of visual attentiveness to such optical stimuli (13). A diagram in Yarbus's *Eye Movements and Vision* could help to illustrate. It shows the motions of the viewer's eye when looking freely at an image compared to when the viewer had particular tasks to accomplish (Fig. 16.1).

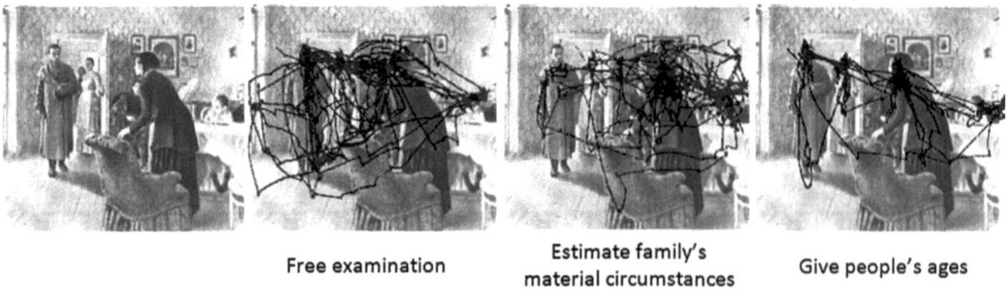

Fig. 16.1 Tracked eye movements for different tasks in Yarbus' *Eye Movements and Vision.* (Image from Yarbus (1967), here modified. Original includes seven patterns, slightly different text, and none of the patterns are superposed upon the painting)

One impression these patterns might give us is that our eyes are from the beginning always in a state of continuous motion, so we can see how it could be that our eyes are both tending toward a stimulus while simultaneously being drawn to it. Hence, we need not portray eye motion behavior as being dragged around from place to place by the external stimuli alone, but instead the motions and the stimuli are causally coupled. This is further apparent when we note that the eye movements were directed according not just to the content of the image (as the image remained the same for all the tasks) but also in accordance with the viewer's interests. So, moving to the framed paintings in the background is both the image calling to our attention while at the same time it is our eye seeking such things, when we are interested in the family's material circumstances.

Thus in this case, Merleau-Ponty is referring to the causal influence the response has on the way its stimulus is given to it. Clark seems even to take his interpretation one step further to remind us that in the previous example, the animal is likewise responding to its perceptions of our motions, and so we are reacting to "worldly events which are at the same time being continuously responsive to our actions" (Clark 1997, p. 171). But, it is not necessary for both parts to perceive the other; in the least they need to be mutually affective. However perception facilitates this affectability, because it provides an interface that acts as

> *an open conduit allowing environmental magnitudes to exert a constant influence on behavior*. Sensing is here depicted as the opening of a channel, with successful whole-system behavior emerging when activity in this channel is kept within a certain range. What is created is thus a kind of new, task-specific agent-world circuit. (Clark 2008, p. 16)

This process is a matter of deperceptualization or dephenomenalization, where we gradually cease noticing our perceptual interface. Clark notes how this commonly happens with tool use. When first using the tool, we notice the point of contact between ourselves and it. A beginning wall painter for example will feel the texture of the brush handle and its imbalance in the hand. After practiced use the painter ceases noticing the brush and instead just perceives the texture of the painting surface, like the dryness that slows the brush motion or the sheen that increases its glide. It is as if the painter's nerves grew into the handle, then through the bristles, to now touch the wall itself, pushing the interface further away from the body and deeper into the external world. This is a phenomenon Clark calls *technological transparency*.

So, when constant adaptive interaction causes us to no longer sense the implement we are using, it has become "transparent." Prior to that phase it is "opaque" technology, which means it is highly visible or noticeable in our use of it. It trips us up and requires skills and capacities that do not come naturally (Clark 2003, p. 37). But the tool gradually converts to transparent technology as it becomes "so well fitted to, and integrated with, our own lives, biological capacities, and projects as to become [...] almost invisible in use," because we and the tool have become one composite problem-solving system (37–38). Thus, "the artist's sketch pad and *the blind person's cane* can come to function as transparent equipment, as may certain well-used and well-integrated items of higher technology, a teenager's cell phone perhaps" (38, emphasis mine).

Clark in numerous cases refers to the blind person's cane or more generally to a stick used for the same purpose of feeling-out the world. He directly cites Merleau-Ponty's *Phenomenology of Perception*, and we will later examine that text in more detail. For now we will see more precisely how this example works for Clark, that is, how it illustrates the way that perceptual interfaces become transparent and pushed deeper into the external world. He writes, "fluently using a stick, we feel as if we are touching the world at the end of the stick, not [...] as if we are touching the stick with our hand. The stick [...] is in some way incorporated [...] (see Merleau-Ponty [*Phenomenology of Perception*])" (Clark 2008, p. 31). When using the stick, there are two key interfaces, "the place where the stick meets the hand and the place where the extended system 'biological agent + stick' meets the rest of the world" (31). Yet, when the stick and the blind person cooperate as a seeing machine, the phenomenal data sensed at the hand/stick interface is no longer regarded as telling us about the stick itself but rather about the world the stick touches. New human-machine interface technologies also work this same way, and so our nervous activities increasingly extend deeper into the world, and into one another, as these technologies continue advancing (31).

Clark explains that our brain's neuroplasticity is what allows for external implements to become integrated transparently into our own bodily and cognitive systems. Through neuroplastic processes, "human minds and bodies are essentially open to episodes of deep and transformative restructuring in which new equipment (both physical and 'mental') can become quite literally incorporated into the thinking and acting systems that we identify as our minds and bodies" (30–31). To further illustrate neuroplasticity, Clark discusses other cases of sensory substitution that are like the blind person's cane. There was a system pioneered in the 1960s that created dynamic tactile maps to allow blind people to sense things at a distance as if they had vision. They wore a camera on their head and a grid of nails on their back. The camera translated the visual data of whatever came before the person's head into analogous patterns of nail stimulation from the grid. The subjects first only felt vague tingling sensations but after practicing goal-driven activities like walking and eating, they "stop feeling the tingling on the back and start to report rough, quasi-visual experiences of looming objects and so forth" (35). Because the subjects voluntarily controlled the camera's direction, they could experiment to explore how visual data corresponded to the tactile impressions, which allowed their brains to neuroplastically "rewire" and accommodate their workings to the new sensory interface (35–36).

This sort of recalibration is seen in studies done with primates that also learned to use such tools. In one case monkeys used a rake to snag distant food. There are bimodal neurons that dually respond to both the tactile sensations near their hands while as well to the visual data for what they see in their hand's vicinity. Yet, after mere minutes of using the rake to reach for food, these same neurons then began associating the sensations in the hand with the visual data at the end of the stick. The monkeys' brains "rewired" so that they could "feel" what the rake was touching (38, citing Maravita and Iriki 2004, p. 79). Similarly another study examined how our brains distinguish space beyond our grasp (far space) from the space within reach (near space), but when using the stick as a tool, it "causes a remapping of far space to near space. In effect the brain, at least for some purposes, treats the stick as though it were a part of the body" (Berti and Frassinetti 2000, p. 415, as quoted in Clark 2008, p. 38).

So far these examples involve perceptual interfaces. Recently there have been developments in sending information signals directly from and to the brain using neurally implanted electrodes. Again, in these cases, neuroplasticity allows the brain to reconfigure its workings so to integrate external prosthetics into one's body-schema. Clark discusses one such important breakthrough. In this experiment, a monkey handles a joystick that measures both the strength of the monkey's grip and the direction of its hand motions. This translates into changes in the position and size of a dot cursor on a computer screen (Fig. 16.2).

The monkey is trained firstly to move the cursor to a target area, then secondly to grip the joystick pole hard enough so that the circle expands to a targeted size. Thirdly, the tasks are combined, simulating virtually the motor action for reaching and grabbing an object. All the while during this "pole control" phase, researchers recorded the monkey's relevant neural activity by means of electrodes inserted into its brain, so to determine which neural behaviors correlate with the particular changes in cursor movement. Then, in the following "brain control" phase, the researchers disconnect the joystick wiring. On the basis of the recorded correlations, now only the monkey's brain states determine the cursor's motion, so the monkey quickly ceases using its arm and merely uses its brain. Once the monkey adapts to these new conditions, the researchers then add a robotic arm into the loop. The monkey now is no longer directly controlling the screen cursors. Instead, its brain states control the position and grip of a robotic arm, whose parameters are then secondarily read and displayed on the screen. But the robot arm, being an actual mechanical device, responds more slowly than the cursor did when directly

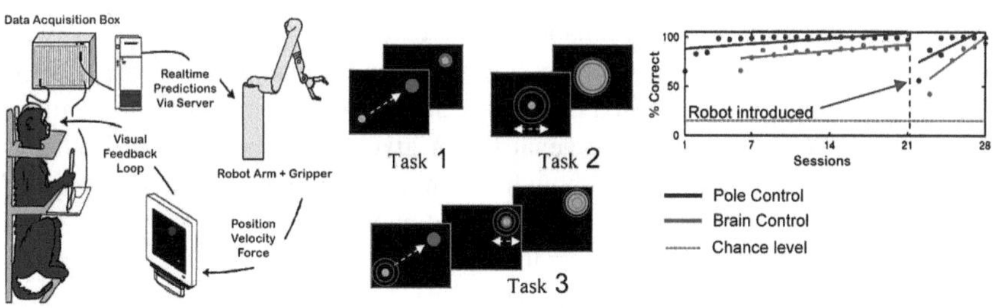

Fig. 16.2 Diagrams from Carmena et al.'s brain-machine interface study. *Left panel* shows a simplified brain-machine circuit. *Center panel* displays the viewed tasks. *Right panel* shows the initial break then increase in fluency with the added robotic arm. (Image from Carmena et al. (2003), here modified. Original circuit diagram includes additional components not relevant to our treatment, namely the "ANN and Linear Fit," "LAN," and "Client." Also the tones were modified for conversion to black and white)

controlling it. So, at first the monkey loses a notable amount of fluency in its now indirect control of the cursors. However, very quickly it adapts to the new mechanical conditions (Fig. 16.2, right panel).[2] The researchers conclude by proposing that

> long-term operation of such a device by paralyzed subjects would lead, through a process of cortical plasticity, to the incorporation of artificial actuator dynamics into multiple brain representations. Ultimately, we predict that this assimilation process will not only ensure proficient operation of the neuroprosthesis, but it will also confer to subjects the perception that such apparatus has become an integral part of their own bodies. (Carmena et al. 2003)

3 Medical Prosthesis

There has been recent research into therapeutic prosthesis that examines the phenomenological dimension of the patients' adaptation to their prosthetic device. And like Clark, a number of these studies explain the process of transparency on the basis of Merleau-Ponty's phenomenology, specifically citing the blind person's cane example. Craig Murray, for example, reports on surveys he conducted with medical prosthesis users, many of whom experienced the full integration of the device into their body schema (Murray 2004, 2008). For example, a recent amputee who had to adjust to the malfunctioning mechanics of his shortened leg explained, "the brain had not yet become accustomed to the change in mass [...] but now it's not so noticeable" (Murray 2004, p. 967). Similarly, prosthesis users then must adjust once again after first acquiring their new device when having to invest much of their attention and effort to learn how to use it. As one patient explains, the "mechanics" of the activity become "automatic": "once moving, in general, it's pretty much a matter of well I want to go from here to there, and I just walk. It's intuitive now" (968). A man who wore a prosthetic leg for 27 years became so accustomed to it that when it was off, his body still acted mechanically as if it were still on. "I [...] got up, and forgot I did not have my limb on. I fell on the floor [...]" (968). And, the process of acclimation involves the perceptual interface between body and device fading from awareness: at first "it feels unnatural, so you're aware of it. That feeling [has] decreased over the years, so perhaps in some ways I'm less aware then" (968). This dephenomenalization gives them the impression that no part is missing from their body: "though I've not got my lower arm, it's as though I've got it and it's part of me now" (970). And another explains, "my prosthesis is an extension of my body. (I can actually 'feel' some things that come into contact with it, without having to see them. [...]) It must 'feel' as close to not being there as possible" (970). In fact, despite doctors' predictions, one user could feel the ground through his prosthesis: "I do sense it [the ground] with the prosthesis on. It is a

[2] The researchers also report they found the same results when adding the robotic arm in the pole-control phase.

general awareness of the ground. As I walk, I can feel my heel land, and the foot move forward to the toes" (971). An example we will return to later is of a man who did not want a device looking like a hand. He wanted something more practical, an attachment fixed to his arm that allowed him to insert any of a number of various tools: "I wanted a socket for a swim fin, bike breaking device, things to allow me to be more active and productive" (971).

Building in part from Murray's findings, Frederick Mills offers an extensive treatment of Merleau-Ponty's phenomenology of the body to provide the theoretical basis for more successful prosthesis use. What is of interest to us here is his explanation for how sensorimotor feedback enables the prosthetic device to become transparent and integrated into the patient's body schema. Sensorimotor feedback "is a dynamic relationship between the adaptive body and environmental stimuli," and when it occurs "at the interface of the prosthesis and the environment," incorporation of the device could be more likely (Mills 2012, p. 4, 6). One way this feedback loop can be more successfully closed is by "targeted reinnervation" techniques (6). When performing amputation, instead of cutting the neural tracts with the incision, they can be removed intact from the severed limb and reattached at the end of the stump. Any sensations at this new location feel as if they come from the absent appendage. Some patients were then given a prosthetic limb with electronic touch sensors that converted tactile information into mechanical stimulations topically administered to the reinnervated nerve regions. The patients could then indirectly feel what the prosthesis was feeling. According to the researchers, "this may help amputees to more effectively incorporate an artificial limb into their self image, providing the possibility that a prosthesis becomes not only a tool, but also an integrated body part" (Marasco et al. 2011, quoted in Mills 2012, p. 6). Reinnervated nerves also have been used successfully to direct the prosthesis' movement (Kuiken 2006).

Recently there have been developments promising even greater advances in neuroprosthesis. In 2008 monkeys with neural implants operated a robotic arm to pick up food and bring it to their mouths (Velliste et al. 2008). In 2011 chips were used to record rats' memories and functioned in place of their biological memory. These chips could even be fitted for human use (Berger et al. 2011). Also that year there was a study where monkeys were given one set of neural implants for controlling a virtual arm and yet another one for receiving artificial touch signals, opening the possibility that robotic neuroprosthetic limbs can be both directly controlled and felt by the brain (O'Doherty et al. 2011). Then in 2012 two human quadriplegics with brain implanted sensors successfully used robotic arms to perform simple tasks like grasping and bringing drinks to their mouths (Hochberg et al. 2012). Cochlear implants, which send electrical signals into the nerves in the ear to replace lost hearing abilities, have been in use for some time, and there are currently neuroprosthetic eye implants that can restore some basic visual capabilities (Caspi et al. 2009). In addition, there have been numerous advances in brain emulation. By creating computer simulations of human neural dynamics, it is conceivable that the lost functioning of damaged parts of one's brain could be restored with computing equipment (Markram 2006).

4 Merleau-Ponty and Prosthetic Embodiment

Since Merleau-Ponty's stick example and the theories it illustrates form the theoretical basis for much research on prosthesis, I will analyze them in greater detail before examining the alternate model of the body. For Merleau-Ponty, the blind person's use of a cane is an example of "the *organic* relationship between subject and world." Like Clark's and Chalmers's extended cognition, "the active transcendence of consciousness" for Merleau-Ponty is carried "into a thing and into a world by means of its organs and instruments" (Merleau-Ponty 1962, p. 176, emphasis mine). And, there is a bidirectional integration of body and world that accompanies the process of the cane becoming a transparent extension of one's body.

> To get used to a hat, a car or a stick is to be transplanted into them, or conversely, to incorporate them into the bulk of our own body. (166)The blind man's stick has ceased to be an object for him, and is no longer perceived for itself; its point has become an area of sensitivity, extending the scope and active radius of touch, and providing a parallel to sight. (165)The pressures on the hand and the stick are no longer given; the stick is no longer an object perceived by the blind man, but an instrument with which he perceives. It is a bodily auxiliary, *an extension of the bodily synthesis*. (176, emphasis mine)

Merleau-Ponty explains that likewise our gaze is "a natural instrument analogous to the blind man's stick," because it ranges over objects as if "questioning" them (17).

Our bodily synthesis with the world for Merleau-Ponty is a phenomenal fusion with the things we perceive, which results from us becoming perceptually "sympathetic" to them so to better sense them. Upon hearing something, parts of our ear apparatus vibrate at the same frequency as the sound they are sensing. So when expecting some sensation, we "surrender" a part of our body or even our body entirely to what we are sensing (Merleau-Ponty 1962, p. 246). Consider if we reach out to feel something smooth. To do so, our hands will adopt a particular "degree," "rate," and "direction of movement" that is appropriate for feeling that object's given type of surface. Were we to feel something rough or with a different shape, our hands would have taken on a different comportment toward the object:

> [M]y hand, while it is felt from within, is also accessible from without, itself tangible [...] Through this crisscrossing within it of the touching and the tangible, its own movements incorporate themselves into the universe they interrogate, are recorded on the same map as it; the two systems are applied upon one another, as the two halves of an orange. (Merleau-Ponty 1968, p. 133)

Our sympathetic relation places us into a "pre-established harmony" and "kinship" with the thing we sense (133). Thus:

> [T]he sensor and the sensible do not stand in relation to each other as two mutually external terms [...] my gaze pairs off with color, and my hand with hardness and softness, and in this transaction between the subject of sensation and the sensible it cannot be held that one acts while the other suffers the action. (Merleau-Ponty 1962, p. 248)

For Merleau-Ponty, our perceptual integrations with the world are a matter of us fusing with them, becoming one "flesh" by means of a "reversible" "chiasmic" relation: "the body sensed and the body sentient are as the obverse and the reverse, or again, as two segments of one sole circular course which goes above from left to right and below from right to left, but which is but one sole movement in its two phases" (Merleau-Ponty 1968, pp. 137–138). To explain what he means with this circular relation, we will first find an interpretation of his meaning for our chiasmic relation with the world. He offers an image for this reversible relation where we and the object of our perception are both seeing and seen. When we hold-up two mirrors to one another, they produce an infinite series of images set one within the next, which produces an entirely new image. The mirrors then form a coupling that is "more real than either of them" (139). And we become able to see ourselves as from the outside, because we exist within the object of our perception, being "seduced" and "captivated" by it "so that the seer and the visible reciprocate one another and we no longer know which sees and which is seen." This relation of sensibility, which in a way makes us anonymous, is what Merleau-Ponty calls "flesh" (139). It is not just the matter making up us and the world; it is rather the "coiling over of the visible upon the seeing body, of the tangible upon the touching body" (146). We lend our body to the things we sense so that they may inscribe themselves upon us so to give us their resemblance.

We find in his working notes on the chiasm more clues as to what he means with this metaphor. The chiasm, he writes, is what allows us all to belong to the same world, to the same body, all while we maintain our opposing relations (the "for-Oneself for-the-Other antithesis"). In the chiasm, there is more than just a "me-other rivalry" between us and the other things in the world; there is also a "co-functioning": "We function as one unique body" (215).

So, let's note the features of our chiasmic relation with the world in order to better conceptualize Merleau-Ponty's unique meaning for it: 1. there is an overlapping of related parts, yet 2. the parts still maintain their individuality, but 3. there is ultimately an integration of the parts into an interwoven fabric or "flesh" of the world. We often times see the chiasmic structure characterized as: *ABBA*. In Merleau-Ponty's case, there is an overlapping at work. To visualize it, let us draw from a diagram in Barry Dainton's "Time in experience: Reply to Gallagher." Here he gives helpful illustrations for different forms of temporal continua. One diagram displays a sort of continuum resulting from an overlapping of superposed temporal parts (Fig. 16.3).

In one sense, Merleau-Ponty is saying that when we perceive the world, we are sharing that part of us which sympathizes with the things we are sensing, as in the case of our hands pre-conforming to the conditions that the object sets for our feeling it. As we said, this contact is like two mirrors facing one another. In Dainton's diagram, the two *B*'s are considered superposed because we think of there being a procession from left to right, with the two *B*'s happening simultaneously. My use of the diagram will not have this temporal meaning. I could have placed all the blocks in a straight row, like the letters in *ABBA*. But, this other staggered arrangement depicted above better allows us to represent the crisscrossing

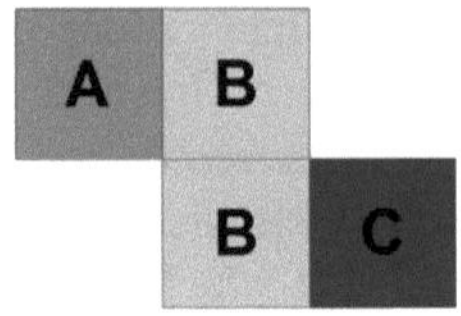

Fig. 16.3 Dainton's diagram of overlap by superposition. [Image modeled after Dainton (2003, Fig. 9)]

and coexisting that merges sensing and sensed all while making the differences between their roles ambiguous. This was what makes us reside together in one flesh. Recall also that the two "reversing" segments are a part of "one sole circular course which goes above from left to right and below from right to left" (138). This circular course could be the bidirectional relation of ambiguity that itself is the flesh we live in (Fig. 16.4). One difference between my diagram and Dainton's is that we have *A* on both sides. This is because the dual "motion" of the sensation interweaves both sides into one flesh, marked with a *C*. So, the two sides are different by being on either pole of the relation. Yet, they are not distinguished insofar as they are both already of the same flesh. It is in this way that we might keep the chiasmic structure's representation as *ABBA*. The *A*'s are the sensor and the sensed, both interwoven into the same flesh. The *B*'s then are the sympathizing places of contact where one mirrors the other. And finally, their double motion of sensing and being sensed weaves them together into one flesh, *C*.

Merleau-Ponty's organic model of bodily embeddedness in the world on the one hand explains the way prosthetic devices integrate into our body schema, but on the other hand seems to be at odds with this notion of the human body becoming more like machines made of very dissimilar parts. I turn now to Deleuze's and Guattari's theory of the machine, and I propose that their model be adopted in place of Merleau-Ponty's organic one, with their example of the mounted archer replacing the blind person's cane.

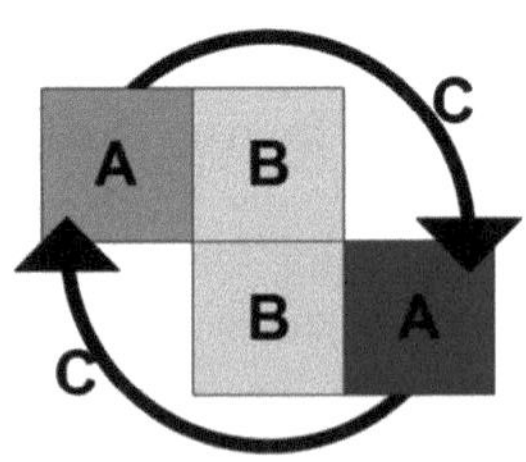

Fig. 16.4 My diagram of Merleau-Ponty's chaismic flesh

5 Machinic Embodiment

When discussing organicism in cinematic montage, Deleuze notes that one feature of the organism is "unity in diversity, that is, a set of differentiated parts" (Deleuze 1986, p. 31). Machines for Deleuze are also made of diversified parts, but they are not necessarily "unified." Rather, they are linked up without being assimilatory.

> Machine, machinism, "machinic": this does not mean either mechanical or organic. Mechanics is a system of closer and closer connections between dependent terms. The machine by contrast is a "proximity" grouping between independent and heterogeneous terms. [...] The machine, in requiring the heterogeneity of proximities, goes beyond the structures with their minimum conditions of homogeneity. (Deleuze 2007, p. 104)

To better grasp how machines can function despite the heterogeneity of their parts, we turn briefly to the appendix of Deleuze's and Guattari's *Anti-Oedipus*, titled "Balance-sheet for desiring-machines." Here Deleuze and Guattari speak of an absurd sort of machine in literature and art, which mis-operates "through the physical impossibility of the organization of the working parts, or through the logical impossibility of the mechanism of transmission" (Deleuze and Guattari 2009, p. 91). They note how for example Man Ray's painting *Dancer/Danger, Impossibility* is a machine whose constituent mechanisms operate against one another (Fig. 16.5).

Humans are component parts of machines. In the case of *Dancer/Danger*, we are to think in the first place that the gears' whirling is to express the twirling of a Spanish dancer. But, the impossibility of the machine's workings is to convey the idea that a machine by itself could never perform something as non-mechanical as human dancing. Yet, the machine does express something about the motion. Implied in its entitled workings are the human dancer's motions. Even though she is not shown, her necessity for completing the dance is implicit. This illustrates the need for humans to be a part of "desiring machines" (91–92). For our purposes, we are concerned more with the mechanics Deleuze and Guattari are employing here rather than with the issue of desire. They go on to say that humans become components to machines when we communicate our functioning by recurrence to the other parts of the machine, all under the specific conditions of our functioning. They

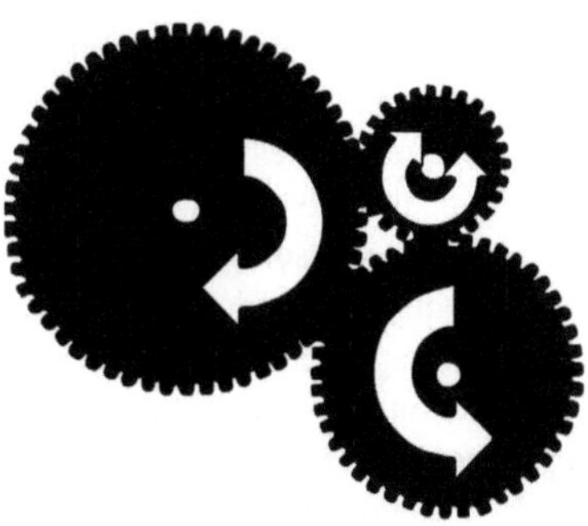

Fig. 16.5 Diagram depicting part of the machinery in Man Ray's *Dancer/Danger, Impossibility*, 1920

have us consider for example a mounted archer. What do a horse, a man, and a bow and arrow have to do with one another? Their functioning is unrelated, except when on the steppes where war is waged. The recurrence of the horse's trot communicates its functioning to the man, whose recurrent pulling of his arm communicates to the recurrent springing of the bow and arrow. Normally, such recurrent functions would be meaningless to one another. Why should a horse care about a man's arm pulling back and forth? Why should the man care about the horse's feet moving up and down? But, when they communicate the differences of their functioning under the conditions of war on the steppes, they together incoherently form a lethal war machine. In machines, then, "heterogeneous elements are determined to constitute a machine through recurrence and communications" (91–92).

Deleuze and Guattari distinguish tools from machines. A tool might have parts that make contact and that communicate motion or force, but unlike machines, a tool's parts are not really functionally independent and heterogeneous from one another. Also, there will be a possibility that a tool is usable in certain situations. Yet, in the operation of machines it is more of a matter of them having a probability that its parts might reconfigure under different functional relations or be used in ways that are unforeseeable. And finally, when we see something as a tool, we think of it in terms of how all its parts integrate and work together for a common purpose ("the functional synthesis of a whole"), but when regarding something as a machine, we understand it with respect to how its parts work heterogeneously and incoherently ("real distinctions in an ensemble") (92–93).

We will use their next example, the Greek phalanx, to better grasp the inter-workings of the heterogeneous parts as springing-up out of the conditions of their functioning. Deleuze and Guattari write, "Hoplite weapons existed as tools from early antiquity, but they became components of a machine, along with the men who wielded them, under the conditions of the phalanx and the Greek city-state" (93). The reason the phalanx is machinic is not because it is like a gear in the army machine, nor is it because the phalanx itself has gears, like the pike's fulcrum and the marching legs. Rather, one reason it is a machine is because these men and their mechanically-related parts enter formation within the conditions of the heterogeneous machinery of their social and political circumstances. Being a citizen of a Greek city-state has nothing to do with wielding a long pike. They do not associate at all. However, neither of the two would have been able to sustain itself if both their heterogeneous functions were not combined. These civic conditions and the war machinery supporting them are inseparable.

We normally think of machines and mechanisms as repeating a function, and the overall effectiveness of the machine we often regard as being the result of the mechanical parts maintaining their assigned function. But, this is not really a machine, because its production is limited to manufacturing only one thing redundantly. Instead, a more proper machine would have the capacity for new productions, and this would result from it being able to reconfigure itself and also its functional relations with the functional mechanisms around it. In fact, as early cyberneticists John von Neumann and W. Ross Ashby observe, machine systems with the capacity to reconfigure their own workings are more able to maintain themselves in the face of unpredictably changing environments (Ashby 1954, p. 110; Neumann 1966, p. 73), and recent studies further confirm this using more complex robotic machinery (Meng and Jin 2011, p. 144; Johnson 2008, p. ix, 22).

So along with the machine's power to connect with things around it and the power of its parts to connect together, it also has the power to form new connections and hence to break those already in function (Deleuze and Guattari 2009, p. 96). Thus machines have a

> capacity for an unlimited number of connections, in every sense and in all directions. It is for this very reason that they are machines […]. For the machine possesses two characteristics or powers: the power of the continuum, the machinic phylum in which a given component connects with another, the cylinder and the piston in the steam engine […], but also the rupture in direction, the mutation such that each machine is an absolute break in relation to the one it replaces, as for example, the internal combustion engine in relation to the steam engine. Two powers which are really only one, since the machine in itself is the break-flow process, the break being always adjacent to the continuity of a flow […]. (96)

So machines on the one hand connect heterogeneous parts, like a train engineer being connected to his levers and the engine parts they operate, which connects his body to long kilometers of surface on the earth and to the people he interacts with on both ends. But also, on account of the fact that machines operate by the incoherence and heterogeneity of their parts, these connections on the other hand very easily can break and in fact machines often operate most properly when their connections do sever. So, the teams of inventers and engineers who worked with mechanical parts to design and produce the internal combustion engine not only made use of the flexibility allowed by the incoherence of mechanical parts to break their connections and produce new arrangements, but also they broke the course of development in engines and set it along on a new path, and they broke the train engineer's functional habits and connections to the steam powered parts of his usual engine (96). Machinery understood in this broader sense tells us of a higher sort of mechanical productivity, one that produces new mechanical connections, rather than manufacturing the same product over and over without variation. Now if production is really the primary function of machines, would not more effective machines be ones without a fixed purpose?

To explain the non-associativity of machine parts, Deleuze and Guattari compare the visual relations in Dadaist and Surrealist artworks. The relations between images in Surrealist art often follow a "flow of association" and hence are not like the unassociated relations of Dada (Rubin 1978, p. 116). And Surrealist images, although made to look somewhat unusual, are still recognizable, like in dreams. "An object might be dreamed of as distorted, its perspective wrenched, but it is always an object familiar to us in our waking life" (113). In Dadaist works, if the parts still cause us to have associations, then even so, for the most part, these associated images found on another level of awareness did not themselves associate with one another. In Surrealism, however, we see the opposite. While the different images might seem logically incompatible, their associated images still might weave together and integrate in a way that could possibly make some sort of vague and "irrational" sense on another level of our consciousness.

For example, consider Man Ray's Dadaist work *L'image d'Isidore Ducasse*. He was inspired by a line in Isidore Ducasse's *Les chants de Maldoror* (written under his pseudonym Comte de Lautréamont): "the chance encounter of a sewing machine and an umbrella on a dissection table." Man Ray gives a "literal representation of the metaphor": He "undoubtedly assembled the appropriate objects—dissecting table, umbrella, and sewing machine; he made them 'pose' in order to photograph them" (Hubert 1988, p. 192). The parts of this work do not cohere together. Yet somehow it works on our brain. Even the associations each part gives us also seem not to integrate with each other. Now instead, we consider a Surrealist work, Giorgio de Chirico's *The Song of Love*, which depicts the head of a Greek statue, a surgical glove, a green ball, and a train. William Rubin explains that although these objects themselves do not associate, the images associated with them "cross-fertilize" each other (Rubin 1978, pp. 131–132). So, the surgical glove might make us think of Western medicine, coming from the ancient Greeks, like in the Greek statue, and the Greeks appreciated pure forms, like the sphericity of the ball. And, the knowledge of these Western-originating sciences led to technological advances seen much later in the steam engine, for example. Also, the ball and the glove both call to mind rubber, and the glove makes us think of hands that would sculpt the statue or play with the ball. The coherence of the associations is vague and elusive, but think of the affects it gives us. We feel as though there is some harmony to it all, even though on the surface none can be explicitly found.

Deleuze and Guattari elaborate on Dada's anti-associativity by making use of what they consider the "anti-Oedipal" and the "schizoanalytic." They note how free association inevitably leads our thinking to Oedipal representations. It is almost as if there is something Oedipal about associations themselves. Perhaps it is the fact that associations are like mechanisms governing regimented representation. In a way, there is a sort of restrictive power acting on our mental associations. And if we struggle to resist it, we are only entering into a fight with a governing force. Would it really be healthiest, then, to replace our psyche's troubled associations with other ones, when all associations structurally involve an enforced regimentation incapable of new productions? What if instead of manipulating our associations, we made use of psychic mechanisms that operate by means of non-associative connections?

> Let us return to the necessity of breaking up associations: dissociation not merely as a characteristic of schizophrenia but as a principle of schizoanalysis. The greatest obstacle to psychoanalysis, the impossibility of establishing associations, is on the contrary, the very condition of schizoanalysis – that is to say, the sign that we have finally reached elements that enter into a functional ensemble of the unconscious as a desiring-machine. It is not surprising that the method called free association invariably brings us back to Oedipus; that such is its function. Far from testifying to a spontaneity, it presupposes an application, a mapping back that forces a preordained ensemble to associate with a final artificial or memorial ensemble, predetermined symbolically as being Oedipal. In reality, we still have not accomplished anything so long as we have not reached elements that are not associable, or so long as we have not grasped the elements in a form in which they are no longer associable. (Deleuze and Guattari 2009, p. 103)

Deleuze and Guattari then quote Serge Leclaire: "What is involved, in brief, is the conception of a system whose elements are bound together precisely by the absence of any tie, and I mean by that, the absence of any natural, logical, or significant tie," "a set of pure singularities" (103, quoting Leclaire, "*La realite du desir*"). So for example, if we analyze our dreams for associations, these associative mechanisms are not really productive, and they do not constitute a machine. However, Deleuze and Guattari describe a method by Dolfi Trost which can render dream analysis machinic:

> [I]n order to retrace the dream thought [...] it is necessary to break up the associations. To this end, Trost suggest [sic] a kind of à la Burroughs cut-up, which consists in bringing a dream fragment into contact with *any* passage from a textbook of sexual pathology, an intervention that re-injects life into the dream and intensifies it, instead of interpreting it, that provides the machinic phylum of the dream with new connections. [...] the passage *selected at random* will always combine with the dream fragment to form a machine. And no doubt the associations re-form, close up between the two components, but it will have been necessary to take advantage of the moment, however brief, of dissociation. (102)

Recall how the Surrealist associations integrated while the Dadaist ones did not. Dadaism is machinic because its parts function together non-associatively, but Surrealism is associative and Oedipal. Real machines, however, are "a set of really distinct parts that operate in combination *as being really distinct* (bound together by the absence of any tie)." We find such machines in the works of kinetic sculptor Jean Tinguely and cartoonist Rube Goldberg (104).

In Jean Tinguely's machinic artworks, we have heterogeneity of parts and functions, all for seemingly a purpose that has nothing to do with anything else at all, nothing other than pulling us into it, conjoining us to it so that we together make a bigger machine without a pre-established purpose. In his "Cenodoxus" *Altar* kinetic sculpture, all the parts connect together mechanically, but these conjoined parts are heterogeneous to another one, for example the human and animal skulls rotating in conjunction with a Madonna figurine aimlessly tracking from one side to the other (Fig. 16.6). Here is how Deleuze and Guattari describe the heterogeneity of the mechanical parts' functions, whose incoherence is what opens it up for the greatest machinic productivity:

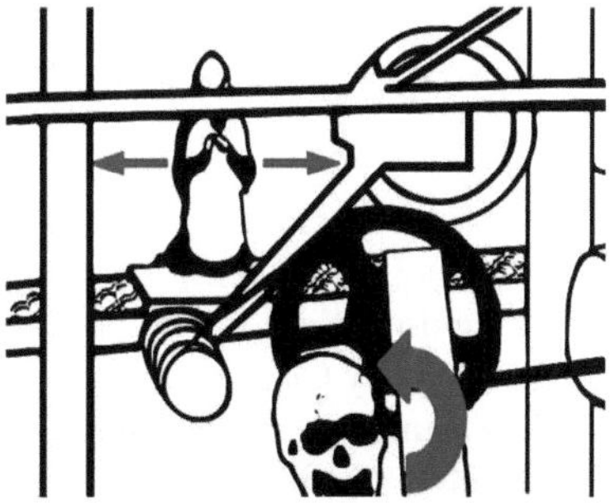

Fig. 16.6 Diagram depicting part of the machinery in Jean Tinguely's "Cenodoxus" *Altar*, 1981

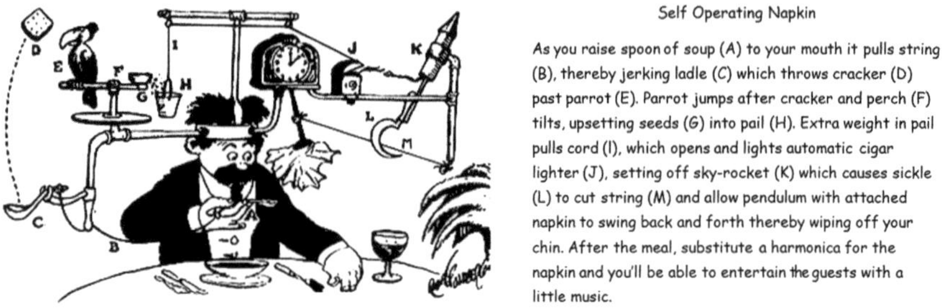

Fig. 16.7 Rube Goldberg's self-operating napkin machine. [Image from Goldberg (1915, text recreated)]

> In Tinguely, the art of real distinction is obtained by means of a kind of uncoupling used as a method of recurrence. A machine brings into play several simultaneous structures which it pervades. The first structure includes at least one element that is not operational in relation to it, but only in relation to a second structure. It is this interplay, which Tinguely presents as being essentially joyful […]. The grandmother who pedals inside the automobile under the wonderstruck gaze of the child – a non-Oedipal child whose eye is itself a part of the machine – does not cause the car to move forward, but, through her pedaling, activates a second structure, which is sawing wood. (104)

Deleuze further explains Dadaist mechanics with Rube Goldberg's machines, because they exhibit "processes of physical causality, which pass through detours, extensions, indirect paths, liaisons between heterogeneous elements, providing the absurd element which is indispensable to the machine" (Deleuze 1986, p. 181). Consider for example Goldberg's machine, "The self-operating napkin" (Fig. 16.7).

According to Deleuze, "each element of the series is such that it has no function, no relationship to the goal, but acquires one in relation to another element which itself has no function or relation…. These causalities operate through a series of disconnections" (181). Notice in particular the bird-cracker mechanism. We anticipate the bird eating the cracker, but this is a matter of probability, which as we noted is a characteristic feature of productive machines. What if the bird flies away or sees more appealing food and eats that instead? And, could there not be a variety of external influences that disruptively enter into the other fragilely connected mechanisms and completely change their operations?

6 Conclusion

The machinic view, then, would not see prosthetic extension as a matter of assimilating one's body to that device's functioning. The parts in the Goldberg machine do not need to reduce their heterogeneity in order to successfully operate together. Andy Clark in fact makes a similar point when responding to an objection to the extended mind hypothesis. Adams and Aizawa think that the causal processes involved in external cognitive systems are too dissimilar to internal ones for both to be analyzed together under one science of cognition (Adams and Aizawa 2001, pp. 51–52). Yet, Clark notes that even internal processes that Adams and Aizawa consider to be undoubtedly cognitive could in fact involve a "motley crew" of causal mechanisms "with not even a family resemblance (at the level of actual mechanism) to hold them together." For example, watching sports involves motor mechanisms, but imagining a lake does not (Clark 2010, p. 51).

> In the light of all this, my own suspicion is that the differences between external-looping (putatively cognitive) processes and purely inner ones will be no greater than those between the inner ones themselves. But insofar as they all form parts of a flexible and information-sensitive control system for a being capable of reasoning, of feeling, and of experiencing the world (a "sentient informavore," if you will) the *motley crew of mechanisms* have something important in common. (51, emphasis mine, Clark's emphasis removed)

What is important with regard to prosthesis is not our body parts' assimilations to the device but rather that we and the prosthesis as a conglomerate machine successfully create new shared interface connections. Try for yourself if you wish. Take a pen in your hand, close your eyes, and use it to feel around your immediate space to detect the objects in your vicinity. While doing this, how concerned are you with perceiving the pen itself and accommodating your hand to its properties? Or, do you instead find yourself more focally aware of the properties of the things the stick is touching? So, is it really such a helpful strategy to place emphasis on the body's organic integration with the device rather than on the new disjunctions with the surrounding world that they jointly create? The lesson Frederick Mills gains in his studies of Merleau-Ponty and therapeutic prosthesis integration is that persistence in usage is the vital condition that enables users to eventually come to successfully use their new device. This is especially difficult, because initial frustrations can cause the patients to give up altogether. Our question is then, which view of the body better encourages one to persist in using a prosthetic device despite initial frustrations? Consider if users begin with the view that their bodies are organic rather than machinic, that all its parts assimilate to one another and to the world around it to form one flesh. Might that not make persistence more difficult, since the patients would at first be constantly aware of the heterogeneity of their own flesh with the device's metal and plastic composition and strange manner of operating? What if instead prosthesis users began by viewing themselves as a mishmashed machine, a "motley crew" of parts like eyeballs and brains that is already linking up with foreign things like computers and power tools? Perhaps many of us will need to make this fundamental shift in our self-understanding from an organic to a machinic model, because we could someday face the decision of using robotic neuroprostheses as our organs begin to fail. If we, piece by piece, become more robot than human, what happens when we look in the mirror and see so many robotic devices in places where our body parts once were? If becoming robotic lies in our future, should we not now prepare by beginning to see ourselves as machinic?

This brings us to our second concern: if the robotic prostheses can be made to have greater functioning than their biological counterparts, should we feel compelled to still only use devices whose functioning is limited to the range of normal human capability? Competitive runner Oscar Pistorius, whose carbon-fiber J-shaped prosthetic legs earned him the nickname "Blade Runner," raced against able-bodied runners in the 2012 Summer Olympic games, being the first amputee to do so. Yet, first he had to fight a ban placed on him, which was based on an independent scientific study that determined his legs in certain important ways gave him a substantial advantage over able-bodied runners. And, there are now cochlear implants that allow the users to shut out external sounds and instead receive direct feeds into their nerves from mp3 players or mobile phones, giving them the extra-human ability of hearing these sound sources clearly in noisy environments. Is it not conceivable that as ocular prostheses advance, they could be equipped with telescopic or microscopic vision? Or, that prosthetic limbs be much stronger than the biological ones they replace? Or, that the computer chips implanted in the brain to treat failing memory actually enable photographic recollection? These technologies lie on our doorstep, and they imply a vision of the human body as a machine with replaceable parts. The patient in Murray's studies who wanted a socket on his arm for plugging in various tools, one being a swim fin, seems to already have this machinic view of his body. But, he never got his attachment; the doctor could not comprehend why anyone would want various odd new tools instead of something that looks like a natural hand. Nonetheless, this sort of posthuman capacity for machinic alterations and additions is where we are headed. As a result of our analyses here, we can see there is ample reason to reconsider the Merleau-Pontian theoretical basis for prosthesis integration and to experiment instead with a Deleuzo-Guattarian machinic one.

References

Adams, F., & Aizawa, K. (2001). The bounds of cognition. *Philosophical Psychology, 14*(1), 43–64.

Adams, F., & Aizawa, K. (2010). Defending the bounds of cognition. In R. Menary (Ed.), *The extended mind* (pp. 67–80). Cambridge: MIT.

Ashby, R. W. (1954). *Design for a brain*. New York: Wiley.

Berger, T. W., Hampson, R. E., Song, D., Goonawardena, A., Marmarelis, V. Z., & Deadwyler, S. A. (2011). A cortical neural prosthesis for restoring and enhancing memory. *Journal of Neural Engineering, 8*(4), 1–11.

Berti, A., & Frassinetti, F. (2000). When far becomes near: Re-mapping of space by tool use. *Journal of Cognitive Neuroscience, 12*, 415–420.

Birnbacher, D. (2008). Posthumanity, transhumanism and human nature. In B. Gordijn & R. Chadwick (Eds.), *Medical enhancement and posthumanity* (pp. 95–106). Dordrecht: Springer.

Carmena, J., Lebedev, M., Crist, R. E., O'Doherty, J. E., Santucci, D. M., Dimitrov, D. et al. (2003). Learning to control a brain-machine interface for reaching and grasping by primates. *Public Library of Sciences: Biology, 1(2),* 193–208. (Image taken from the on-line version and used in accordance with its open access, unrestricted use allowance. Available: http://www.plosbiology.org/article/info:doi/10.1371/journal.pbio.0000042).

Caspi, A., Dorn, J. D., McClure, K. H., Humayun, M. S., Greenberg, R. J., & McMahon, M. J. (2009). Feasibility study of a retinal prosthesis: Spatial vision with a 16-electrode implant. *Archives of Ophthalmology, 127*(4), 398–401.

Clark, A. (1997). *Being there: Putting brain, body, and world together again*. Cambridge: MIT.

Clark, A. (2003). *Natural-Born cyborgs: Minds, technologies, and the future of human intelligence*. Oxford: Oxford University.

Clark, A. (2008). *Supersizing the mind: Embodiment, action, and cognitive extension*. Oxford: Oxford University.

Clark, A. (2010). Memento's revenge: The extended mind, extended. In R. Menary (Ed.), *The extended mind* (pp. 43–66). Cambridge: MIT.

Clark, A., & Chalmers, D. (2002). The extended mind. In D. Chalmers (Ed.), *Philosophy of mind: Classical and contemporary readings* (pp. 643–652). Oxford: Oxford University. (Revised reprint).

Dainton, B. F. (2003). Time in experience: Reply to Gallagher. *Psyche, 9*(12), 1–41.

Deleuze, G. (1986). *Cinema 1: The movement-image* (H. Tomlinson & B. Habberjam, Trans.). London: Continuum. Deleuze, G. (1983). Cinéma 1: L'image-mouvement. Paris: Les éditions de minuit.

Deleuze, G., & Guattari, F. (2009). Balance-sheet for "desiring-machines". In S. Lotringer (Ed.), *Chaosophy: Texts and interviews 1972–1977* (pp. 90–115) (R. Hurley, Trans.). Los Angeles: Félix Guattari and Semiotext(e).

Deleuze, G., & Parnet, C. ([1987]2007). *Dialogues II* (H. Tomlinson & B. Habberjam Trans.). New York: Columbia University.

Goldberg, R. (1915). Self operating napkin. Wikimedia Commons. On-Line. Available: http://commons.wikimedia.org/wiki/File:Professor_Lucifer_Butts.gif.

Haugeland, J. (1998). *Having thought: Essays in the metaphysics of mind*. Cambridge: Harvard University.

Hochberg, L. R., Bacher, D., Jarosiewicz, B., Masse, N. Y., Simeral, J. D., Vogel, J., et al. (2012). Reach and grasp by people with tetraplegia using a neurally controlled robotic arm. *Nature, 485*, 372–375.

Hubert, R. R. (1988). *Surrealism and the book*. Berkeley: University of California.

Johnston, J. (2008). *The allure of machinic life cybernetics, artificial life, and the new AI*. Cambridge: MIT.

Kuiken, T. A. (2006). Targeted reinnervation for improved prosthetic function. *Physical Medicine and Rehabilitation Clinics of North America, 17*(1), 1–13.

Marasco, P. D., Kim, K., Colgate, J. E., Peshkin, M. A., & Kuiken, T. A. (2011). Robotic touch shifts perception of embodiment to a prosthesis in targeted reinnervation amputees. *Brain, 134* (3), 747–758.

Maravita, A., & Iriki, A. (2004). Tools for the body (schema). *Trends in Cognitive Sciences, 8*(2), 79–86.

Markram, H. (2006). The blue brain project. *Nature Reviews Neuroscience, 7*, 153–160.

Menary, R. (2010). The extended mind in focus. In R. Menary (Ed.), *The extended mind* (pp. 1–26). Cambridge: MIT.

Meng, Y., & Jin, Y. (2011). Morphogenetic self-reconfiguration of modular robots. In Y. Meng & Y. Jin (Eds.), *Bio-inspired self-organizing robotic systems* (pp. 143–171). Berlin: Springer.

Merleau-Ponty, M. (1962). *Phenomenology of perception* (C. Smith, Trans.). London: Routledge.

Merleau-Ponty, M. (1963). *The structure of comportment* (A. L. Fisher, Trans.). Boston: Beacon.

Merleau-Ponty, M. (1968). *Visible and the invisible* (C. Lefort (Ed.). A. Lingis Trans.). Evanston: Northwestern University.

Mills, F. B. (2012). A phenomenological approach to psychoprosthetics. *Disability and Rehabilitation, 35*, 1–7. (Early online).

Murray, C. D. (2004). An interpretative phenomenological analysis of the embodiment of artificial limbs. *Disability and Rehabilitation, 26*(16), 963–973.

Murray, C. D. (2008). Embodiment and prosthetics. In P. Gallagher, D. Desmond, & M. MacLachlan (Eds.), *Psychoprosthetics* (pp. 119–130). London: Springer.

O'Doherty, J. E., Lebedev, M. A., Ifft, P. J., Zhuang, K. Z., Shokur, S., Bleuler, H., et al. (2011). Active tactile exploration using a brain–machine–brain interface. *Nature, 479*, 228–231.

Rubin, W. S. (1978). *Dada and surrealist art*. London: Thames.

Shores, C. (2012). Body and world in Merleau-Ponty and Deleuze. *Studia Phaenomenologica, 12*, 181–209.

Velliste, M., Perel, S., Spalding, M. C., Whitford, A. S., & Schwartz, A. B. (2008). Cortical control of a prosthetic arm for self-feeding. *Nature, 453*, 1098–1101.

von Neumann, J. (1966). *Theory of self-reproducing automata*. Urbana/London: University of Illinois.

Yarbus, A. L. (1967). *Eye movements and vision* (B. Haigh Trans.). New York: Plenum. (Public domain image from Wikimedia Commons. On-Line. Available: http://commons.wikimedia.org/wiki/File:Yarbus_The_Visitor.jpg.

Chapter 17
From "Enhancement Medicine" to "Anthropotechnology"

Sylvie Allouche

1 Introduction

Techniques developed within medical practice seem to be more and more easily exported into contexts where the medical, which is to say therapeutic, aim is disputable or even explicitly denied. One very clear example of this would be the use of erythropoietin (EPO) to enhance athletic performance. This situation has progressively led to a broadening of the scope of medicine in order to include these extended applications, and we now regularly encounter the term "enhancement medicine." My purpose here is to dispute the legitimacy of this expression and suggest its replacement by the term "anthropotechnology."

In order to advocate for the use of this neologism, I will mainly rely on a discussion of concepts, emphasising the difficulties raised by the use of the disputed expression. At some key-stages of my argument however, I also rely on the methodology developed during my PhD (Allouche 2012), whose main strategy was to make use of science fiction to build philosophical arguments. I shall begin by saying a few words about this methodology.

An earlier version of this paper has been published in French under the title "*Des concepts de médecine d'amélioration et d'enhancement à celui d'anthropotechnologie*" (Allouche 2009).

S. Allouche (✉)
Département de Formation Humaine & Laboratoire de Biologie Générale (UMRS 449, EPHE), Université Catholique de Lyon, Université de Lyon, Lyon, France
e-mail: allouche.sylvie@gmail.com

D. Meacham (ed.), *Medicine and Society, New Perspectives in Continental Philosophy*, Philosophy and Medicine 120, DOI 10.1007/978-94-017-9870-9_17

1.1 Using Science Speculation to Do Philosophy

My PhD research consisted of analysing forms of interventions in and on the human body that appear in science fiction, and marginally in what I call "science speculation," focusing my study on interventions presenting a minimal degree of scientific plausibility (at least from our present standpoint). By the term "science speculation," I mean speculation based on science as it appears not only and principally in the genre of science fiction, but also in non-fiction: scientific papers (Clynes and Kline 1960), philosophical essays (Habermas 2001), futurology books (Kurzweil 2005), etc.

I should also specify that I make a distinction between the notions of "world" and "universe," where "universe" means the object built up by a fictional work, which provides a point of access, a window, on the set of possible worlds described by the universe. I admit that there is always (except perhaps in ad hoc borderline cases such as "M_0 is the unique world described by the universe U_0"), an infinity, or a whole *spectrum* of possible worlds referred to by a given universe U_x. My principal methodological hypothesis, therefore, consists of considering the universes built by science fiction as describing alternate worlds or alternate versions of our world, which can help us in the task of understanding it. This is, in fact, what thought experiments are supposed to do when, for example, they provide situations that compel us to clarify our moral intuitions, as Sidney Shoemaker suggests in his seminal work *Self-knowledge and self-identity* with regard to his own thought experiments:

> The question of what most people would say if the imagined events occurred is of course a factual question, and not a question for philosophers to decide. But something can be said, of a philosophical nature, about what would be the case if such events were to happen and if nearly everyone were to agree that a change of body had taken place (Shoemaker 1963, p. 246).

Derek Parfit, in *Reasons and persons*, points in the same direction: By considering these cases [...] [w]e discover our beliefs about the nature of personal identity over time. Though our beliefs are revealed most clearly when we consider imaginary cases, these beliefs also cover actual cases, and our own lives (Parfit 1984, p. 200).

To come back to science fiction, a large number of the worlds explored by the genre deal with speculative future evolutions of our world, which often leads people to think that science fiction is quintessentially the genre of the future. In fact, science fiction is not reducible to this,[1] but this is not the place to explain why, especially as I plan to feed my present reflection from this subsection of the genre. More precisely, I rely on one of its key procedures, which consists of departing from a given technology, or a combination of several technologies, and imagining

[1]See for example the 5th International Science Fiction Conference in Nice, organised in March 2005 on the theme "Science fiction in history, history in science fiction" (Terrel 2005).

their various philosophical stakes and consequences, in terms of ethics, politics, psychology, sociology, etc.

In this exercise of science speculation, reflection on the philosophical aspects of enhancement medicine forms such an important part that it is impossible to give a full account of it. But even if I cannot here explore all the relevant fiction in all its interesting details, my argument will try and show, following Hottois and Missa (2002) and Jérôme Goffette (1992, 1996, 2006), that if we really want to encompass what is at stake in the contemporary revolution of medical practice, the concept of enhancement medicine, though acceptable, is too limited, and that we would be better off replacing it with a broader one: "anthropotechny," which I divide into "anthropotechnics" and "anthropotechnology."

2 First Objection to the Concept of Enhancement Medicine

To begin with, what do we mean by enhancement medicine? If I analyse the concept, it seems to designate a set of medical interventions, the goal of which is to enhance the state of a person in relation to a particular function. However, this concept raises two problems, the first being that the notion of enhancement medicine, if we mean medicine in a strict sense, seems to be a contradiction in terms, and the second lying in the difficulty of determining an absolute sense of what an enhancement is. But before exploring these two issues in detail, it is necessary to clarify the conception of medicine I am utilising here, which is broadly inspired by the theses of Georges Canguilhem in his seminal text *Le normal et le pathologique* (*The Normal and the Pathological*, 1966). In this book, which is an expansion of his 1943 doctorate in medicine, Canguilhem emphasizes among other things the importance of an individual's subjective perception of her or his own states over a narrow positivistic understanding of medicine focused on the objective signs of health and illness.

2.1 Medicine and Norms

The traditional goal of medicine appears to be taking care of human beings, whether by means of the complete cure of their condition, whatever it might be, or, if a complete cure cannot be attained, by the establishment of the physiological conditions deemed to be the best possible under the circumstances. Thanks to the "scientification" of medicine that began during the XIXth century, and the increasing means of intervention that it has produced, more and more possible ways of transforming the human body have developed, to an extent where the classical medical dimension appears to be less and less recognisable. This allows us to see and foresee the passage from a curative medicine, with a regulative idea (in a sense broadly inspired by Kant 1787) of returning to an initial or normal state, to an enhancement medicine, where the regulative idea is to go further, in a positive sense, than this initial or deemed normal state; hence the notion of enhancement.

A first difficulty raised by the concept of enhancement medicine, therefore, emerges from the difference between the "initial" state and "deemed normal" state. It does seem that we have to make a distinction between the return to a previous norm that the individual has already known—the curative process properly understood, where the initial state defines the norm—and the establishment of a norm that the individual has never known, but which is considered valuable or normative for their species; for example, if one proposes to give or return sight to a congenitally blind person.[2] Even if it is perfectly conceivable that a blind person who has become sighted might ultimately ask to return to their initial state (that is, to be blind again), it seems that, for a certain set of "species normal" and perhaps normative features or functions, we do not think that there is a problem in acknowledging the medical nature of the corrective intervention.

But it is also obvious that other characteristics are more problematic, and questions regarding their medical dimension are familiar as, for example, when the "normal size" for a breast or a penis is at issue. With regard to blindness, we might cite the fascinating story by Wells (1904) "The Country of the Blind", in which a character lives for several years in a totally isolated society of blind people, who do not even understand the idea of sight. In the end, he must choose between marrying the woman he loves and keeping his sight, as the blind community has decided he has an illness which simply needs to be cured:

> "His brain is affected," said the blind doctor. [...] "Now, *what* affects it? [...] *This*," said the doctor, answering his own question. "Those queer things that are called the eyes, and which exist to make an agreeable soft depression in the face, are diseased, in the case of Bogota, in such a way as to affect his brain. They are greatly distended, he has eyelashes, and his eyelids move, and consequently his brain is in a state of constant irritation and destruction. [...] And I think I may say with reasonable certainty that, in order to cure him completely, all that we need do is a simple and easy surgical operation – namely, to remove these irritant bodies. [...] Then he will be perfectly sane, and a quite admirable citizen." (Wells 1904 [2003], p. 202)

In the original story Bogota finally escapes, but in the recent French adaptation for the theatre *Le pays des aveugles* by Nino d'Introna (2012), the ending remains open, and the spectator is left free to imagine that Bogota might choose to have his eyes removed. From a more academic perspective, there is, for example, Robert A. Crouch's paper, "Letting the deaf be deaf. Reconsidering the use of cochlear implants in prelingually deaf children" (1997), which addresses the same kind of issue.

[2]The problem is very simply reflected here by the term one chooses to use, as each proceeds from a different assumption on the nature of the intervention: is it a cure ("returns") or an enhancement ("gives")? In the second case however, it would probably be necessary to talk about "individual enhancement"; my former colleague at the University of Bristol, Heather Bradshaw (2011), advocates the use of the term "morphological change," which avoids introducing such potentially disputable assumptions.

In any event, acknowledging the key role that the notions of "norm," "standard," or "normal" ought to play when one tries to think in medical terms, I shall divide the cases of medical action into four classes. Note that for the first three classes the chronological notions of "initial state" and "subsequent state" are sufficient for distinguishing between the classes, as they deal only with comparisons of the various medical states of a particular individual throughout their lifetime. It is only the fourth class of medical actions that relies on the comparison between medical states of different individuals, and which requires the concept of norm. This concept, therefore, can be retrospectively applied to the previous three categories at a second stage. The notion of "normal state" replaces "initial state" in this case all the more easily because it is the former phrase that is commonly used in current language.

2.2 Classes of Medical Action

2.2.1 First Class: Return to the Individual Norm

The central idea of medicine is the following: I start from an initial state in which I am in good health. I then become ill, or I am the victim of an accident that creates a certain incapacity and/or a certain suffering (which might itself be the cause of the incapacity), or lesser negative effects (sickness, discomfort, etc.). Simply put, medicine ideally allows me not to suffer any more, and to be able to do the same things as before (walk, jump, ride a motorcycle, etc.). This is, put rather crudely, the most common perception of medicine. But this central core is linked to a whole series of situations which differ from it.

2.2.2 Second Class: Establishment of a New Individual Norm

In some cases, the initial state cannot be fully attained; there remains an "after-effect" (a weak ankle or knee for example); some of these effects may be of positive value (immunisation to a disease once it has been contracted); in such cases it can be said that the recovered health condition is better than the initial one. Or sometimes, medicine simply compensates externally for the effects of a disorder, as when corrective lenses are prescribed to treat myopia. In this second class of cases, the patient's condition is stabilised and they can continue to live in their new state, without the condition imposing any definite limitation on their life expectancy, apart from the ordinary processes of aging.

2.2.3 Third Class: Impossibility of Establishing a New Individual Norm

There is, however, a third class of cases, in which medicine cannot cure nor compensate the departure from the previous norms and the patient cannot be stabilised in a new state of health. In which case medicine can still provide care until the anticipated death, perhaps postponing it and offering palliative care.

2.2.4 Fourth Class: Reestablishment of the Species Norm (or Whatever Is Thought to Be Such in a Certain Social and Historical Context)

Finally, a fourth class includes cases of differences that are understood as deficiencies, possibly resulting in abnormalities or disabilities, present at birth. In the other classes, what had been designated as the initial state was implicitly used as the norm, but in cases of such inborn deficiencies the initial state is precluded from use as the standard.

This creates a problem: when the norm to be reached was defined by the particular individual in a previous state, it was relatively easy to determine, but as soon as there is no initial state that may serve as a standard, the physician must necessarily refer to a norm in idea[3] (which is not necessarily thought as an "ideal norm"), insofar as the standard the doctor aims to reach never had any empirical existence in a previous state of the patient. And as every body is singular, in the sense that it would be absurd to trace back its norm to the history of another body, the standard to which doctors refer when justifying a "correction" is necessarily an abstraction: in other words an idea. This idea is then more or less easily identifiable, according to the case under scrutiny, and partly variable from one culture or historical period to another—see the paradigmatic case imagined by H.G. Wells cited above.

However, within the varying range of possible norms, we can assume that there is, at least, a sort of hard core, a general standard of humanity as a species, which can serve as the backdrop for all possible variations of individual norms, as identified in the previous three classes. As I am myself a member of a certain (Western European[4]) culture at a certain moment of its historical development, and as my purpose here is not to express any personal opinion, but to try and reflect the current use of language and subsequent practises of which I am aware in the field of medicine, obstetrics and surgery in particular, it is probably difficult to escape all cultural bias on the topic. Having said that, I shall try to suggest some more positive content of this "backdrop of all possible variations": generally speaking, we consider that it is "normal" to be born, for example, with four limbs and no more, with one and only one sex, and generally with a certain type and range of physical and

[3]"In idea" as in Plato's texts, for example *The Republic* IX 592a: "I understand; you mean that he will be a ruler in the city of which we are the founders, and which exists in idea only" (Plato 4th c. BC, p. 287).

[4]See "The American-Western European values gap. American exceptionalism subsides" survey (Pewglobal.org 2011–2012), which shows the importance of being specific about this.

mental characteristics. Individuals born without one of the features intuitively accepted as forming the normal type of human being, even when they are in no danger of dying prematurely, are generally considered as possibly in need of a corrective medical intervention.

There are however all sorts of "gray areas" where, inside a single culture in the same period of time, people do not agree, or even strongly disagree, as to whether or not some morphological differences need to be medically corrected. I have already mentioned Robert A. Crouch's paper. But we may also mention a certain number of members of the "deaf community," who try to alert the general public as to what might be involved with new genetic technologies at our disposal. There is the case, for example, of the 2010–2012 project on "Deafhood and Genetics" funded by the British Leverhulme trust, and led by Paddy Ladd and Steve Emery from the Centre for Deaf Studies at the University of Bristol. On the welcome page of the website, they explain their goals as follows:

> We will investigate Deaf and hearing peoples' fears that, if left unchecked, genetic technology could encourage the development of eugenicist social policies. For example the Human Fertilisation and Embryology Bill (2008) means that couples who wish to try and ensure deaf genes are not passed on when they want a family, now have the support of law for this. There are real fears that laws like these will be extended as genetic technology develops (Deafhoodgenetics.co.uk 2010–12b).

The scope of the project was also thought to be broader than solely deaf community issues, because "ultimately these developments affect everyone. If the UK becomes a society where diversity is rejected and eugenics is widely accepted, then some of the ethical principles which people have taken pride in for centuries will have been jettisoned" (Deafhoodgenetics.co.uk 2010–12a).

2.3 *From Curative Medicine to Enhancement Medicine*

In fact, from the moment we admit that the norm of medical action is not necessarily given by a previous state of the patient, two sets of problems appear.

2.3.1 First Set of Problems: Corrections that Actually Enhance

It may happen that the means available for a corrective intervention results, relative to a particular function, in a better state than the one provided by nature; for example, more resistant artificial teeth, or swifter legs, as in the now famous case of Oscar Pistorius, at least according to the International Association of Athletics Federations (IAAF), which did not initially allow him to run against "able-bodied" athletes in the 2008 Beijing Olympics, for the reason that his prostheses were giving him an unfair advantage. As Anne Marcellini and her colleagues recall:

> Peter Bruggeman, Professor at the Institute of Biomechanics at Cologne University was engaged to lead a team to carry out experiments to in/validate any potential performance advantage for Oscar Pistorius (typically referred to as "boosting") resulting from the use of the "Cheetahs." He concluded that there was a "mechanical advantage" of more than 30 % for an athlete using these prostheses over athletes without prostheses. [...] Based on Bruggeman's study IAAF held that [Pistorius] would no longer be authorised to take part in competitions run under IAAF rules (2008). (Marcellini et al. 2012)

But this decision, announced in January 2008, was immediately challenged by Pistorius:

> [He] filed an appeal to the Court of Arbitration for Sport (CAS) in Lausanne, Switzerland. On 16 May 2008, the CAS upheld the appeal filed by Pistorius and concluded in a press release that: "[...] On the basis of the evidence brought by the experts called by both parties, the Panel was not persuaded that there was sufficient evidence of any metabolic advantage in favour of a double amputee using the Cheetah Flex-Foot. Furthermore, the CAS Panel has considered that the IAAF did not prove that the biomechanical effects of using this particular prosthetic device gives Oscar Pistorius an advantage over other athletes not using the device." (Smith and Thomas 2012)

Pistorius then qualified for the August 2011 World Athletics Championships, in Daegu, South Korea. His relay team won silver. He was also chosen to be a member of the South African Olympic team and so became "the first double leg amputee to participate in the Olympics having competed in the 400 m; Pistorius went on to reach the semi-finals in the individual 400 m and the final of the 4 × 400 m relay" (Smith and Thomas 2012).

Even if Pistorius' blades were ultimately judged not to be giving him unfair advantage, his case spectacularly made manifest a whole range of conceptual and ethical issues regarding disability, technology and enhancement, which science fiction had already begun to explore. One of the best-known examples of this exploration is probably Steve Austin, the protagonist of Caidin's novel *Cyborg* (1972), later adapted into the television series *The Six Million Dollar Man* (Johnson 1973–1979). More recently, we might mention Geordi La Forge's "visor" in the *Star Trek: The Next Generation* series (Roddenberry 1987–1994), which allows him to have a different perception of his immediate environment that is, in some respects, superior to natural vision.

2.3.2 Second Set of Problems: The Norm of What?

But a second set of problems emerges, when it becomes rather difficult to say that the norm followed does pertain to that of the human species. In one possible case, the solicited medical intervention appears as dictated by a socio-cultural norm, as in the striking example mentioned by Arthur Frank in his 2004 paper "Emily's scars: surgical shapings, technoluxe, and bioethics":

> In March 2003, *Vogue* ran a story in its "beauty, health & fitness" section [...] titled "The Flawless Foot" (Lamont 2003). The story interviewed several New York podiatrists whose surgical practice includes shaping women's feet so that they can fit into and can look good

wearing designer shoes. [...] As *Vogue* told the story, surgical practice is being pushed by patient-consumers, who in turn are being pushed by shoe designs. Thus *Vogue* quoted a "Manhattan-based podiatrist and podiatric surgeon" who said: "until recently, my patients would have surgery only to relieve painful foot deformities like ingrown toenails and plantar warts. Now they come in for a consultation, pull a strappy stiletto out of their bag, and say 'I want to wear this shoe'" [Ibid.] (Frank, 2004, pp. 20–21).

Later, mentioning some observations made by one the podiatrists named Suzanne Levine, Frank draws a comparison between Martin Heidegger's critique of modern technology and these practices. In the same way that, according to Heidegger, "the water becomes 'standing reserve' for the power plant and the trees standing reserve for the sawmill" (Frank 2004, p. 21),[5] Levine, says Frank, "presents the foot as standing reserve for surgery [...]. But she then broadens the frame as she presents the practice of surgery as standing reserve for fashion" (Frank 2004, p. 21).

If in this case, the artificiality of the demand (which does not necessarily imply its illegitimacy) appears obvious, there are numerous cases that raise the question of whether we have a trustworthy criterion by means of which to make the difference between human species norms and socio-cultural ones. Should we take into account the average? But which one? Of humanity? Of a subset of it? And how do we decide which subset to choose? How do we know that it is not too small, or perhaps too big? Or should we, instead, favour the tradition followed by a certain culture? But cultures also have subcultures, and an individual might belong to a culture without wishing to follow its standards, etc.

This last remark leads, in fact, to the second case I have in mind, which is one in which a person asks for a medical intervention, not with reference to any pre-existing collective norm, whether classified as natural or socio-cultural, but by appealing to an individual norm without an antecedent, usually by reference to a projected state of happiness, or to the right of autonomy, this last concept being exactly what is at stake here: the power of an individual to produce and follow their own norms ("auto"-"nomos"). I am thinking now of a whole spectrum of cases,

[5]Frank seems to misunderstand Heidegger here. In fact, in Heidegger's text, the transformation of nature in "standing-reserve" does not apply to the sawmill, to which Heidegger refers on the contrary in order to contrast benign traditional technology and "monstrous" modern one: "And certainly a sawmill in a secluded valley of the Black Forest [can be] compared with the hydro-electric plant on the Rhine River. But [...] [t]he revealing that rules in modern technology is a challenging [*Herausfordern*], which puts to nature the unreasonable demand that it supply energy which can be extracted and stored as such. But does this not hold true for the old windmill as well? No. Its sails do indeed turn in the wind; they are left entirely to the wind's blowing. But the windmill does not unlock energy from the air currents in order to store it. In contrast [...] the river is dammed up into the power plant. [...] In order that we may even remotely consider the monstrousness that reigns here, let us ponder for a moment the contrast that is spoken by the two titles: 'The Rhine,' as dammed up into the *power* works, and 'The Rhine,' as uttered by the *art* work, in Hölderlin's hymn by that name. [...] The revealing that rules throughout modern technology has the character of a setting-upon, in the sense of a challenging-forth. [...] Whatever is ordered about in this way has its own standing. We call it the standing-reserve [*Bestand*]" (Heidegger 1953, pp. 101–105).

which are, sometimes for clinical reasons, sometimes for strategic ones, understood as medical, usually in relation to the all-encompassing label of "psychological beneficence"; for instance, the numerous rhinoplasties that are conducted for reasons far more complex, in terms of identity, than questions of malformation or aesthetics, as in the following case: "another wants to eliminate the resemblance with his father, of whom he has the same nose, and from whose influence he has difficulties to free himself" (Faivre 1989, p. 109; see also Dull and West 1991). But we can also mention, still in the field of plastic surgery, interesting cases like those of Maria Jose Cristerna, the Mexican "vampire woman" tagged "the most modified female in the world" (Huffingtonpost.com 2012), or, before her, the French artist Orlan who underwent plastic surgery for artistic purposes (Orlan 1997; Allouche 2005).

So, we end up with all these various cases, and a growing number of the same kind, in which physicians are led to apply their knowledge to situations in which the definitional goal of medicine, which is to say, therapy, is at least questionable. But the need that has progressively emerged to gather all these cases under a single label has led to the emergence of the notion of "enhancement medicine," which has been used by various actors of the field (see, for example, Greely et al. 2008; Wolbring 2008; Bostrom and Roache 2010).

The expression, then, clearly suggests that what is so designated must not be understood as something different from medicine in general, but more like a subspecies of it, similar to regular medicine's various specialties: dermatology, gynaecology, psychiatry, etc. Enhancement medicine would then only differ from traditional medicine because medical techniques are applied with another goal in mind than the one that was prevalent beforehand. But in this interpretation, the difference is not thought of as having any strong impact, because enhancement medicine is conceived as being in perfect continuity with what physicians have always done until now: after the deterioration of someone's health condition (D), the physician used to ensure its improvement until the return to the initial state (I), or a close approximation of it. Similarly, the "enhancing doctor" only ensures, given the same initial state (I), the establishment of a better, enhanced one (E). This enhanced state is then in the same relationship with the initial state (I) as this last one was with the deteriorated one (D). In other words: I/D = E/I, so enhancement of human bodies is just an extension of what medicine has always been doing.

2.4 Critique of the Notion of Enhancement Medicine

If we can easily guess how, in order to account for an indisputable evolution of medical practice, spontaneous conceptual creation has consisted, instead of revolutionising the conceptual architecture on which medicine was built, in adding some kind of appendix, I believe that it would be of interest for us to consider an in-depth reflection on what this appendix (enhancement medicine) actually implies. For there are only two possibilities: either one considers that the knowledge and techniques are truly what defines medicine, and that, consequently, the goal previously associated with it (the reestablishment of a norm) was simply too narrowly conceived—it seems that this is the direction towards which the phrase "enhancement medicine" points; or one considers that medicine is properly defined by its traditional goal and not its means, and that, consequently, any non curative use of medical techniques removes us from the sphere of medicine and takes us into another area, which still needs to be defined.

In fact, the situation appears even more complex, insofar as the emergence of the phrase "enhancement medicine" seems to be an erroneous response to the medical profession's desire to remain faithful to the primary vocation of medicine: even when practising "enhancement," professionals still want to be "doctors," they still want to be in the realm of care, at least the legitimizing and never achieved care of the soul, through care of the body, and more specifically a care that does not forget the first principle of medical ethics: *primum non nocere*.

To conclude this point, I shall assume, that if one considers that medicine is primarily defined by its purpose and not by its means, as a technique or an art of restoring a previous state or one deemed normal, any change, whether or not it is presented as enhancing, beyond this normal or previous state seems inconsistent with the very idea of medicine. The confusion stems from the fact that the techniques for improving human performances currently borrow from the techniques previously restricted to the medical field, and in which only people who are to become doctors are trained. This is the reason why, rather than being genuinely rooted in things as they are, the concept of "enhancement medicine" seems to be a transient concept that accounts for an indeed current tension, but one which ought to be replaced, in order to give way to a more satisfying and lasting concept.

3 Second Objection and Transition to the Concepts of Anthropotechny and Anthropotechnology

3.1 Problems Raised by the Very Concept of Enhancement

3.1.1 What Makes a Modification an Enhancement, and Who Decides?

A second issue raised by the concept of "enhancement medicine" comes from the highly relative and subjective qualification of enhancement, which also points toward quite serious ethical problems. Speaking simply of enhancement suggests that there might be some sort of objective criterion of it; but what might this criterion be, such that it allows someone to say that, for example, healthy Virginia_1 at moment m_1 is an improved version of Virginia compared to healthy Virginia_0 at m_0? It seems quite difficult to talk about enhancement, firstly in an absolute sense, not relative to a function, or even a particular task, and secondly without an explicit indication of whose point of view it is from which Virginia_1, or a particular ability of Virginia$_1$, is considered to be better than Virginia$_0$ or the previous state of the ability in question. In this respect, the question that begins each consultation of the cosmetic surgeons in the TV series *Nip/tuck* (Murphy 2003–2010) "Tell me what you don't like about yourself" is quite enlightening.

Philosophers like Allen Buchanan argue that enhancement is always function/capacity relative.[6] And indeed, from the very beginning of his 2011 book, *Better than Human: The Promise and Perils of Enhancing Ourselves*, Buchanan insists on precisely this issue:

> Before we go any further, I have to emphasize a simple point. An enhancement is an improvement of some particular capacity, but not necessarily something that makes us better off *overall*. For example, if your hearing were greatly enhanced, it might not improve your life. It might make you miserable, because you might not be able to concentrate due to all the noise. That's why it is better to talk about enhancing capacities rather than enhancing people (Buchanan 2011, p. 6).

But even this focus on capacities might not be precise enough, and enhancement might need to be considered as task-relative, as I briefly suggested above. This latter solution would probably be all the more in line with Canguilhem's position, in the sense that enhancement would not be "about function in some general sense but about specific demands placed on the organism by the environment" (Meacham, personal communication 2013). In any case, the very concept of enhancement appears to be problematic, because of the implication it seems to make that there is an absolute reference background against which an enhancement can be defined.

3.1.2 An Enhancement Relative to What Context?

More fundamentally, the way enhancements are usually discussed proceeds from too narrow a vision of what the human condition is, usually grounded in the assumption that this condition is more or less stabilised in its current state of affairs: for example, the fact that humanity is now living on a certain planet with definite types of atmosphere, temperature range, radiation protection, "epidemiographical balance," overall economical organisation, etc. But these living conditions, which is to say, the demands placed on humans by their environment, may vary greatly—and what is considered to be an enhancement will vary accordingly.

It is easy to see how the particular form of thought experiment provided by science speculation can help us to develop our concepts better in this instance. One can, in fact, find in various texts of the genre examples of human modifications that seem difficult to subsume under the simple notions of improvement or enhancement. One of the most striking cases is probably the prospect of modifying our bodies in order to facilitate extra-terrestrial exploration, as imagined, among many others, by James Blish in his novel *The Seedling Stars* (1956), or Clynes and Kline (1960) in their seminal paper "Cyborgs and Space". But there is no real sense in

[6] I am grateful to Darian Meacham for bringing this point to my attention.

speaking of enhancement when talking about modifying the metabolism of humans in order for them to survive without protective suits on other planets or in space, especially if, as in Blish's universe, the alterations are not reversible. Alternatively, we would need to speak of enhancement with respect to a such and such situation; it might be simpler to speak of "adaptation" or something similar from the outset.

Another range of possible states of the world that undermines the use of "enhancement" as generic term comprises those that imagine a radical change in the conditions of human existence on Earth itself, as in the case of a global epidemic. One can find, for example, a whole series of novels that hypothesise various kinds and degrees of sterility epidemic spreading in the human species, and as many varied responses from the human community: for instance in *Where Late the Sweet Birds Sang* (1976) by Kate Wilhelm, *The Handmaid's Tale* (1985) by Margaret Atwood, *Chroniques du Pays des Mères* (1992) by Élisabeth Vonarburg, *The Children of Men* (1992) by P.D. James, *Inherit the Earth* (1998) by Brian Stableford, *Maximum Light* (1998) by Nancy Kress, etc. The prospect of global climate change also provides a fruitful starting point, as in J.G. Ballard's *The Drowned World* (1962), John Barnes' *Mother of Storms* (1994) or Kim Stanley Robinson's "Science in the Capital" trilogy (2004, 2005, 2007). The various technological and political solutions proposed in these novels and others in order to deal with the envisaged problems are, once again, difficult to label as enhancements without further precision.

To conclude this point, if one wants to think about new applications of medical techniques and use concepts that are robust and durable enough to incorporate the potential evolutions of the issue at stake, then it appears desirable to reflect, from the outset, on the things that the term enhancement aims to designate, within a broader conception of what the possibility of technical intervention on human bodies implies. Rather than sticking to the ideas of improvement or enhancement, I therefore propose to use, following Gilbert Hottois and Jérôme Goffette, a (relative[7]) neologism which consists in linking together the two Greek words "*anthropos*" and "*techne*." I then arrive at three general concepts: "anthropotechny," "anthropotechnics" and "anthropotechnology," which I detail in the next section. The general umbrella concept is "anthropotechny," which is then partitioned into "anthropotechnics" and "anthropotechnology." "Anthropotechny" refers to the overall set of possible technical modifications of the human body. "Anthropotechnology" refers to its part based on modern scientific methodology as it has developed since the XVIIth century. "Anthropotechnics" refers to all the other practices of non-therapeutic interventions in the human body that exist in various human cultures.

[7]See Schunck de Goldfiem (1948) for a previous use of "anthropotechnie" and Goffette (2010) for a general history of the term.

3.2 *Anthropotechny, Anthropotechnics, Anthropotechnology*

3.2.1 Construction of the Three Concepts

In order to build the concept of anthropotechny and its derivatives, we must start from the classical thesis according to which humanity is essentially characterised by its ability to conduct technical actions in the world. More specifically, human beings transform, to greater or lesser extent, things in the world[8] in order to meet certain goals they assign to themselves, provided that these goals must be understood in a very general sense, and thus also cover all kinds of efforts to respond to varying environmental demands. Among those technical actions, some of them do, in fact, concern human bodies, with the crucial difference for a particular individual between their own body and those of others—see the notion of "*corps propre*" in works of French phenomenologists like Maurice Merleau-Ponty or Paul Ricœur (Ricœur 1990; Allouche 2007). The technical action on the human body can then be ordered a priori[9] according to the same variety of goals that command actions upon any other part of the world. However, different refined classifications have gradually emerged in various human cultures, between interventions that are considered legitimate, recommended, tolerated, mandatory, etc. on the one hand, and those that are illegitimate, impermissible, not recommended, forbidden, etc. on the other.

In the midst of all these possible interventions is a particular class defined by its specific purpose, namely the restoration of the human being to a state considered compliant to a certain standard, essentially given by nature. Insofar as medical action answers a powerful human need, whose legitimacy is widely if not universally agreed upon, techniques at its disposal have developed exponentially with the advent of scientific medicine in the XIXth and XXth centuries.

As a consequence, humanity now possesses a whole series of "anthropotechniques" developed and taught only from the medical perspective. This situation creates a tension around these techniques, so deeply understood as medical that they are commonly thought of, not only by doctors but also by philosophers, and therefore exist for the wider public, only under this particular vocabulary of medicine.

In his 2006 book, Jérôme Goffette defines "anthropotechny" (in French "*anthropotechnie*") as the "art or technique of extra-medical transformation of human beings by intervention on their physiology" (Goffette 2006, p. 69). Following

---

[8]And by doing so change the environment itself: in other words, the question of humanity's destiny is always also an ecological one.

[9]That is, by deduction from the initial concepts, rather than by first looking into existing practices, which have not necessarily actualised all possibilities yet. The a posteriori methodology can serve for ulterior verification, and this is, in any case, the one already mostly used by current analysts of human enhancement… and perhaps one of the reasons why, by being a bit too much focused on empirical data, they miss the opportunity to see "the big picture"—although that is not the case with Goffette, who also uses an inductivist approach, but whose interest was from the beginning triggered by science fiction (personal communication, 2013).

the general thesis developed by Goffette, I advocate that it is now time, in philosophy and beyond, to acknowledge the fact that the demand for the use of medical anthropotechniques for non-medical purposes exists, and that this demand will, in all probability, not only grow, but also be particularly profitable for the professionals who answer it. Where I depart slightly from Goffette's position is that I do not believe that anthropotechny should be considered as a discipline alongside medicine. Indeed, I think that anthropotechny must be conceived as the generic discipline, inside which one finds medicine, and non-medical anthropotechny (which follows all the other goals that can be assigned to the artificial modification of the human body). It is, I hypothesise, mainly for reasons of cultural history, which I briefly consider in the next section, that medicine has long occupied the entire field of anthropotechny. But medicine was in fact the tree, or rather the grove, hiding the forest of the many other possible goals of anthropotechny.

In this construction, therefore, medicine appears as a region of anthropotechny, part of which is "anthropotechnical," and the other "anthropotechnological." It goes without saying that the border between anthropotechnics and anthropotechnology is not strictly defined, and depends on the understanding one has of the reach of science. While most of us would classify make-up and leech therapy as what I call anthropotechnics, and EPO doping and pacemakers as anthropotechnologies, where some anthropotechniques should be placed is likely to be disputed, but it is not my intention to discuss that here.

3.2.2 Why Differentiate Between "Anthropotechnics" and "Anthropotechnology"?

But what is exactly the purpose of making such a distinction between "anthropotechnics" and "anthropotechnology"? One of my reasons is simply an effort to parallel the most current use of the already existing vocabulary of "technique" and "technology," and more specifically the use of "technology" as a suffix in a growing number of new fields of applied sciences, as in "biotechnology," "nanotechnology," "neurotechnology," "mnemotechnology," etc. But in reality, I am far from certain that the designations I have settled upon here are the right, which is to say the most intuitive, ones. Indeed, I hesitated between "anthropotechnics" and "anthropotechnique," which would be the word used in French anyway; but there is also the fact that I used "anthropotechnique", as it were, spontaneously when talking about particular forms of anthropotechny in the plural—probably, I realise now, to account for the parallel between "medicine" and "medical techniques" on the one hand, and "anthropotechny" and "anthropotechniques" on the other. In any case, how words (substantives and adjectives) based on the root "techne" are used in current language appears, upon closer inspection, especially inconsistent, all the more so when one tries to cross-reference French and English. See for example the following parallel series (numbers correspond to Google.co.uk results in August 2013):

Techny 752,000 (Techny neighbourhood in Illinois)	Technie 98,200	Technics 31,800,000 (Technics brand)	Technique 344,000,000	Technology 1,710,000,000	Technologie 136,000,000
Mnemotechny 56,900	Mnemotechnie 148,000 Mnémotechnie 12,400	Mnemotechnics 93,000	Mnemotechnique 217,000 Mnémotechnique 145,000	Mnemotechnology 6030	Mnemotechnologie 4930 Mnémotechnologie 4850
Anthropotechny 6	Anthropotechnie 1990	Anthropotechnics 15,400	Anthropotechnique 6430	Anthropotechnology 2630	Anthropotechnologie 3860

So, beyond any definite prescription with regard to words, what is really important here is to hold together the three, and even four, concepts at hand. For, and this will be my second and deeper reason for advocating these distinctions, the various forms in which debates on technological progress tend to crystallise, regardless of whether they deal with human enhancement or other applications of science (nuclear power, cloning, genetic modification, synthetic biology, geo-engineering, etc.), strategic assumptions are usually made, although not often explicitly discussed per se, as to whether the technology in dispute is a "game changer" (see Heidegger's paradigmatic argumentation about windmills and hydroelectric plants in note 7) or whether "there is nothing new under the sun."

As a matter of fact, the latter position ("nothing new under the sun") plays a prominent role in the "human enhancement" debate as it is framed by this very label of "human enhancement," prevalent in the Anglophone debate. I could give dozens of examples of this, but in reality, a whole paper needs to be devoted to demonstrating this point (to "*débroussailler*" the various uses which have developed from the initial "techne" root, as sketched above), so I will content myself here with reiterating the fact that this is precisely how Buchanan kicks off the 2011 book mentioned above:

> Michelle's boyfriend Carlos tells her she shouldn't take Ritalin. He says, "It's cheating and besides it might be dangerous." Michelle replies: "Calm down. It's just a cognitive enhancement drug – a chemical that helps me think better – it's not cocaine. Don't be hypocritical. You take a cognitive enhancement drug too – probably in dangerously high doses – namely caffeine. And don't think you're fooling me. You say you've quit, but I know you sneak a cigarette now and then when you're up late studying. I can smell it in your hair. Look, caffeine and nicotine both help you stay alert and think more clearly; that's why many people use them. So if I'm cheating, so are you and a lot of other people. Besides, if you're worried about unfair advantages, why pick on cognitive enhancement drugs? Just being at this university gives us a huge advantage. What do you think education is? It's cognitive enhancement. Or what about the fact that both your parents are really smart and have PhDs?" (Buchanan 2011, pp. 3–4)

So by choosing the somewhat awkward denominations of "anthropotechny," "anthropotechnics" and "anthropotechnology," I am trying to provide a conceptual framework that allows us to think about the continuity of technical activity without dissolving out its discontinuity, and vice versa. I recognise however, after about ten years of practising the different denominations in French and English, that from a purely practical point of view, it is usually simpler—and shorter—to use "anthropotechnie" as Goffette does, to designate all those practices whose convergence was not until recently visible by lack of a common label, whereas "medical anthropotechny" had already a name, "medicine." And if one wishes to rely on Google's results, it seems that "anthropotechnics" is the word gaining ground in English.

In any case, if the anthropotechny under consideration aims to restore a human being to a previous state or one considered normal, then it is medicine; the rest is non-medical anthropotechny. Anthropotechny then appears as the fundamental concept, currently undergoing a phase of transition, perhaps even of "unconcealment,"[10] by means of which the awareness arises that medicine is overwhelmed from everywhere by goals that are not its owns, and thereby allows for the emergence of the distinct concept of anthropotechny, hitherto more or less confused with it.

3.3 Is It Ethically Acceptable to Unconceal the Concept of Anthropotechny?

So while it may be conceptually interesting to order distinctions in this manner, a further question arises concerning the ethical and political desirability of making public and advocating such distinctions.[11] It may, indeed, be the case that one of the reasons why the concept, and therefore the very existence of anthropotechny, and more specifically of anthropotechnology, has been obscured for so long by medicine, which seemed to sum up all the anthropotechnological possibilities, is that it provided the solution in advance, by simply not raising them, of an inexhaustible field of ethical dilemmas; or, more importantly, to avoid the conduct of interventions intuitively considered as unethical, whose possibility was however opened up by medical technology. Unnamed things, especially when they are in the realm of unrealised possibilities, have more difficulty than others in coming into existence: see Norman Daniels' catchphrase argument "we cannot ethically get there from here" in answer to the question of his paper entitled "Can anyone really be talking about ethically modifying human nature?" (Daniels 2009, p. 38).

The absence of naming and conceptualization (the taboo nature?) of anthropotechnology might, then, have served a certain ethical and political function for a time. However, regardless of the position one takes on this issue, the by-now large body of essays about the non-medical applications of technologies developed by today's medicine seems naturally to challenge the appropriateness of this enduring absence.

In terms of strict conceptual requirements, which is to say, of the simple quest for truth that steers philosophical research, it therefore seems to me that we need to

[10]Cf. Heidegger's concept of "unconcealment" ("*Unverborgenheit*") precisely in "*Die Frage nach der Technik*" (1953), and also his other works.

[11]See in particular the scandal provoked in 1999 in Germany by the Heideggerian Peter Sloterdijk's paper on the same subject, in which he uses the term "anthropotechnik" (Sloterdijk 1999).

put an end to this lack of recognition of the concept that might bear the name of anthropotechnology. And on an ethical and political level, I accept the risk that naming and conceptualising something might sometimes be a way to legitimise it. For is it not the very gamble of science and philosophy to believe that truth, its quest and deployment, are good in themselves?

And anyway, with the current domination over the field of the especially biased vocabulary of "enhancement," even outside the English language, the worry I used to have appears now resolutely outdated, and it seems all the more important to try and promote what I think is a better vocabulary for a better philosophical reflection—which is, I understand, exactly the kind of things "analytical philosophy" initially set out to do.

4 Conclusion

The first part of my argument was designed to show why the concept of "enhancement medicine" was certainly admissible, but limited, and ultimately unsatisfactory in the long run. It is a transitional concept, undoubtedly valid to describe a temporary state in the evolution of medicine, but philosophically unacceptable by virtue of this very transitory nature. I then argued that medicine could be advantageously understood within a broader concept, that of anthropotechny, which I have divided into anthropotechnics and anthropotechnology.

If the heart of this argumentative set was already based on the examination of speculative cases, allowing me to provide a glimpse of what could be offered by the philosophical analysis of science speculation, it still remains to show how this methodology can be used in the analysis of the ethical issues of anthropotechnology, and how it can help to build better philosophical concepts.

One might retort that the right moment to philosophize about new technologies is when they emerge, that we already have a hard time with current problems, and, in consequence, that we should satisfy ourselves with Hegel's famous phrase: "The owl of Minerva takes flight only as the dusk begins to fall" (1821). But even if this "contemporanist strigid" position is indeed legitimate and provides useful studies, it seems that the type of speculative insight that I invite could be minimally understood as complementary. Is it what Norman Daniels was suggesting in the paper previously mentioned, when he wrote in its final sentence "I should stop because I want to leave the ethics of science fiction to others" (Daniels 2009)? Maybe not, as this last remark could just be an echo of the ironical undertone that lingers somewhat throughout the essay, beginning with its title, and also its first lines: "The organizers of a conference I was recently invited to asked speakers to examine what is involved ethically in modifying human nature through genetics. One possibility is that their invitation deliberately engaged in hyperbole in order to stimulate more interesting papers" (Daniels 2009). But notwithstanding this interrogation, if a rational reflection can be conducted on the issues raised by *possible* technological transformations of human beings, genetic ones included, who will do it, if not philosophers? Rather than owls, I therefore invite philosophers to turn themselves into bionic or GM eagles at their pleasure, and to manage to acquire enough altitude before dusk falls.[12]

References

Allouche, S. (2005). "La Caresse" ou l'hybride comme œuvre d'art. Que peut-on savoir de l'art du possible? À partir d'une nouvelle de Greg Egan. In F. Dupeyron-Lafay (Ed.), *Détours et hybridations dans les œuvres fantastiques et de science-fiction* (pp. 15–28). Aix-en-Provence: Publications de l'Université de Provence.

Allouche, S. (2007). 'Identité, ipséité et corps propre en science-fiction: Ricœur, Parfit, et Egan', *Alliage, 60: Que prouve la science-fiction?*, 86–99. Available: http://www.tribunes.com/tribune/alliage/60/Allouche.html.

Allouche, S. (2009). Des concepts de médecine d'amélioration et d'*enhancement* à celui d'anthropotechnologie. In J.-N. Missa & L. Perbal (Eds.), *"Enhancement": éthique et philosophie de la médecine d'amélioration* (pp. 65–78). Paris: Vrin.

Allouche, S. (2012). *Philosopher sur les possibles avec la science-fiction: l'exemple de l'homme technologiquement modifié* (PhD thesis, sup. J. Mosconi & S. Laugier). Paris: Université Paris 1 Panthéon-Sorbonne.

Allouche, S. (to be published). Fiction du futur et anthropotechnologie. In G. Hottois & J.-N. Missa (Eds.), *L'humain et ses préfixes: une encyclopédie de l'humanisme, du transhumanisme et du posthumanisme*. Paris: Vrin 'Pour demain'.

Atwood, M. (1985). *The handmaid's tale*. Toronto: McClelland & Stewart.

Ballard, J. G. (1962). *The drowned world*. New York: Berkley.

Barnes, J. (1994). *Mother of storms*. New York: Tor.

Blish, J. (1956). *The seedling stars*. New York: Gnome Press.

Bostrom, N., & Roache, R. (2010). Smart policy: cognitive enhancement and the public interest. *Contemporary Readings in Law and Social Justice, 1*, 68–84.

Bradshaw, H. (2011). *Defining enhancement, disability and therapy: How technology affects identity and the ethical implications of this* (PhD dissertation). Bristol: University of Bristol.

Buchanan, A. (2011). *Better than human: The promise and perils of enhancing ourselves*. Oxford: Oxford University Press.

Caidin, M. (1972). *Cyborg*. New York: Arbor House.

Canguilhem, G. (1966). *Le normal et le pathologique*. Paris: PUF.

Clynes, M. E., & Kline, N. S. (1960). 'Cyborgs and space', Astronautics, September 1960. In C. H. Gray, H. Figueroa-Sarriera, & S. Mentor (Eds.), *The cyborg handbook* (pp. 29–33). New York: Routledge.

Crouch, R.A. (1997). Letting the deaf be deaf. Reconsidering the use of cochlear implants in prelingually deaf children. *The Hastings Center Report, 27*(4), 14 21. doi:10.2307/3528774.

Daniels, N. (2009). Can anyone really be talking about ethically modifying human nature? In N. Bostrom & J. Savulescu (Eds.), *Human enhancement* (pp. 25–42). Oxford: Oxford University Press.

Deafhoodgenetics.co.uk (2010–12a). Deafhood and the research project. http://www.deafhoodgenetics.co.uk/index.php/deafhood-and-the-research-project.

Deafhoodgenetics.co.uk (2010–12b). Welcome. http://www.deafhoodgenetics.co.uk/index.php/welcome.

[12]I would like to thank Brian Stableford for having kindly proofread this text.

d'Introna, N. (2012). *Le pays des aveugles* (drama adapted from H. G. Wells' short story). Lyon: Théâtre Nouvelle Génération/Centre Dramatique National de Lyon.
Dull, D., & West, C. (1991). Accounting for cosmetic surgery: The accomplishment of gender. *Social Problems, 38*(1), 54–70. doi:10.2307/800638.
Faivre, I. (1989). La chirurgie des apparences: un rite corporel contemporain. *Ethnologie Française, 19*(2), 107–110. doi:10.2307/40989106.
Frank, A. W. (2004). Emily's scars: Surgical shapings, technoluxe, and bioethics. *The Hastings Center Report, 34*(2), 18 29. doi:10.2307/3527682.
Goffette, J. (1992). *De la biomédecine à l'anthropogénie—Essai de clarification épistémologique et éthique* (Master's thesis, sup. J. Gayon). Dijon: Université de Bourgogne.
Goffette, J. (1996). *De la biomédecine à l'anthropogénie—Réflexion épistémologique et éthique* (PhD thesis, sup. J. Gayon). Dijon: Université de Bourgogne.
Goffette, J. (2006). *Naissance de l'anthropotechnie*. Paris: Vrin.
Goffette, J. (2010). Anthropotechnie: cheminement d'un terme, concepts différents, *Alliage, 67*. http://revel.unice.fr/alliage/index.html?id=3318.
Greely, H., Sahakian, B., Harris, J., Kessler, R. C., Gazzaniga, M., Campbell, P., et al. (2008). Towards responsible use of cognitive-enhancing drugs by the healthy. *Nature, 456*(7223), 702–705. doi:10.1038/456702a.
Habermas, J. (2001). *Die Zukunft der menschlichen Natur. Auf dem Weg zu einer liberalen Eugenik?*. Frankfurt: Suhrkamp Verlag.
Hegel, G. W. F. (1821). *Grundlinien der Philosophie des Rechts*. Berlin: Reimer.
Heidegger, M. (1953). Die Frage nach der Technik. In M. Heidegger (1954) *Vorträge und Aufsätze* (4th ed., 1978, pp. 9–40). Pfullingen: Neske (W. Lovitt, Trans.). The question concerning technology. In C. Hanks (Ed., 2010), *Technology and values: Essential readings* (pp. 99–113). Oxford: Blackwell.
Hottois, G., & Missa, J.-N. (2002). *Species technica*. Paris: Vrin.
Huffingtonpost.com (2012). "The vampire woman" is the "most modified" female in the world on "Taboo" (video). http://www.huffingtonpost.com/2012/09/24/vampire-woman-most-modified-taboo-video_n_1908605.html.
IAAF (2008). Oscar Pistorius—Independent scientific study concludes that cheetah prosthetics offer clear mechanical advantage. http://www.iaaf.org/news/printer,newsid=42896.htmx.
James, P. D. (1992). *The children of men*. London: Faber & Faber.
Johnson, K. (1973–1979). *The six million dollar man* (TV series). USA: ABC.
Kant, I. (1787). *Critik der reinen Vernunft. Zweite hin und wieder verbesserte Auflage*. Riga: Johann Friedrich Hartknoch.
Kress, N. (1998). *Maximum light*. New York: Tor.
Kurzweil, R. (2005). *The singularity is near: When humans transcend biology*. New York: Viking Penguin.
Lamont, E. (2003). The flawless foot. *Vogue*, 437, 442, 444.
Marcellini, A., Ferez, S., Issanchou, D., de Léséleuc, É., & McNamee, M. (2012). Challenging human and sporting boundaries: The case of Oscar Pistorius. *Performance Enhancement & Health, 1*(1), 3–9. doi:10.1016/j.peh.2011.11.002.
Murphy, R. (2003–2010). *Nip/tuck* (TV series). USA: FX.
Orlan, (1997). *De l'art charnel au baiser de l'artiste*. Paris: Jean-Michel Place.
Parfit, D. (1984). *Reasons and persons*. New York: Oxford University Press.
Pewglobal.org. (2011–2012). The American-Western European values gap. American exceptionalism subsides. http://www.pewglobal.org/2011/11/17/the-american-western-european-values-gap.
Plato (4th c. BC). *The Republic* (B. Jowett, Trans.). In Plato (1989) *The Republic and other works* (pp. 7–316). New York & Toronto: Random House.
Ricœur, P. (1990). *Soi-même comme un autre*. Paris: Le Seuil 'Points Essais'.
Robinson, K. S. (2004). *Forty signs of rain*. New York: Bantam.
Robinson, K. S. (2005). *Fifty degrees below*. New York: Bantam.
Robinson, K. S. (2007). *Sixty days and counting*. New York: Bantam.

Roddenberry, G. (1987–1994). *Star trek: The next generation* (TV series). USA: Paramount.

Schunk de Goldfiem, J. (1948). *Anthropotechnie. De la science de l'homme à l'art de faire des hommes*. Paris: Calmann-Lévy.

Shoemaker, S. (1963). *Self-knowledge and self-identity*. Ithaca, NY: Cornell University Press.

Sloterdijk, P. (1999). *Regeln für den Menschenpark. Ein Antwortschreiben zu Heideggers Brief über den Humanismus*. Frankfurt: Suhrkamp.

Smith, A., & Thomas, N. (2012). The politics and policy of inclusion and technology in Paralympic sport: Beyond Pistorius. *International Journal of Sport Policy and Politics*, *4*(3), 397–410. http://dx.doi.org/10.1080/19406940.2012.745893.

Stableford, B. (1998). *Inherit the Earth*. New York: Tor.

Terrel D. (Ed.). (2005). *Cycnos, 22(1 & 2): La science-fiction dans l'histoire, l'histoire dans la science-fiction* [Proceedings of the 5th International Science Fiction Conference of Nice, March 2005]. http://revel.unice.fr/cycnos/index.html?id=427, http://revel.unice.fr/cycnos/index.html?id=361.

Vonarburg, É. (1992). *Chroniques du Pays des mères*. Montréal: Québec/Amérique.

Wells, H. G. (1904). The country of the blind. *The Strand Magazine*, *26*(160), 401–415. http://www.gutenberg.org/files/37484/37484-h/37484-h.htm#The_Country_of_the_Blind. In J. Huntington (Ed., 2003) *The H.G. Wells reader: A complete anthology from science fiction to social satire* (pp. 187–205). Lanham MD: Taylor Trade Pub.

Wilhelm, K. (1976). *Where late the sweet birds sang*. New York: Harper & Row.

Wolbring, G. (2008). The politics of ableism. *Development, 51*(2), 252–258.

Index

D. Meacham (ed.), *Medicine and Society, New Perspectives in Continental Philosophy*, Philosophy and Medicine 120, DOI 10.1007/978-94-017-9870-9

MIX
Papier aus verantwortungsvollen Quellen
Paper from responsible sources
FSC® C105338

If you have any concerns about our products,
you can contact us on
ProductSafety@springernature.com

In case Publisher is established outside the EU,
the EU authorized representative is:
Springer Nature Customer Service Center GmbH
Europaplatz 3, 69115 Heidelberg, Germany

Printed by Libri Plureos GmbH
in Hamburg, Germany